NEUROSCIENCE RESEARCH PROGRESS

HUMAN BRAIN THEORY

INFORMATION-COMMUTATION DEVICE OF THE BRAIN AND PRINCIPLES OF ITS WORK AND MODELING

NEUROSCIENCE RESEARCH PROGRESS

Additional books in this series can be found on Nova's website under the Series tab.

Additional e-books in this series can be found on Nova's website under the eBooks tab.

NEUROSCIENCE RESEARCH PROGRESS

HUMAN BRAIN THEORY

INFORMATION-COMMUTATION DEVICE OF THE BRAIN AND PRINCIPLES OF ITS WORK AND MODELING

ANDREY S. BRYUKHOVETSKIY

NOVA BIOMEDICAL

New York

NOTICE TO THE READER

The Publisher has taken reasonable care in the preparation of this book, but makes no expressed or implied warranty of any kind and assumes no responsibility for any errors or omissions. No liability is assumed for incidental or consequential damages in connection with or arising out of information contained in this book. The Publisher shall not be liable for any special, consequential, or exemplary damages resulting, in whole or in part, from the readers' use of, or reliance upon, this material. Any parts of this book based on government reports are so indicated and copyright is claimed for those parts to the extent applicable to compilations of such works.

Independent verification should be sought for any data, advice or recommendations contained in this book. In addition, no responsibility is assumed by the publisher for any injury and/or damage to persons or property arising from any methods, products, instructions, ideas or otherwise contained in this publication.

This publication is designed to provide accurate and authoritative information with regard to the subject matter covered herein. It is sold with the clear understanding that the Publisher is not engaged in rendering legal or any other professional services. If legal or any other expert assistance is required, the services of a competent person should be sought. FROM A DECLARATION OF PARTICIPANTS JOINTLY ADOPTED BY A COMMITTEE OF THE AMERICAN BAR ASSOCIATION AND A COMMITTEE OF PUBLISHERS.

Additional color graphics may be available in the e-book version of this book.

Library of Congress Cataloging-in-Publication Data

ISBN: 978-1-63484-741-4

Published by Nova Science Publishers, Inc. † New York

CONTENTS

FOREWORD

The reviewed text is absolutely original and the author's spirit hovers at such a height of integrative speculations that any attempts to juxtapose it with previous individual or team generalizations would be unproductive. The author is original and inimitable regarding his key idea; though some of the European and American projects exhibit vertical integrative approaches top-down from global concepts to important details, Andrey Bryukhovetskiy resolutely turns away from the approach in neurobiology nicknamed as "dictatorship of details".

Thank you for the book, for the text, for the project of the Author's Spirit (what else can it be called?). I am grateful to the author for his courage to climb the Everest of our knowledge and guesses of the edges, limits and balance between CNS cells and higher integral tissue, which is more than just nervous cells (an important and correct supposition). I would like to keep within the frames of the biological positivism that unites me with the author at different platforms of creativity.

First of all, about the author. His Spirit reached inestimable thresholds. He, like Joseph Brodsky, achieved milestones in our field; the level of his predictions is invaluable for experts: biologists, neurophysiologists, masters of art and philosophy. But he is knocking at a new door, behind which biology needs new criteria and a new vision of metaphors and predictions. Quantitative measuring remains far behind. The cognitive demands and criteria of the author have reached new bounds; his higher positive language does not search for "new proofs in old stables". The author is trying to enter a new door, behind which new paradigms and a new panoramic vision are requisite for positive metaphors and predictions. The language of quantitative evidence in the scale of brain micromodels was left far behind as it is not suited for the leaps of integrative knowledge. The author proposes bringing a new order to the knowledge.

The method for the globalization of organization and the main codes of brain is revised here. The blanks are explained by the gaps in the knowledge of tissue modules of the brain (regional vascularized tissues, meninges, CSF spaces – all heterogeneous tissue environments between organs of senses and neural networks).

I would like to make small additions that have appeared as a response to the book. In the 1960s a great geneticist from St. Petersburg, Mikhail Lobashev, offered the term "signal heredity" to escape from the first pages of the vegetative biology of cells to the world of our sensory organs. First, it seems to me that the brain is the factory in which the flows of audial, visual and intellectual information are manipulated. The epigenetics of signal systems of nervous cells is associated with local micro-environment obligatorily through multiple functional statuses of the cells and tissues to catalogue all brain signals depending on their origin and functions (as in the immune system).

Second, the novelty and organized behavior of the cells are absent without sense (semantic) information. All immune and neural memory is derived from epigenetics, a huge molecular machine that codes the memory of single cells and whole circuits. New epigenetic memories develop due to the erosion of previous ones, and this is one of the most energy-consuming projects. Ontogenetic competition and the selection of current/operative or long-term memories are the basic script for survival in the information-abundant context. In our epoch of evolution, the main semantic motivation goals dominate in ontogenesis in the formation of new emergent creative behavior, which merely cancels primitive competition in Darwin's college of survival.

The technologies of creativity avoid the word 'us' of the crowd antagonism. All basic instincts stop being driving engine for the creative vision of motivation. As in religion, a new scale of priorities rules social psychology and the new counter-adaptive collective behavior. Other functions of CNS, outside the epicenter of global novelty generation, outside epigenetics, creative existence and breakthroughs, stay inactive in our times.

I am neither an expert in cell neurobiology, nor involved in the discussion of "hot spots" of the brain (2013), but I was astonished and convinced by the arguments of Prof. Bryukhovetskiy on the fragmented fundamental data and vacant gaps in therapeutic approaches (including the absence of clear macro- and micro-targets). And truly, we do not know anything about the epigenetics of CSF, vascular/nerve tissue, etc.

The other thing is how to introduce this theory innovatively and efficiently with clinical and information means. The book does not discuss it, though I am sure the competent author has saved some surprises for the readers.

Good luck, Prof. Bryukhovetskiy!

Respectfully yours,
Prof. Vadim Repin, PhD
Corresponding member of the Russian Academy of Medical Sciences
and the Russian Academy of Sciences
October 10, 2013

INTRODUCTION

ABSTRACT

The goal of the range of multi-scale international research initiated in the second decade of the 21st century is understanding the organization of the human brain. Neuroscientists, neurologists and experts in neurocomputers are looking for the answers to the main challenges of neuroscience: "How is the brain organized?', "What is consciousness and thinking?", "Where are the mind, intellect and memory located in the brain?" It is supposed that if humankind finds answers to these challenges, most brain diseases will become curable, advanced platforms for the super-fast processing of data will be established, artificial intelligence will be developed, a new generation of super-powerful brain-like computers will appear and the brain-computer interface will become real. But are we able to understand how the brain operates and how it is organized at our contemporary level of science? Can contemporary neuro-research, which relies on the system approach, explain the information and cybernetic principles of the operation of the brain? There is no unambiguous answer. Available fundamental evidence on the anatomy and physiology of the human brain does not allow for understanding its informational organization, the information-commutation interconnections of a whole brain and the way the brain processes the information. These considerations induced the author's theoretical studies and revision of available fundamental knowledge about the brain, which resulted in the development of an alternative viewpoint on the informational organization of the human brain and principles of its operation and to present an alternative vision of the architecture and module structure of the brain from the perspective of informationology. The author proposes a new insight into the mechanisms of the development of the symptoms and syndromes of brain disease, novel understanding and physical meaning of some of the brain's functions (memory, consciousness and thinking) and their disorders. The information approach was used as an innovative method of study in the sphere of research and critical analysis of available discrepant facts about the brain and served as the main tool for 'theoretical neurology". It is clear that "theoretical neurology" - just like "theoretical physics" - is becoming one of the most important fields of science, allowing for the development of a theory of the brain's operation and for the prediction of novel evidence first, and for the consequent detection of them in the clinic or in the laboratory, instead of adjusting new findings to the existing morphofunctional concept of the brain. A short history of the term "theoretical neurology" is given, as well as a description of its scientific content and borders.

Keywords: understanding of the human brain, challenges of neuroscience, system approach in neuro-research theoretical neurology

The idea to write a book came to me after I first read the Human Brain Project report to the European Commission dated April 2012 [1]. The report seemed absolutely fascinating. Every detail impressed; from the funds allocated by the European Commission (€1.19 billion) to the authors' deep scientific conviction of the feasibility of "neuromorphic" and "brain-like" biotechnologies, as well as a whole range of inconceivable information-communicative biotechnological platforms to simulate a virtual brain, neuro-computing and neuro-robotics. If it were not for the list of 300 renowned experts, I would have thought it was a script from a science fiction film, or a joke. My "neurological" mind could not accept the innovative ideology of the project, and was riddled with contradictions and doubt. On the one hand, I could not understand how the rational and conservative EU could have allocated over €1 billion for rather conventional research on the human brain based on an outdated scientific framework from the 20th century, i.e., the system approach. Who could have become so interested in the issue of fundamental brain research that they had allocated a huge sum of money to the abstract science, and why? On the other hand, none of the current innovative communication and information technologies supposedly in development fit the Procrustean framework of contemporary European neurology with its clichéd topical morphofunctional orientation and conservatism. What has changed? Who among the European experts in neurology had become the main ideologue and flag-bearer of this ambitious, challenging and future-oriented plan?

One has to find the answer to the main question: how will novel breakthrough communication and information biotechnologies of the 21st century be developed using the standard facilities of clinical neurology? Obviously, breakthrough innovations of the new century can hardly be developed using outdated tools and methodology. This would be either a methodological and technological error or an error of judgment. I even suspected that Europe might also have its version of Russia's *Skolkovo* project, in which the science is an excuse for money laundering.

However, the more I understood the concept of the project, the more I admired the grandeur of the idea and the selfless intentions of the European scientists. Strict hierarchy, systematicity, non-standard design and an ambitious approach to the multilevel research of the human brain made a deep and strong impression on me. I enjoyed the logic of the tasks and the beauty of the radically new concepts and design of neurocomputing technologies that would follow the principles of brain functioning. Apparently, the cooperation of neurologists and mathematicians had provided a sound scientific basis for cataloging the available histological, anatomical and cytological data and the evidence of the most advanced visualizing techniques within the framework of electronic atlases of brain. The approaches of systematicity of the conducted research and system analysis of all available data run like a common thread through the whole project and attest to the high level of its research.

Apart from admiration and curiosity, however, I still felt the urge to object to the range of technical and technological inconsistencies I noted in the project and to discuss their understanding of the work of the brain and methodological approaches that seemed to me to be outdated and incorrect. I would also like to point to the inconsistencies and scientific misconceptions in some theoretical assumptions and constructs. I came to the conclusion that if my opinion radically differs from the collective voice of enlightened Europe and scientifically advanced America, only a clear statement in writing can become a forcible argument for the validity and consistency of my views. I am not sure if I have succeeded in bringing my ideas to my readers, but I have done my best by writing this book. I started writing it as a conversation and dispute with the European experts in the neurosciences, trying to prove my ideas with the schemes and examples. But then the process captivated me completely and my own theories occupied my mind so that I kept thinking over key theoretical challenges of neurology and looking for the answers to eternal questions of neurosciences, day and night. The deeper I studied the issue, the deeper was my understanding that contemporary neurology and neurosciences are in a dead-end and cannot find the way out. We are stalemated by the paradoxes and mismatches in the development of high technology computerized diagnostics in neurology (CT, spiral CT, MTI, Functional MRI, PET, MEG, etc.) and the obsolete and backward theoretical basis of neurology, which is unable to explain new scientific evidence received by novel diagnostic methods. The more I investigated the issues of contemporary theoretic neurology and neurosciences, the clearer it became that we had very vague ideas of how the human brain was organized. It must be admitted that neurologists, neurosurgeons and neuroscientists have declared their impotence but the banner of neurological research has been promptly picked up by the physicists, chemists, and mathematicians who have continued to study the brain, devoting all of their abilities, with great mathematical accuracy and a high level of abstraction. They have applied all of the known mathematical and physical theories to the brain and transformed old problems of neurology into new challenges of theoretical physics and applied mathematics. They offer a body of versatile theories, concepts and hypotheses on brain organization and functioning and have interspersed them with mathematical calculations and physical evidence to substantiate them. The titles of novel theories of the brain have started to sound like the fields of theoretical physics: the quantum theory of consciousness [2], the holographic brain model [3], the theory of mathematical dynamic neurocommunication [4], the theory of dynamic integration [5], etc. Unfortunately, it has not helped us much to understand the brain. On the contrary, new theories have contributed to the general confusion by their mathematical wording and exacerbated it by adding the terms and formulas of control theory, graphs of system constructions and goal trees to the mixture of anatomical, histological, biophysical and neurophysiological terms and concepts.

It therefore seemed to me to be of great importance to understand what was true and what was pseudo-science pretending to offer the fundamental principles of the human brain's functioning. Obviously, a fresh look at the problem must be taken; a novel breakthrough methodology is required. But the key thing that must be done today is a global revision of the available data and concepts of the brain and the separation of the wheat from the chaff, i.e., we need to understand what can be left and what should be thrown away as irrelevant.

First of all, I studied the methodology of the European and American experts. Surprisingly, the more deeply I studied it, the more I was convinced that their methodology belonged to the past century and was outdated.

The goals and tasks that the European experts set themselves challenge all previous global scientific research. The goals of the Human Genome Project, started in the past century and accomplished in 2006, are incomparable with the hopes and expected results of the Human Brain Project. The European experts succeeded in wording the scientific needs of contemporary neurosciences and bringing them home to the highest authorities of the European commission, so that the necessity and feasibility of the project was not questioned.

This prompts us toward the supposition that the main role in the project was not played by the doctors and neurobiologists, but by the army generals and specialists in computation. It may be that the demand for large-scale research on the brain was not motivated by the essential needs of EU Commissioners to examine the human brain, or to use the evidence obtained thereby in the struggle against the aging of the European population and Alzheimer's disease. In fact, this intense interest in neuro-research is associated with the big-league politics and changes in the global balance of power in the international arena. The main incentives for the Human Brain Project seem to be the following:

First, it is obvious that in the 21st century, international parity and the security of any country has shifted from the sector of nuclear deterrence and military and industrial confrontation to the sphere of *innovations and critical biotechnologies*: nanotechnologies, bioengineering (molecular, peptide, tissue engineering, etc.) technologies, cell, genome, and post-genome technologies of robotics and program control, etc. Innovative military biotechnologies do not lead to the total elimination of humankind, unlike nuclear weapons, but the power of psychological, psychophysical and devastating action on living systems surpasses any previous weaponry. Any lag in the generation of new knowledge and the accumulation of fundamental evidence can be critical even for well-developed countries, threatening their sovereignty and even existence. Hence, large-scale research projects are a forced measure to maintain the biotechnological balance, economic and social priority, technological deterrence and strategic parity. Large-scale research projects give the EU and the USA strategic economic and biotechnological advantage over their partners and potential enemies.

Secondly, the initiative by highly developed states to study the human brain is an attempt to overcome the technological deadlock in the development of computing and artificial intelligence. Evidently, human brain research will promote the development of artificial intelligence systems. To date, the progress of computing machines, observed in the past 50 years, encountered a major obstacle that will be very hard to overcome; namely, the Power Wall. According to Moore's law, the only way to enhance the capacity of computers is to increase the number of processors. However, this leads to increased energy consumption, entailing an increase in the net costs of all operations. Expansion of the architecture of computers causes entropy increase due to the high risks of separate components' failure. In contrast, the human brain functions at minimal energy consumption. It consumes about 30 watts, i.e., a thousand times less than the smallest computer. That is why the development of energy-saving technologies can offer a solution in the studies of brain functioning. To find the solution for the Power Wall, the European experts considered it necessary to change the whole paradigm of computation. A new computation paradigm can be based either on the principles of quantum mechanics or neuromorphic technologies using algorithms of the operation of the human brain, which is able to perform asynchronous and stochastic calculations and process petabytes of data in milliseconds, which is impossible for all of the computers on Earth combined.

Thirdly, the turn to large-scale brain research projects is associated with economic stimulation of the ambitious plans for leadership and job creation. Such projects have become the method to overcome economic and social crises: "…every dollar we invested to map the human genome returned $140 to our economy," - said Barak Obama in 2013 – "Today, our scientists are mapping the human brain to unlock the answers to Alzheimer's; developing drugs to regenerate damaged organs; devising new material to make batteries ten times more powerful."

Now is not the time to gut these job-creating investments in science and innovation. Now is the time to reach a level of research and development not seen since the height of the Space Race. And today, no area holds more promise than our investments in American energy. … "We can't afford to miss these opportunities while the rest of the world races ahead. We have to seize them. I don't want the next job-creating discoveries to happen in China or India or Germany. I want them to happen right here, in the United States of America" [6].

Such a statement from the national leader of a highly developed nation with the first economy in the world and experience in large-scale research projects must have a solid financial and technical basis on which to implement these ambitious intentions. However, the European Union is ahead of the US in this sphere and the claims of the US President contain a fair amount of sense. These claims should set us thinking, too – us, the scientists who work in Russia, and our politicians. Our government and the President should consider the development of similar projects and the provision of favorable conditions for the next discoveries and inventions to be made in Russia, as neither our neighbors nor partners take us seriously.

Fourthly, all neuro-technologies developed in the project are dual-purpose. The goals of these projects are not only the mapping of brain activity, as claimed in the US BRAIN Initiative or European Commission declaration, but fundamental biotechnological studies of the principles of brain operation and the principles of program functioning of different brain areas. The novel biotechnologies of human brain control and management will rely on the systemic principles and functional models of the brain.

The project tasks include the development of novel military neuro-technologies of brain remote control by the implantable micro- and nano-systems of electronic chips and, conversely, control of the robotics linked with these brain-implanted microchips; the development of a brain-computer interface to enhance the mnestic and intellectual potential of a human and the immediate implementation of brain-computer interface in primates and humans for military purposes. Obviously, the military biotechnologies of the human brain control developed over the next decade by our European neighbors and American partners will provide an opportunity to control our military capacity and natural resources even without destructive warfare and invasions. Those who can rule human brains will rule the world!

All of the above characterizes the incentives and reasons for the initiation of large-scale research projects by highly developed states. The Human Brain Project is the first project of integrated European economic leaders. In April 2013, the US President Barak Obama proposed the BRAIN Initiative, a similar project, with 3 billion US dollars per ten years' funding [7]. So, the next ten or twelve years (the period when the brain research will be accomplished) guarantee us grand scientific breakthroughs in neurosciences and neurocomputing, as their novelty is already assured.

All this taken together has prompted me to analyze the current state of affairs in the neurosciences and state my own point of view on the immediate situation in contemporary neurology. My vision differs from the concepts of European and American brain research presented in their reports. We think differently in Russia. Unfortunately, there is no national methodology or strategy in neuro-research so far in this country. One has to be established from scratch. That does not mean that nothing is being done in Russia in this sphere. I presume that our leading academic research institutes and centers (the Scientific Research Institute of Neurology of the Russian Academy of Medical Sciences, The Scientific Research Institute of Neurosurgery of the Russian Academy of Medical Sciences, The Institute of Human Brain and other specialized institutions) are working on these issues of theoretical neurology, but they do not make their results public. However, the Minister for Health, Veronika I. Skvortsova, being the Professor of Neurology, has approved a strategic biotechnological platform for the development of contemporary neurology and other fields (oncology, regenerative medicine, highly technological medicine, etc.). Analysis of the promise of an approved strategy for neurology and neuroscience development leaves a rather sad impression of the developmental perspectives of neurology in Russia. The proposed platform is far from the ideology and methodology of the European and American approach to the development of the science. The offered platform is so formal that an innovative approach and opportunity to make scientific and technological breakthroughs can hardly be expected.

I would like to stress that in this book I am not trying to juxtapose my own knowledge and understanding of the strategic development of neurology with the fundamental knowledge of the leading experts in neurosciences, neurology and neurocomputing in Russia, not to mention Europe and the US. It merely seems to me that the methodology of European and American neuroscientists suffers from some inaccuracies that result in a misunderstanding of the basic components of the multilevel system of the human brain. This has led me to clarify my own ideas, which include not only my observations of the inaccuracies that I noted in the projects but also my perception of the methodological approaches and recommended toolkit for such neuro-research. Also, I wanted to formulate the theoretical bases of an information approach applied to the neurosciences as a new methodology of scientific search and analysis of neuro-research data, while also presenting my position on the necessity and practicability of the application of the information approach as an alternative to a system approach in neurology and neurosciences. The key point is that following my theoretical investigation of neurology, I have developed my own alternative integrated information-commutation theory of the organization of the brain and its functioning. To my mind, the opinion of the Professor of Neurology, trained both in neurology and psychiatry with 30 years' experience of clinical practice, not funded by any organization, can yet be of interest to those well-supported by the European Union, the US or Russian government.

For a long time I could not make up my mind what title to give to the book that reflects my theoretical view on the development of neurology and explains my methodological approach to neuro-research. The final version "Theoretical Neurology" seemed as boundless as the history of human brain studies. Neurology, as the basic medical science of the healthcare system, has existed for over two centuries and is one of the most fundamental, rigidly structured branches of medical science. The generation of theoretical, experimental and clinical evidence of neurologic science is acknowledged to be the classics of topical diagnostics for all contemporary medicine. From the end of the 19th century till the era of X-rays, magnetic resonance and computer tomography (end of the 20th century), fundamental theoretical neurologic knowledge of the topography of the brain and spinal cord provided the means to diagnose a wide range of diseases of the nervous system and to perform complicated neurosurgical interventions. Theoretical scientific breakthroughs in neurology have led to the development of several interdisciplinary branches in neurology: neurosurgery, psychosurgery, neurocybernetics, neurobionics, neurophysiology, neuropsychology, etc.

In the book we will not examine the history of neurological theories, or discuss the theoretical fundamentals of topical diagnostics of neurological disease and the methods to determine lesions in the brain, as the number of fundamental studies dedicated to these issues is abundant. Neither shall we dwell on the clinical aspects of general and specific neurology, as their details are set in the manuals and guides in clinical neurology and neurosurgery. Nor will we retell and rewrite well-known facts of general and specific neurology in our interpretation, presenting them as the theory of neurology.

The concept of such a monograph permits a perception of neurology from the perspective of brand new genome and post genome research and approaches multidimensional synthetic and systemic neurobiology, critique of nervous diseases diagnostics and therapy, discussion of methodological approaches to nervous diseases diagnostics and therapy, evaluation of novel developing areas of neurology, so that I can present my own understanding and perception of the most important issues and challenges of neurosciences, and offer my own ideology and methodology for neuro-research, which seems to correspond to the technocratic set-up of science development in the 21st century.

Evidently, neuroscience has appeared and is developing as a methodological and technical tool to investigate the work of the brain in health and in various pathologies, and reflects the level of the development of all science and methodology today. Contemporary theoretical basic and applied neurological evidence on anatomy, histology, cytology neuro- and psychophysiology, psychology and the cognitive functions of the brain and nervous system-related diseases is so huge, multifaceted and incomprehensible that a single lifespan would hardly be enough to look through all of it. These materials are voluminous manuals, guides, references and monographs dedicated to various aspects of neurological science and practice. Today we seldom read the books on the neurology and psychiatry of the previous century, admiring their detailed description of clinical pictures. Unfortunately, this knowledge does not provide us with anything useful for the novel development of new branches of neurology. In my book I do not negate all systems of previously acquired knowledge but I want to discuss only fundamental and methodological aspects of contemporary neurology within the framework of the science-intensive term *theoretical neurology*. This term was taken as a basis for this work and for its title.

The term was first heard at the XVIIth World Congress of Neurology in London, 2001, when the chairman Prof. Richard Hughes spoke about the vital problems of contemporary neurology and its priorities in a new century. The clinical content of a proposed term astonished me. One would think, what is new in this term? Neurology as a clinical science has earned considerable luggage of fundamental and theoretical knowledge about nervous system morphology, about the anatomy and physiology of conducting pathways, about information transfer in the brain and spinal cord, methods of topical diagnostics of pathological states and data on the treatment of nervous diseases. As students, we used to hear that only the clinical picture must be the main tool for a doctor of any specialty, and for clinical neurologists, it is the main thing. As Peter Duus cited Alf Brodal: “To receive significant results from the clinical work, the neurologist has to understand the main principle of nervous system organization and to have good knowledge of its structure and function” [8]. In other words, if you know anatomy well, then you are a top-rated neurologist able to make topical diagnosis correctly and to detect a lesion in the brain. But time changed everything. Today brain investigation with MRI and CT permits the detailed localization of any brain lesion and the verification of it with topical diagnosis. No one demands a fantastic memory and logic in order for a neurologist to be considered an excellent diagnostician. Nevertheless, that did not help in the search for therapy for nervous diseases. And the reason for this is in the lack of an accomplished and well-articulated theory of the brain's workings on the whole and at various levels of its biological organization. This is the meaning and the content Prof. Hughes embedded into the term "theoretical neurology". It was born of the necessity to develop a basically new theory of brain work, deep neurobiological investigation and the theoretical apprehension of the fundamentals of brain functioning in health and disease. The leading experts in neurology who participated in the Congress came to this conclusion after deep analysis of the state of things in neurology in the 20th century. At the very beginning of the millennium they wanted to look back at what had been achieved and to step to the next level of the processing and analysis of available information: theoretical consideration and integration of scientific evidence under a new theory. Since then, at various international congresses, I have heard much about the necessity of revising current theoretical concepts of the brain and spinal cord and an urgent need to establish an integral theoretical platform to coordinate neuro-research. First, these words seem like the rhetoric and grandiloquence of the coryphaeuses of modern neurology and do not draw much attention to them. I presumed that if you have nothing to talk about, then you can talk about theoretical neurology. To my big surprise, in April 2012 the flagship report of the Human Brain Project again mentioned the term "theoretical neuroscience" [1]. By that time European neuroscience had formulated the conceptual position of leading neurologists, neuroscientists and experts in neurocomputing on the necessity of establishing an academic institution involved in the issues of theoretical neuroscience as the main intellectual and technological driving force in the development of a novel concept of the brain work and a functional tool for conducting neuro-research. The European experts concluded that without determined theoretical and methodological framework, the fragmentarity in neuroscience data and research was impossible to overcome. Theoretical neurosciences must involve coordinated programs of theoretical brain research concentrated on the mathematical principles underlying the relationships between different levels of brain organization and the methods of information acquisition, presentation and storage. The experts working on the problem decided to establish the European Institute for Theoretical Neuroscience, a public academic institution which will play the role of an incubator for new approaches and support the participation of the scientists not involved in the global neuro-research of the EU and the US.

Today, in the opinion of leading European neurologists, neuroscience is extremely fragmented and its biological data demonstrate only slight earthliness. The absence of the theory does not permit the application of the knowledge on the brain to medicine or neuro-computation. Hence, theoretical neuroscience should include coordinated programs of research and solutions in strategically chosen themes important for the neuroscience goals: mathematical methods to obtain simplified models of complex brain structures and dynamics; the patterns of coordination of training events and memories for synaptic plasticity; large-scale models of bridging behavior data and visualization data, as well as mathematical descriptions of neural calculations at different levels of brain organization.

So, in this book I wanted to talk about the present and future of theoretical aspects of neurology and neurosciences. I am deeply convinced that the formation of basic novel theories of neurology presented as laws, principles, postulations, formulas and regularities of brain work can provide a scientific foundation for further neuro-research and understanding of brain functioning.

In the first chapter we critically, and in a somewhat biased and exaggerated manner, dwell on the state of things in contemporary clinical neurology, discuss paradoxes and discrepancies in the neurosciences that have appeared due to the uneven development of neural diagnostics, misbalance of therapeutic and neurosurgical toolkits for the adequate therapy of neural diseases and the complete absence of a theory that would explain the fundamentals of brain functioning.

In the second chapter we describe contemporary academic views and available opposing concepts of the brain offered by contemporary neuroscientists by the second decade of the 21st century. We wanted to demonstrate different viewpoints on the farmework of brain functioning, the principles and mechanisms of its work and structure, objectively and open-mindedly. The chapter is rather long, though the list of concepts is not complete, as one-third of them are purely metaphysical and hardly require academic analysis and the other one-third does not permit an understanding of the authors' ideas. I included only the works whose ideas seemed understandable to me. In some of them the sense is so carefully hidden under the wording that the ideas and principles of brain work remain unperceived.

The third chapter of the monograph describes almost all global projects of brain research, their goals and objectives and the content of the main program activities. Moreover, we tried to formulate the goals of a new global project based on the principles of the information approach.

In the fourth chapter we show the methodology and possible applications of the system approach as the basic toolkit for neuro-research, and discuss what hopes are raised by the European and American experts on this methodology of scientific research. In the chapter we concentrate on the positive advantages of the system approach this methodology provides in the global projects' goal and objective setting. By the end of the chapter we attempt to demonstrate and prove an important fact to the reader, that the methodology used in the 20th century was a driving engine of scientific and technical progress in all spheres. Meanwhile, in the 21st century this methodological approach turns out to be a deterrent of progress due to its rigid regulations, bulky graphs and constructions and the small information capacity of the technologies. The diagnostic and research equipment of the 21st century yields such huge arrays of biological data that their excessive quantity demands a new toolkit for their processing, storage and analysis, detecting key and controlling information, as well as system work with the already available data of adjacent databases and competing data.

In the fifth chapter of the book I share my own views and describe existing mathematical concepts of the methodology of modern information approach in the science and attempt to adapt it to the tasks of neuroscience. In my book *Transplantation of Nervous Cells and Tissue Engineering in Nervous Diseases*, published in 2003, I was already trying to bring information theory to the attention of neurologists and neurosurgeons. That book has a chapter dedicated to the ideology, methodology and implementation of the information approach in the transplantation of nervous cells and tissue engineering; as well as this, I explained in the book the advantages of the methodology of information approach in brain research as compared with the system approach. Unfortunately, but for a few "mentally deficient" pseudoscientists dealing with bioenergetics, bioinformatics and extrasensorics, nobody understood me. Mostly, the neurologists in the discussion preferred to talk about clinical issues and cell technologies, avoiding that issue. Their explanation was that it was all technically complicated, unclear and hard to understand, especially its use in neurology. The only support was offered by two professors of mathematics from Moscow Physical and Technical University. These people understood me and my ideas did not seem insane to them. My second attempt to explain the essence of the information approach to brain research is presented in the fifth chapter of this monograph. My hopes are optimistic because of the flagship report of the Human Brain Project. Today I am sure that there are people among the neuroscientists and neurocomputing specialists who will understand what I am trying to say. Moreover, I think they will use my theoretical assumptions to enhance their own solutions.

The sixth chapter offers the fundamentals of the information-communication theory of the brain that I developed for the discussion. The chapter declares new fundamental principles of information organization and functioning of human and mammal brains. Undoubtedly, the material requires specification and refinement and cannot be accepted as absolute truth. These are my personal scientific and intuitive ideas about the brain. My starting point was an old academic principle that the work does not have to be right to be classical and influential. I wanted to present my own opinion, which differs from the conventional, and to look alternatively at the well-known anatomy of the human brain and functions of subarachnoid and subdural CSF spaces. I present a functional chart of the information organization of the brain and have attempted to display the brilliancy of the design of a perfect mechanism of the brain's extraneural data processing. I have put to paper my rather rebellious ideas that the brain is not the substrate of intelligence, but only a bioorganic switch-board for the processes that happen extraneurally, outside the brain parenchyma. I am not able to provide weighty arguments to prove it, at least so far. These are only my ideas and I share my understanding of information processes with the readers. All of this reminds me of the words of Alan Turing, a pioneer of computer science, in his work *Computing Machinery and Intelligence*. The description he gives to his feelings is very exact and quite close to mine: "The reader will have anticipated that I have no very convincing arguments of a positive nature to support my views. If I had I should not have taken such pains to point out the fallacies in contrary views. Such evidence as I have I shall now give." [9] I found myself in a very similar position and could hardly state that something was really so. However, this theory provides me with the explanation of a range of facts that have not been explained so far by clinical neurology and psychiatry: why is memory affected in traumatic brain injury? Why is it that reflex activity can be automatic, but if we want to, we can control it with our minds? For the first time I can explain to myself what "brain engrams" are, their physical and information meaning. It seems clear why hypnosis works and the thought is material. Information-commutation theory gives logical and clear (to neurologists) answers to very complicated questions, and lets us understand both common and complicated processes, such as sleep, control and simultaneous performance, and many other questions that bother us with their mysteries. Simple explanations of complicated processes offered by the information-commutation theory bring to our minds the words of the Ukrainian philosopher Hryhoriy Skovoroda, who thanked God for making the attainment of what is necessary easy, and for making everything that is hard to get unnecessary.

In the seventh chapter I analyze and compare different methodological approaches to brain research: the European methodology of systemic multilevel approach to brain structure investigation and the methodology of the information approach that we offer. How successful the process of comparative analysis was can be evaluated by the readers, but it definitely was very exciting. With the scrupulosity and meticulousness of a school teacher I picked the flaws and errors out of the Human Brain Project methodology. I was close to reading a lecture to its authors about the fundamentals of information science and to explaining that the "information" notions cannot be mixed with "anatomical" and "psychological" elements of the tissue, as well as reproaching them for combining the non-combinable in their system, but I abstained, having seen a long list with 300 names of the specialists. So I avoided critical comments and tried to stick to the facts and methodological discrepancies without any emotional evaluation.

In the eighth and ninth chapters of the monograph we discuss the data, tools and technologies used to achieve virtual modeling of brain, as well as opportunities and perspectives of mathematical modeling as the basic research tool for the development of multilevel information structures and virtual 3D models of the brain in health and in disease. In these chapters we demonstrate the methodology and principles for 3D brain modeling and the main sources of the data for mathematical modeling. Moreover, these chapters contain theoretical speculations, arguments and academic suppositions on the methods and technologies of magnetome-based biocontrol of the functions of intact and injured brain and possible novel approaches to the magnetome-based therapy of nervous diseases.

The tenth chapter offers the discussion of the promises of theoretical neurology and my viewpoint on the reasons and developmental mechanisms of some complexes of neurologic symptoms; it demonstrates a brief history of neurocomputing and shows our opinion about the implementation of academic advances of theoretical neurology and opportunities to translate theoretical constructs of mathematics, neurocomputing and artificial intellect. Here we dwell on the available solutions to the human brain-computer interface, advantages and flaws of microchip implants to the brains of mammals and humans as well as our own methodology and technology to develop a non-contact magnetome-based brain-computer interface. The chapter also describes the future of such scientific achievements and information approach concepts in theoretical neurology, clinical neurological practice and other neurosciences.

In the conclusion we discuss the methodology of the information approach in contemporary neuro-research as an alternative to the current system approach of neurosciences, and analyze its advantages over system approach ideology, as well as discussing the academic results and theoretical investigations resulting from using new methodology in theoretical neurology.

The author expresses his gratitude and appreciation to the Director General of the FGBU Federal Research and Clinical Center for Specialized Types of Medical Assistance and Medical Technologies of the Federal Medical Biological Agency of Russia, Professor O.P. Kuzovlev, PhD, MD, for the opportunity to present the novel concept at the Major Academic Council and ideological support in publication of the monograph. The author is grateful to his wife, Nelly V. Triklinovich, for her assistance in writing the book. Her mathematical training and software engineering experience made her the first reader, the first opponent, and the first reviewer of the author's theoretical concepts, thus polishing and improving them till they were brought to order and understandability for an individual with a medical and technical background. The author also thanks his secretary and translator, Maria V. Zhukova, for her assistance in preparing foreign material for the book.

I would be glad to receive criticism and proposals on my book. Please do not hesitate to contact me at my e-mail address: neurovita-as@mail.ru.

Chapter 1

NEUROLOGY AND NEURAL RESEARCH IN THE EARLY 21ST CENTURY

ABSTRACT

The introductory section of the chapter discusses the paradoxes of the evolutionary development of contemporary neurology and imbalances in the ideology of neuroscience that result from the discordance of computerized highly technological diagnostics and existing methods of reconstructive surgical manipulations. Contemporary diagnostic imaging of the brain (CT, MRI, MEG, PET, etc.) allows for highly accurate description of lesions in the brain, but that does not have any real meaning or continuation in the treatment. The chapter attempts to give a critical and honest, although a bit biased, evaluation of the state of things in contemporary clinical neurology. We propose looking at the conservatism of contemporary neuroscience in general, and of neurology in particular, from the perspective of the technological opportunities of the working places of specialists from other fields (ophthalmologists, ENTs, dentists, etc.). The absence of scientific theory that would explain the fundamentals of the brain's operation is demonstrated. Today, speaking about the perspectives of neurology, neuroscientists do not formulate the patterns, principles or scientific laws, but speak of possible directions in the solution to the problem of the development of neuroscience and neurology. The author proposes several novel solutions for the development of neurology that will lead to new theories of the human brain and new rules of brain management. Eight paradoxes of contemporary neurology are presented that contribute to the therapeutic ineffectiveness of the neurologists, neurosurgeons and psychiatrists. These paradoxes led to the growth of the cases of neurological diseases in arithmetic progression, while the costs of their treatment grow exponentially. The European Union spends about € 80 billion on the treatment of cases of organic brain disorders annually. To conclude the chapter, the necessity for revising the available evidence and knowledge is validated, as well as the search for missing facts and the call for a unified theory of the human brain organization.

Keywords: the issues of clinical neurology, paradoxes of neuroscience, revision of knowledge and evidence about the brain, computerized working place for neurologists

As already mentioned in the Introduction, every epoch has its own scientific basis and its own technologies that characterize the level of scientific and technical progress in every branch of science. This certainly applies to the neurosciences in general, and neurology in particular. If one opens any textbook or manual in neurology, one is sure to find a statement that neurology is among the most rapidly developing branches of medicine, and the claim that new methods of advanced diagnostics and therapies for the management of neurological patients have appeared recently. Russian neurologists D.R. Schtulman and O.S. Levin in their manual "Neurology: A Guide for Medical Practitioner" [10] came to the conclusion that the "scope of curability in neurology has significantly expanded and the perception of neurologists as poor practitioners is unfounded". But has the state of neurological science and the recovery rate of neurological patients really changed by the second decade of the 21st century? Let us look closely and assess the real situation in neurology in an honest and unbiased way.

We will start from the very beginning; that is, from the method of neurological examination. Neurologists in the 21st century are still equipped with the same tools – a hammer, a light, a pin or a needle and a brush – that they were given a hundred years ago. One may well ask what can have changed in the classical neurological examination. To my mind, in the 21st century, a hammer, a light, a pin and a brush ought to have been replaced by a computerized working place equipped with video recorders, neuro-computing analyzers of the data received from the muscles, as well as devices to evaluate movement coordination with electric and magnetic stimulators, etc. If we look at the dentist's surgery, or that of an ENT specialist, ophthalmologist, or oncologist, we will see the progress that has been made in these fields and realize that the so-called "advances" of contemporary neurology have been relatively negligible. As a matter of fact, academic conservativism, technical illiteracy and the reluctance of neurologists and psychiatrists to accept technological change and innovations explain why a computerized working place for neurologists and psychiatrists has not yet been developed; and why all of the evidence from the primary assessment and follow-up remains subjective and informal, presented as personal judgment, intuition and description. Today, it is absolutely possible to develop the appropriate software and enter the data on topical diagnostics for neurologists to use in their practice.

One may object that today neurology can boast an array of diagnostic tests to assess the neurological condition of a patient across a range of nervous diseases; for example, to evaluate a coma we use the Glasgow coma scale; to evaluate independence, the FIM score is employed; or for spinal cord injury there is the ASIA scale. We know these scales by the names of their authors (e.g., Karnofsky score, Frankel Classification, Eysenck Personality test), but they only record the levels or aspects of neurological deficit, the deficiency of brain functions and the severity of the patient's disability. They are sufficient to evaluate the condition of the patient, but do not show the state of the brain in complex and the consequent changes in neurological state. To reflect the current state of the brain and to follow it up one needs batteries of tests and scales that require much time and effort and which can hardly be conducted in the course of the neurologist's daily routine. Therefore, it is apparent that the development of a computerized working place for a neurologist with video recording, computer processing of neurological examination data and automatic topical diagnostics for computer modeling of the brain is absolutely necessary and will be in high demand in the next decade.

Another important aspect when we assess the achievements of neurology is its effectiveness in treating neurological diseases. Unfortunately, contemporary neurology is characterized by a very low efficiency of the therapy of nervous diseases with considerable organic deficiency. Dear colleagues, can anybody name one serious neurological disease that we are now able to cure in the second decade of the 21st century? Can anybody name at least one major organic disease of the brain for which neurology can claim to have an effective therapy? Can we cure amyotrophic lateral sclerosis or, to be exact, motor neurone disease? No. Can we cure malignant tumors of the brain? Not in least. Moreover, the cost of cancer therapy for brain neoplasms has increased a hundredfold, while efficiency remains practically the same as in the 19th century. Is the number of lethal outcomes of hemorrhagic and ischemic strokes drastically different from the statistics of the 1970s and '80s? The difference is only slight; moreover, we can observe an opposite trend: the number of severely disabled people is increasing, as is the number of those who have no prospects of recovery after a stroke or after a highly technological life-saving neurosurgical intervention.

Supposedly, we can help in spinal cord injury cases. However, a spinal cord injury is still a life sentence with little or no chance of returning to a previous productive life. Annually, the US government spends about 2 billion dollars on the treatment of spinal cord injuries with a complete absence of functional restoration. Then, perhaps, neurology can demonstrate positive outcomes in the treatment of diffuse axonal injury of the brain resulting from severe traumatic brain injury? Unfortunately not. Any consequences of severe traumatic brain or spinal injury remain a blind-alley process with low rates of recovery. Is there at least one type of dementia for which neurology and psychiatry can help reverse intellectual-mnestic deficiency? Regretfully, contemporary neurology and psychiatry are helpless here. Maybe neurodegenerative diseases such as Parkinson's, Huntington's, and Alzheimer's diseases can be cured? We have been telling our patients that we have conquered Parkinson's disease and that we have an adequate substitutive pharmacological therapy. However, it has now become obvious that pathogenetic substitutive pharmacological therapy of Parkinson's disease is methodologically incorrect. This is only a symptomatic therapy that, if administered for a long time, leads to conditions under which the involved cells of striatal and pallidal areas of the brain stop secreting dopamine; in five to ten years of the therapy the body builds up a tolerance and the therapy becomes inefficient. The neurologist is helpless again, and the patient starts looking for new doctors and new treatments; sadly, to help them after our long therapy is almost impossible. All of this is unfortunately quite obvious and controversial: non-functioning organs or tissues atrophy. The most illustrative is the immobilization of a broken limb, when we observe the atrophy of non-functioning muscles and nerves caused by inactivity. Somehow this outcome is not obvious when dealing with the nerve tissue of the brain.

The ineffectiveness of current therapies for Alzheimer's and Huntington's diseases is undeniable. The problem of multiple sclerosis therapy remains unsolved as well as that of other autoimmune diseases of the brain and spinal cord. Likewise, we are helpless when faced with an organic defect of the brain caused by hypoxia or severe intoxication.

It can be objected that the neurosurgical interventions of brain trauma are an obvious achievement of neurology. However, if we look more closely, we will see that this is not the case. My personal experience of the treatment of the gunshot and explosion injuries of the brain and spinal cord that were inflicted in various local wars and armed conflicts (Afghanistan, Karabakh, Chechnya) allows me to say that we are as inefficient here as we are in the treatment of nervous diseases. What we actually can do is to reduce the mortality rate from various injuries and destructive factors thanks to novel interventions, organization and tactics of medical assistance, new approaches to primary surgical debridement of head wounds in the battlefield, use of potent broad-spectrum antibiotics, etc. However, we are still unable to restore the functions of the brain once they have been lost.

Undoubtedly, the current vogue is the introduction of brand new methods of imaging (computer tomography, spiral computed tomography, magnetic resonance imaging, computed tomography angiography, dopplerography ultrasound, duplex scanning, etc.), of functional diagnostics of the brain, spinal cord and peripheral nerves (echoencephalography, electroencephalography, brain mapping, EEG, electroneuromyography with transcranial magnetic stimulation and somatosensory evoked potentials, computer magnetoencephalography), and the methods of dynamic neuro-diagnostics (functional MRI, positron-emission tomography of brain, magnetic resonance angiography, micro-neurovisualization, etc.). All this has led to massive amounts of data, fragmented and discrepant information about the brain and spinal cord, both in health and in disease, that reflect brain morphology and functions in different ways but are not integrated into one system.

This discrepancy and the fragmentary nature of the available data on the brain do not provide an integrated picture of its structure and functioning. We keep trying to put a picture together without knowing how the whole picture looks and missing half of the pieces, then we try to compensate for it with our imagination.

As a matter of course we understand that we are dealing with the complex and multicolored picture of the brain structure that obviously lacks some details and elements. At this level of assembling our jigsaw puzzle we see that some parts of it are clear and obvious, while others are still missing or obscure. Consequently, we cannot achieve a complete understanding of the picture, of the plot and storyline; we have only our subjective judgments and guesses that we make on the basis of disparate elements. We do not perceive a whole and have to retrieve the details. Mathematical modeling has the capability to objectively calculate all of the missing components of any system, but as yet we do not have such models. Without any doubt, the data received by contemporary methods of diagnostics (CT, MRI, PET, MEG, EEG) and different scales of neurological assessment have the potential to create such a virtual computer model of the brain of a specific patient, but the results of objective computerized clinical evaluation must take their important place in the development of a virtual model of the brain.

To sum up the aforementioned characteristics of contemporary neurosciences, we have to acknowledge a whole series of paradoxes that exist in neurology today.

1. **Escalation of costs and low therapy effectiveness:** we observe an unreasonable growth in the costs of the therapy of nervous diseases that does not reduce the number of patients suffering from them. The costs of the treatment of neurological patients in Europe keep growing while incidence and treatment rates remain the same. According to the data of the European Commission, the costs of the therapy of neurological patients have doubled over the past 5 years and currently total about €800 billion per year, while the incidence remains almost unchanged.
2. **Population aging and increase in the incidence of neurodegenerative diseases**: the aging of the population in countries with highly developed economies has led to an increase in the incidence of Alzheimer's disease. The data of the Chicago Health and Aging Project showed that the number of cases of Alzheimer's disease will soon double: from 4.7 million in 2012 it will grow to 13.8 million by 2050 [11]. Therefore, by 2050 every 85-th person will suffer from Alzheimer's and we still cannot offer efficient therapy to these patients. Moreover, all of the available

evidence about the pathogenesis of this disease has to be revised and reconsidered as it is inconsistent with the real situation.

3. **The increased number of severe disability rates in the surviving neurological patients.** This paradox of contemporary neurology is characterized by the rapid increase of the number of surviving neurological patients with pronounced organic and psychic deficiency and the outcome into chronic vegetative state, dementia and complete work incapacity. The achievements of neuro-resuscitation in prosthesing vital functions, in the management of medical coma, thrombolysis and excellent anesthetic support to vascular and traumatic neurological patients have resulted in the increased survival rates of patients after severe brain damage (brain traumas, strokes, intoxications) with massive injuries of brain tissue and brain deficiency incompatible with productive intellectual life.
4. **Morphological paradox of neurology**. Refinement of the methods of cytology, histology, immunohistochemical tests of the nerve tissue samples, neuro-imaging of pathology inside the brain (neuroendoscopy, stereotaxis) and novel technologies of radio-diagnostics of nervous diseases (enhanced MRI, spiral CT, CT-myelography, angiography) permit the exact detection of the morphological composition of the abnormal focus, its size and localization and specific characteristics. However, these data are of relatively little significance to the contemporary therapy of the nervous diseases and are used only for diagnostics and evaluation of the dynamics of morphological changes resulting from sanogenesis in the brain. In other words, the exactness of morphological and topical diagnostics of the abnormal focus now does not mean much for the administration of adequate conservative treatment of most nervous diseases. Furthermore, high-precision interventions to excise the most malignant tumors of the brain (glioma, astrocytoma, etc.) using brand new systems of neuro-navigation, microscopy and stereotaxis, chemo- and radiotherapy relying on the morphological data of the tumors are inefficient, as the survival rates of this category of patients have not increased over the past 50 years. Still, the survival median in these cases amounts to 14 months regardless of the character, scope and methods of the highly technological treatment or symptomatic and palliative therapy.
5. **The paradox of functional diagnostics.** In contemporary neurology the methods of functional diagnostics (functional MRI, PET, radioisotope scanning, EEG, quantitative EEG (brain mapping), duplex scanning, ultrasound dopplerography of neck and brain vessels, rheoencephalography, ENMG with somatosensory evoked potentials and visual evoked potentials) have achieved perfection in the description of the disordered functions of the brain and spinal cord. But these extremely precise data can only be used indirectly in the treatment of nervous diseases, and are employed to assess the dynamics of functional changes. The functional diagnostics of brain pathologies should play a more significant role and be more widely used in the therapies and treatments.
6. **The "genetic" paradox.** The methods of genetic diagnostics and genetic engineering describe the structure of genetic defect in almost all nervous diseases, from hereditary disorders to Alzheimer's disease and brain tumors. However, this information lacks any practical therapeutic meaning and is used to diagnose the mutation and as grounds for refusing to provide medical assistance. Thirty years of genetic engineering have given only occasional positive outcomes in some diseases.

7. **Post-genome paradox.** The global introduction of the technologies of system and synthetics neurobiology and post-genome technologies (transcriptomics, proteomics, metabolomics, secretomics, RN-omics, etc.) has passed neurology by and brought only theory and research to the therapy of nervous diseases without any impact on clinical practice.
8. **The paradoxical mismatch between therapeutic tools and the complexity of the research field**: therapeutic treatments in all nervous diseases (pharmaceuticals, vaccines, immune therapy and correction, physiotherapy, radiotherapy, hyperbaric oxygenation, target therapy, neuro-rehabilitation) and neurosurgical approaches, surgical methods and stereotaxic radiosurgery are quite "crude" instruments to employ for restoring the brain; they are incompatible with the complexity of the research field and treated focus in the brain. Consequently, neurologists still remain inefficient.

The list of paradoxes and imbalances between automatized computer diagnostics, the methods of neuro-navigation and microsurgery and the methods of clinical assessment and the limited efficiency of the therapy is a long one. It is apparent that this is the result of vigorous development in contemporary biological and computing technologies, although the genuine reason is the lack of a theoretical basis for neurological research. We do lack a fundamental understanding of how the brain works and functions. Our knowledge about the brain and spinal cord is superficial and does not let neurologists establish conditions that would be favorable for brain/spinal cord self-sanitation. Our knowledge relies on tiered parameters of imaging of the site of injury that are virtually useless for the therapy of the injured brain, and not on mathematical patterns, laws of physics, the physics of information reception, processing and storage and models of how all this works. All technological breakthroughs in the engineering, solid state physics, and aerospace industries have had a theoretical basis. In the sciences (mathematics, chemistry, physics, theory of strength of materials, etc.), the theory comes first, prior to the practice, and it conditions the main practical tendencies of scientific thought. First, the quantum theory was developed, then the Higgs particle (boson) was predicted and only after the construction of the Large Hadron Collider was the particle actually detected. In medicine generally, and in neurology particularly, everything starts from practice and not from theory. Contemporary neurosciences (neurology, psychiatry, psychology, neurosurgery, etc.) developed as a descriptive part of a centuries-long research process accompanied by the reasoning of researchers about the possible character of the observed evidence. The tissue, cellular, molecular and atomic research relied on the *principle of visualization* of the research results by the methods of *objective* visualization accompanied by a detailed description of the properties and characteristics of the studied biological subject, and not its information structure: it only exists if we see it; if we do not see it, it does not and cannot exist. This approach has led to a significant loss of information.

Even today, speaking of the promises of neurology, we formulate only possible ways to solve the problem of neurosciences and neurology development, and do not attempt to question the principles, laws and patterns. What seem to be the possible directions in which contemporary neurology can move forward?

The first direction: *"From neuromorphological diagnostics to morphological neuro-restoration"*. Presumably, therapeutic manipulations should be as close as possible to the underlying morphological substrate of the disease, and the subject of the therapy should be the intratissular restoration of the elements of nerve tissue (neurons, neuroglial cells, endothelial cells, synapses) at the tissue and cell levels.

The second direction: *"From neurofunctional diagnostics to information analysis, neurofunctional regulation and biological management".* Neurofunctional diagnostics should reflect the dynamics of the information processes in cell systems: the correlations must be detected between the functional changes in the brain operation at the macro-level and the systems, information mechanisms of regulation of the cell signaling at the micro-level.

The third direction: *"From the genetic engineering of a nerve cell to the reprogramming of its intracellular signaling and phenotype modification by changing the nerve tissue inductance*". Use of epigenetic signal action on the genome, transcriptome, proteome and metabolome of injured nerve cells for their restoration without genetic engineering modification of the cell karyotype: development of the technologies to biologically control and maintain the mechanisms of intracellular and intercellular signaling of neurons and their networks by wave resonant induction approaches in the nerve tissue and development of cytoregulatory therapy of nervous diseases [12].

The fourth direction: *"From pharmaceuticals to information bio-carriers and bio-manipulators".* Development of a specialized toolkit at the micro- and nano-range for in vivo manipulations at the cellular and sub-cellular levels: cell systems with reprogrammed properties, nanobots, cell manipulators, self-targeting nano-constructions (e.g., liposomes, immunoliposomes, nanocapsules, nanotubes), and information chips for controlled regeneration and intracellular regulation.

The issue of how to compensate for the condition and stabilize the destabilized genome of injured nerve cells or partial compensation must come to the foreground of contemporary neurology, instead of curing the nervous disease. Obviously, the cure of a nervous disease is impossible, as the genome of the nerve cells has already mutated and will hardly disappear; however, the state of the patient still requires compensation and their life quality can be and must be improved. A classic example of turning on and off the mechanisms of compensation and decompensation in neurology is the example of acute cerebral circulation disorder in the case of systemic atherosclerotic vascular disease. In severe cases of atherosclerotic vascular disease the plaques in the neck and brain vessels cannot be removed either conservatively or surgically. In acute blood supply disorders of the brain the patient is admitted to hospital in a severe condition. Without a timely stabilization of general and cerebral hemodynamics, the patient dies, but if a proper vascular treatment and restoration of metabolic homeostasis in the brain tissues are provided, the patient survives, notwithstanding atherosclerotic plaques and ischemic zones in the brain. The concept of compensation-decompensation of neurological conditions should be applied at the cell level of nerve tissue, and the concept of compensation-decompensation of the genome, transcriptome and proteome of a pathological nerve cell should be developed. This is a promising approach for developing new therapeutic strategies for nervous diseases.

Another way to improve treatment in neurology lies in the unconventional therapeutic approach of cell and regenerative technologies. The first attempts of novel cell therapies that involved advances in regenerative medicine (cell transplantology, tissue engineering, etc.) were observed in the early 1990s in a new approach now known as neurorestoratology. Neurorestoratology, as an international theoretical and methodological concept of restoration of a damaged nerve cell at the micro- and nano-level, developed into a new branch of contemporary neurology in 2005-2006 [13]. For the first time, experts who practice cell therapies in neurology, neurosurgery, immunology and neurobiology from 35 different countries began to refer to themselves as neurorestoratologists. This decision was taken at the first meeting of the International Association of Neurorestoratology in Beijing in 2006, when the principle "the nerve cells can be restored" was declared and methods of neurorestoration of the injured brain and spinal cord were proposed. The instrument of neurorestoratology is the application of high (critical) technologies for the online neurorestoration of a damaged differentiated nerve cell:

- Cell therapies
- Gene and genetic engineering technologies
- Tissue engineering
- Biopolymers and elastomers
- Nanotechnologies
- Information technologies

Neurorestoratology set itself the challenge of working out a highly technological toolkit and a set of bioengineering products at the cellular, intracellular, micro- and nano-meter levels: the first experimental samples of cell systems with specific properties and neuro-chips with programmed functions have now been developed.

However, the views of specialists in neurorestoratology are not universally shared by neurologists and neurosurgeons around the world. Today, it seems to be the fashion to be pessimistic on this question, especially for neurosurgeons. Still, everyone understands that something should be done.

In response to the suggestion of the European Commission in 2011, the leading specialists in neurology, neurobiology and neurocomputing examined the opportunities and main directions for reforming the system of contemporary neurology. It took a year to scrutinize and analyze the current state of the neurosciences, the achievements of clinical neurology and diagnostic methods, and to evaluate its real condition, as well as opportunities and perspectives for further development. Their conclusions were even more radical than my speculations. They showed that global and European neuroscience (and neurology in particular) extends across a broad spectrum of diverse scientific disciplines and research communities. Each of them dedicates their activity to a very specific level of the neurobiological organization of brain, studies of a selected area of brain/spinal cord or nervous disease, types or methods of diagnostics and therapy of specific nervous diseases to be best adapted to specific goals and tasks of these disorders. Rapid progress at all levels of contemporary neurology has led to a situation in which all novel data and evidence were fragmented, discrepant and random. No complete data have been gathered for even one living species; neither at the cellular and tissue levels of brain/spinal cord anatomy, nor at the level of cell synapses and functional connections of brain areas. "Even in *C. elegans* – the only species the neuronal circuitry of which has been completely deciphered – we still miss essential information, such as data on neural morphologies. At the physiological level, we do not have a clear, quantitatively accurate picture of physiological response in different types of synapse, cell and circuit. Data on long-range connections between different brain regions is similarly sparse. In the absence of data, we cannot understand the relationships between different levels of brain organization – for instance, the way in which a variant in a specific gene can affect the architecture of an animal's neural circuitry and its subsequent behavior" [1].

European researchers also conclude that to understand the work of the brain we need multilevel data about its structure; we need new evidence to comprehend the interaction of different elements of brain operation and to construct the large-scale models of the brain. Structured cognitive tests combined with magnetic resonance imaging (MRI) and magnetoencephalography (MEG) limit the models of brain neural networks to visual perception, activity evaluation, decision making, information storage, coding and its retrieval from the memory, and analysis of space, numbers and language. Changes in neural networks during embryogenesis, ontogenetic development and the differences between growing up and aging limit the neural networks models in various ages and acquisition of the data for such studies of brain cellular models.

The fundamental multifaceted and complex research performed by leading European experts demonstrates that the available data must be reviewed, while the missing data and evidence must be sought to fill in the gaps among the already known schemes and brain systems, and the fragmentary and separate medical data must be integrated. To sum up, an integrated theory that explains brain organization and the principles of its operation is the key element that is required as soon as possible.

Chapter 2

CONTEMPORARY SCIENTIFIC CONCEPTS OF THE HUMAN BRAIN OPERATION AND ORGANIZATION

ABSTRACT

Contemporary scientific concepts and opposing viewpoints on the brain structure constitute the main content of the chapter. The incentive to write the article was the intention to represent the ideas of various researchers about the framework of the brain's functioning, principle and mechanisms of the brain's operation and organization in an objective and unbiased way. The chapter is rather long and detailed due to the morpho-functional and physical-mathematic descriptions, although it does not include even two-thirds of the concepts of the brain. The third part of the hypotheses and theories is theological and metaphysical and hardly requires scientific analysis and discussion, while the content of other works was not understandable. Of about 400 concepts and hypotheses we could not choose even one useful theory that would be able to unite all data about the brain. Summing up various works of contemporary neuroscientists, most of the researchers come to the same conclusion about the discrepancy, selectiveness and incompleteness of the available evidence, and the need to systemize them, rather than to gather new facts and knowledge. Understanding of the brain can be gained only by synthesis of different theories though their principles and the synthesis of the principles will disclose the principles of the operation of the brain.

Keywords: neuroanatomy, neurophysiology, cognitive functions of the brain, contemporary theory of the brain, morphofunctional organization of the brain, concepts of brain functioning, oscillation theory, theory of the brain

"Understanding the human brain is one of the greatest challenges facing 21st century science" is claimed in the abstract of the Human Brain Project (HBP) report to the European Commission [1]. Three hundred European neuroscientists (neurologists, neuromorphologists, neuropsychologists, neurophysiologists, experts in neurocomputing and neurorobotics and others) estimated a contemporary state of the art in brain research. They came to the conclusion that the technological level of molecular biology, genetics and post-genome research approaches the technological level of computation sciences, thus promising serious breakthroughs in brain understanding. Their scientifically grounded expert judgment permitted speaking of the real opportunity to establish a novel methodology for the research and development of a working model of the brain based on a new information understanding of the brain organization and principles of brain operation. This will provide the solution to all fundamental tasks set in the sphere of advanced innovative neuro-technologies: "If we can rise to the challenge, we can gain fundamental insights into what it means to be human, develop new treatments for brain diseases and build revolutionary new Information and Communications Technologies (ICT)". The idea is so perfectly expressed that one can only quote it, admiring the depth of the academic thought and accurately chosen wording. The collective opinion of scientists is always right, depersonalized and strategically grounded, so that one cannot help but listen to it; and there is always the hope that the collective scientific mind will find the solution that so far cannot be seen on the horizon as even the approaches to it are unclear. Just as it is unclear how to establish revolutionary methodology for the development of the information and communications technologies that will help "understand" the human brain.

What does that mean: "understanding the human brain"? Most probably, it means that the researchers will enter into the fundamentals of brain structure and formulate the main principles of brain functioning. However, to understand something in science one should have an orderly academic theory that explains the essence of the processes going on in the studied object. Unfortunately, to date there is no such theory that would explain the mechanisms of the brain's organization. Our expertise in the morphological and anatomical structure of the brain does not permit us the judgment of its intellectual, mnestic and thinking capacity. Although the neuroanatomists have studied the morphology of the nerve tissue of the brain accurately and meticulously, we cannot explain the nature of reflex and the higher nervous function of humans and animals. Tens of brilliant manuals in brain anatomy and the topical diagnostics of brain injuries, and radio and computer diagnostics of the brain in health and disease give a complete picture of the connectome (connections and communications) of the brain, but somehow these data do not help us to understand the information setup of the brain and its main principles of operation. The detailed guides for the neurophysiological testing of the brain and spinal cord include all contemporary methods of functional tests: EEG, evoked potentials EEG, quantitative EEG (brain mapping), ENMG and ENMG with evoked potentials and transcranial stimulation, magnetoencephalography and positron-emission tomography of the brain. However, that did not add clarity to the framework of the brain functioning and, as before, we do not understand its functional principles.

A notable advance of neuropsychologists was observed in the studies of the localization of the functions in the cortex of the brain, but this did not improve our understanding of the information processes in the brain. There are over four hundred hypotheses and concepts that describe the theoretical principles of the brain functioning, but there is no theory that would integrate all of them and explain the origin of the intellectual-mnestic and higher nervous activity of the humans. Moreover, some researchers came to a disappointing conclusion that the current state of affairs in the understanding of the brain's organization and principles of its functioning is so dissatisfying that "we do not have a broad framework of ideas in which to interpret these different approaches" [14]. Scientists have acknowledged that a huge mass of fundamental and interesting evidence has been gathered, but these data and facts are discrepant and fragmented and permit only an implicit judgment of the brain's functioning; they do not provide an integrated picture of the information and commutation processes in the brain. This fact encouraged the European and American experts to look for the solution in the information and communication neuro-technologies that can be the key to understanding the brain's organization and functioning.

Regrettably, the lack of innovative methodology in brain research prevents us from understanding the fundamentals and the algorithms of memory and intellect functioning, making us unable to get to the core of the mechanisms and patterns of thinking, reflexes and higher nervous activity. Conventional morphofunctional methodology of brain research is not efficient to date. Most of the specialists in neurology and neurosciences hope that the system multilevel approach to the data obtained according to this approach, and computer emulation and visualization of the brain will bring new life to the issue of understanding the human brain as the main tool of intellectual functions.

First, the absence of an integral brain theory was publicly acknowledged by the co-discoverer of the structure of the DNA molecule, Francis Crick, the Nobel Prize winner, in the *Scientific American*, September 1979 [15]. His analytical work about the brain claims that we do not know anything about the brain so we should not believe what we are told about the brain: "What is conspicuously lacking is a broad framework of ideas in which to interpret these different approaches" [14]. Francis Crick clearly stated the absence of the methodology and new theory in neuroscience.

The head of the Redwood Center for Theoretical Neuroscience in Berkeley, California, and the creator of the Palm and Treo, Jeff Hawkins, comments on these words of Francis Crick: "I thought the word framework was great. He didn't say we didn't even have a theory. He says, we don't even know how to begin to think about it -- we don't even have a framework. We are in the pre-paradigm days, if you want to use Thomas Kuhn" [14]. In his talk Jeff Hawkins is brilliantly and impressively convincing in his explanation of the necessity for a good theory of the brain. I would like to quote here a part of his emotional speech: "So why don't we have a good theory of brains? And people have been working on it for 100 years. Well, let's first take a look at what normal science looks like. This is normal science. Normal science is a nice balance between theory and experimentalists. And so the theorist guys say, well, I think this is what's going on, and the experimentalist says, no, you're wrong. And it goes back and forth, you know? This works in physics. This works in geology. But if this is normal science, what does neuroscience look like? This is what neuroscience looks like. We have this mountain of data, which is anatomy, physiology and behavior. You can't imagine how much detail we know about brains. There were 28,000 people who went to the neuroscience conference this year, and every one of them is doing research in brains. A lot of data. But there's no theory. There's a little, wimpy box on top there.

And theory has not played a role in any sort of grand way in the neurosciences. And it's a real shame. Now why has this come about? If you ask neuroscientists, why is this the state of affair, they'll first of all admit it. But if you ask them, they'll say, well, there's various reasons we don't have a good brain theory. Some people say, well, we still don't have enough data, we need to get more information, there's all these things we don't know. Well, I just told you there's so much data coming out of our ears. We have so much information, we don't even know how to begin to organize it. What good is more going to do? Maybe we'll be lucky and discover some magic thing, but I don't think so. This is actually a symptom of the fact that we just don't have a theory. We don't need more data – we need a good theory about it.

Another one is sometimes people say, well, brains are so complex, it'll take another 50 years. I even think Chris said something like this yesterday. I'm not sure what you said, Chris, but something like, well, it's one of the most complicated things in the universe. That's not true. You're more complicated than your brain. You've got a brain. And it's also, although the brain looks very complicated, things look complicated until you understand them. That's always been the case. And so all we can say, well, my neocortex, which is the part of the brain I'm interested in, has 30 billion cells. But, you know what? It's very, very regular. In fact, it looks like it's the same thing repeated over and over and over again. It's not as complex as it looks. That's not the issue.

Some people say, brains can't understand brains. Very Zen-like. You know, it sounds good, but why? I mean, what's the point? It's just a bunch of cells. You understand your liver. It's got a lot of cells in it too, right? So, you know, I don't think there's anything to that. And finally, some people say, well, you know, I don't feel like a bunch of cells, you know. I'm conscious. I've got this experience, I'm in the world, you know. I can't be just a bunch of cells. Well, you know, people used to believe there was a life force to be living, and we now know that's really not true at all. And there's really no evidence that says – well, other than people just have disbelief that cells can do what they do. And so, if some people have fallen into the pit of metaphysical dualism, some really smart people, too, but we can reject all that.

No, I'm going to tell you there's something else, and it's really fundamental, and this is what it is: there's another reason why we don't have a good brain theory, and it's because we have an intuitive, strongly-held, but incorrect assumption that has prevented us from seeing the answer. There's something we believe that just, it's obvious, but it's wrong. Now, there's a history of this in science and before I tell you what it is, I'm going to tell you a bit about the history of it in science. You look at some other scientific revolutions, and this case, I'm talking about the solar system, that's Copernicus, Darwin's evolution, and tectonic plates, that's Wegener. They all have a lot in common with brain science.

First of all, they had a lot of unexplained data. A lot of it. But it got more manageable once they had a theory. The best minds were stumped – really, really smart people. We're not smarter now than they were then. It just turns out it's really hard to think of things, but once you've thought of them, it's kind of easy to understand it. My daughters understood these three theories in their basic framework by the time they were in kindergarten.

And now it's not that hard, you know, here's the apple, here's the orange, you know, the Earth goes around, that kind of stuff.

Finally, another thing is the answer was there all along, but we kind of ignored it because of this obvious thing, and that's the thing. It was an intuitive, strong-held belief that was wrong." [14].

I have included this extensive quotation from the speech of Jeff Hawkins because I greatly admired his unconventional opinion of the deep processes happening in the neurosciences and the methodology of brain research so much that I wanted my readers to know his point of view on our failures in this sphere. It is vitally important to understand the reasons for these failures, to draw an objective picture of the way we have passed and to identify the milestones of scientific knowledge of the brain in the 20th century. The revision of the main scientific theories and methodological approaches is necessary to illustrate how the brain was perceived in the 20th century and how it is perceived today. We need to find a rational kernel in all of the existing theories and integrate these kernels in a chain of logical reasoning with one system-forming factor. The information seems to be the key system-forming factor that integrates and organizes all concepts of the brain. The information comes to the body and the environment from the brain, and it passes through receiving, transferring and subscription receptors of the brain. Being transformed in biophysical and biochemical carriers, all information comes through all of the brain structures and various cerebral material carriers transport it at large distances. Only the information is processed, analyzed, synthesized and is forwarded to executive organs of a human body, and only the information can be the "food" for thought.

We presume that our predecessors were hardly mistaken when they developed their own theories of the brain and tested them in experiments. Presumably, each of them could see only part of the information problem, or a whole problem but from a standpoint of their scientific ideology and scientific approach. It is time to integrate all available facts within the framework of an integral information theory of the human brain and to assemble the jigsaw puzzle of discrepant facts, evidence and research data.

We do not claim to give a complete and versatile description of the issue in this chapter; we will only try to outline the available conventional ideas and main trends in the scientific views of the brain in contemporary neurosciences and theoretical neurology for the past decade. As you know, till the middle of the 19th century, the researchers of the brain were mainly neuroanatomists and neurologists who meticulously described all details of the brain's morphology and the main clinical manifestations of brain injury. When this information was summed up in voluminous atlases and guides, it became clear that it could not explain the main intention of the Creator (God, Nature or Evolution), and a new methodology to acquire knowledge was requisite.

At the beginning of the 20th century, the physiologists became the main theorists in the sphere of brain research. The works of such Russian physiologists as Ivan Pavlov, Alexei Ukhtomsky, neuropsychologist Alexander Luria, neurophysiologists Piotr Anokhin, Konstantin Sudakov and others played a huge role in the development of the theory of the brain. All of these scientists claimed their own theory of the brain's organization and functioning. Relying on the principles of conditional reflex activity of the brain of humans/mammals, Ivan Pavlov, the great Russian physiologist, spoke of the first and second signal systems in the human brain which were based on the alteration of conditioned and unconditioned reflexes in the brain [16]. Conditioned reflex, according to Pavlov (1920), is "a temporary nervous connection of countless agents (sounds, smells, etc.) of the environment that are perceived by the receptors of the human or animal with specific activities of the organs". "The main physiologic function of the hemispheres is in the connection of countless signal conditioned stimuli, in other words, in regular supplementation of unconditioned reflexes with the conditioned ones. Hence, a higher nervous activity is not only conductive but also closing apparatus." In the brain hemispheres the conditioned reflexes open and close; in higher animals the reflex arc becomes more complicated: the analyzer-decomposer adds to the receptor, and the contactor-closer (connection and disconnection of the conditioned reflexes with the unconditioned) adds to the conductor.

Despite a rather primitive representation (excitation, inhibition), the theory of the brain's functioning was revolutionary for the time and gave an incentive for further neuro-research. Alexei Ukhtomsky, a Russian physiologist, revealed the inaccuracy of conventional views on reflex activity that allegedly had only protective meaning for the organism and aimed at the elimination or arrest of excitation and stimulus. He accentuated that the receptors of a living being could not develop if the reflex system protected them from approaching the stimulus. Using the example of the extensor reflex, Ukhtomsky stated that, primarily, the reflex system gave way to the reactions of approaching the environment, thus permitting its identification, while protective and negative reactions had the secondary priority. The principle of dominance was formulated by Ukhtomsky (1922) as the main principle of brain functioning [17]. The dominance is the leading focus of excitation in the central nervous system (CNS). This persistent dominance acquires the meaning of the leading factor among other centers: it accumulates excitation from other sources and inhibits the reaction of other centers to the impulses that are targeted at them. First the theory of Ukhtomsky was outlined in his dissertation in 1911, and then it was accomplished in 1922. The theory revealing general patterns of behavior of an organism in the environment had not only biological but also philosophical significance. Surprisingly, it is still usable and some contemporary neurologists employ it in their clinical routine and interpretation of the research [18]. Contemporary psychologists have accepted it as a physiological basis and pre-condition of behavior. The dominance is a working principle or main rule for the nervous system activity that governs any reflex reaction of the body. The dominance is characterized by the following: the excitation increases in the center which becomes domineering; excitation is characterized by the persistence; it cannot be brief. The dominating center is able to accumulate excitations. Excitation in the dominant center correlates with the inhibition of other reflex mechanisms that are not involved in the dominant reaction. According to previous physiological views, a nervous center is something unchangeable, statistically stable and with a definite and singular quality of excitation. Alexei Ukhtomsky showed that the quality depended on its states; in other states, the same center can acquire an absolutely different meaning in a body system. These ideas of Ukhtomsky were confirmed by the experiments with cross-sutured nerves that were well-known to physiologists. At the same time, *a nervous center is not a locally bound part, but presents something like a constellation, an array of the associated areas* (Ukhtomsky called it the "constellation of the centers"), which can be distributed rather loosely, and united not only by regular pathways, but also by the uniform working action. The dominance plays a significant role in the formation of reactions to the environment.

However, the main theoretical breakthrough in the ideas of brain functioning is associated with the holographic concept of the brain and the holographic nature of the mind, which still remain relevant today. The holographic principle of brain functioning was defined by the neuroscientist Karl H. Pribram in the late 1940s; he formulated the fundamental principles of the holographic identity of memories in a series of independent experiments on memory. Karl Pribram came up with the idea of the holographic model of the brain while working on a mystery of where and how the memories were stored. Multiple experiments by Pribram showed that before localization, the memory disperses through the brain. His scientific views underwent considerable changes under the influence of Karl Lashley's research. A series of experiments on rats in the 1920s led Lashley to the conclusion that they were not able to erase the memories of the complicated tasks for which the rat had been trained before surgery, regardless of what part of the rat's brain was removed. The only problem was that nobody could detect the mechanism that would explain that strange "all in one" nature of the memory storage. Karl Lashley, together with Karl Pribram, conducted a series of experiments with rats and appeared unable to answer the question of where the memory was localized in the brain. Later, in the '60s, Pribram came across the concept of holography from David Bohm, the physicist, and thought it to be an explanation for the mystery. Pribram proposed that neural holograms were formed by the diffraction patterns of oscillating electric waves within the cortex [19]. It is important to note the difference between the idea of a holonomic brain and a holographic one. Pribram does not suggest that the brain functions as a single hologram. Rather, the waves within smaller neural networks create localized holograms within the larger workings of the brain. This patch holography is called holonomy or windowed Fourier transformations [20].

The theory of Karl Pribram explained how a human brain can store huge volumes of memories despite weighing no more than 1.5 kg (the brain of Albert Einstein weighed 1.23 kg [21]). It has been established that the human brain is able to memorize about ten billion bits of information during the average lifespan – the amount of information approximating 5 sets of Encyclopedia Britannica. Moreover, it was found that apart from other opportunities, the holograms display an amazing capacity for information storage; multiple images can be registered on one surface changing the angle of two laser waves directed at a photosensitive layer. It has been proved that $1cm^3$ of the surface can contain up to ten billion bits of information.

The unique ability of the brain to restore necessary information out of a huge bulk of memories becomes clear if we presume that the brain functions according to holographic principles. If somebody asks you what comes to your mind when you mention zebra, you would not go deep into alphabetical files to answer, because you would immediately produce such associations as “stripes”, “looking like a horse” and “an African animal”. One of the most amazing features of the human brain is that every part of the information initiates cross-associations with other parts of it in no time, which is typical for holograms, as every part of the information has limitless connections with its other parts. And this, probably, is the most important example of the system of interconnections.

Memory storage is not the only neurophysiological mystery explained by the holographic theory of brain. Another is the way in which the brain transfers the flow of frequencies (light, sound, etc.) from organs of senses to the specific world of our sensations. Best of all, the frequencies are coded and decoded by holograms. According to Pribram, a hologram can function as a lens, a transferring device which is able to transform vague outlines of frequencies into a clear image. Karl Pribram thought that the brain, just as the lens, used holographic models to mathematically transform the frequencies, received by the organs of senses, into the internal world of our sensations. A major part of the experiments confirms that the brain functions according to holographic principles. The theory of Pribram gained support among neurophysiologists and was widely used for its theoretical constructs.

Piotr Anokhin, an outstanding Russian physiologist, supported the holographic theory of the brain of Karl Pribram. In his own theory of the functional systems of the human brain he saw a holographic basis of the brain functioning in the formation of the acceptor of the result of an action. He demonstrated that the *goal-directedness is one of the principles of brain functioning*. All of Anokhin’s theory of functional systems is based on the notions of the result and the hierarchy of the results achieved in the goal-directed behavior. The “problem” of any organism is the achievement of certain results in goal-directed behavior. Hence, the notions of a “problem” and a “goal” are bridged by the notion of a “problem” in mathematical theories and the theory of functional systems. A formal model of the brain work that follows out of this interpretation is the consequence and hierarchy of “weak” formal systems [22].

Piotr Anokhin proposed the principle of anticipatory reflection of reality and probabilistic prognosis as the principle of prediction. The opportunity to predict follows out of Anokhin’s principle of anticipatory reflection of reality: “There is one universal pattern in the adaptation of organisms to the environment that vigorously developed through evolution of a living world: extremely rapid reflection of slowly evolving events of the external world”. Alexei Krechmer offered a physical interpretation of the principle of anticipatory reflection of reality. The principle of anticipatory reflection of reality is specified and manifested in the notion of "probabilistic prognosis" introduced by Feighenberg [23] and used by Pavel Simonov in the information theory of emotions. The only explanation for the prediction (or prognosis) phenomenon can be the model of when the energy comes to an intellectual receiver at a different speed. The proof of this thesis relies on several statements: 1) all the world is flows of energies; 2) there are many levels in the flows of energy that have different force and speed (acoustic, optic, etc.); 3) the energy of different flows can be unified according to the force and time parameters; 4) unified signals can change the conductive structure of the formation (Hebbian synapse). The proof is quite easy. The model: the flows of energy from the sources have different speeds, forces and levels (modalities). These flows get to various receptors, where they are transformed into a unified signal. As far as the signal (stimulus) from the same sources reaches different receptors at different speeds, there appears an opportunity to unify them and to describe the patterns of the signals with different modality. For this these patterns must be memorized. But, according to the fourth statement, when unified signals are combined, the conductance inside an intellectual formation changes; that is, the structure changes too. And, if the set of signals repeats, it causes a response, which is manifested in the preparation to receive the next signals. Hence, the goal and the result of "activity" is the integrated estimate of the state of the system boundary. Then the phenomenon of prognosis is the prediction of the system boundary, and its model or physical sense is the comparison (correlation, evaluation) of energy flows by the channels with different speeds [24, 25].

Relying on Anokhin's theory of functional systems, Konstantin Sudakov, a Russian physiologist (1996-2012), worked out the theoretical insight about the information aspects of system activity of the brain. It was claimed that the information models of discrete *information system-quanta, represented as holographic images* of psychic activity, are developed under the influence of the information equivalents of original needs and their satisfaction during the formation of cerebral architectonics of the functional systems that determine behavior and psychic activity at the morphofunctional structures of the acceptor of the action result. Konstantin Sudakov accentuated the key role of dominating motivations in the development, and anticipatory extraction of the information system-quanta of the psychic activity from the memory, as well as studying the role of emotions in the information evaluation of the system activity of the brain. The researcher supposed that parameters of achievements of adaptive results through backward afferentation are imprinted on the structures of the acceptor of action results in the form of specific holographic images [27].

As we can see, the scientific ideas of Karl Pribram received a new life in the works of contemporary neurophysiologists, although in due time they were also caught up by other researchers and allowed for the development of a new approach to brain functioning. In the late '60s and early '70s research was initiated that was destined to change all of our views on the human brain acquired in the course of the history of science, bringing the Nobel Prize to Roger Sperry from the California Institute of Technology [27]. Robert Ornstein received world fame for his works about the brain waves and function specialization [28]; his work was continued by Eran Zaidel. Briefly, Sperry and Ornstein found that two hemispheres of the brain, joined by an intricate nervous network of corpus callosum, were mostly responsible for different types of intellectual activity. They formulated the theory of the brain's asymmetry.

In most people the left hemisphere is responsible for logical actions, words, digits, argumentation, analysis, etc. Prof. Zaidel, who continued the work of Sperry in the California

Institute of Technology, discovered that each of the hemispheres had more "abilities" than the other, as it was supposed earlier, and that each of them was capable of a broader range of actions [29].

The theory of the brain's asymmetry was further developed in the 1960s and '70s within the framework of a structural-functional model of brain organization proposed by Alexander Luria [30], as the main substrate of psychic activity. According to this model, the brain can be subdivided into three structural-functional units: a) energetic, or the unit of regulation of brain activity (I block); b) the unit of reception, processing and storage of exteroceptive information (II block); and c) the unit of programming, regulation and control after psychic activity (III block). Every higher psychic function is affected by all three units. The first unit consists of non-specific structures of the middle brain, diencephalic regions, limbic system, and mediobasal regions of the frontal and temporal cortex. The first unit provides the general activation background against which all psychic functions develop and supports the general tone of the CNS, which is necessary for any physic activity. The first unit is directly associated with the memory processes (in their modal unspecific form), with registration, storage and processing or information with different modalities. It is the substrate of various motivational and emotional processes and conditions. Limbic structures of the brain (visceral brain) participate in the regulation of emotions and, primarily, elementary emotions: fear, pain, pleasure, anger; as well as in the regulation of motivated states and processes associated with different body requirements.

The first unit of the brain perceives and processes different interoceptive information about the internal state of the organism and regulates these conditions with neuro-humoral and biochemical mechanisms. The nuclei of the cerebral nerves locate in the reticular formation of the brainstem; they conduct excitation from the organs of senses to vasomotor and respiratory centers. The upper part of the first unit contains higher vegetative centers that regulate the functions of internal organs.

The second unit is the unit that receives, processes and stores the exteroceptive information; the unit includes the main analyzing systems: auditory, visual and kinesthetic. This unite provides for the modal specific processes, analysis and synthesis of the input information and different gnostic types of psychic activity. The involvement of the tertiary cortical fields permits complex types of psychic activity, i.e., symbolic, verbal and intellectual.

The third unit of the brain is the unit of programming, regulation and control of the psychic activity; it activates motor, premotor and prefrontal cortical areas of frontal lobes.

Higher centers of the vegetative nervous system (VNS) are located in the frontal cortex. The function of the VNS is twofold: 1) to provide the relative stability of the internal medium of the body in the changing environment and its internal state; and 2) to provide adjusting reactions in a changing environment, especially in the case of a hazard to the organism. The reactions of stress, fear and anger develop in such situations.

According to the concept of Luria, every psychic activity has a definite structure: it starts from the motifs, intentions and plans and later turns into a specific program of actions that includes the "image of the result" and the notion of the methods needed to accomplish the program, which is then fulfilled with the help of certain operations. The psychic activity is completed with the phase of comparison of the result with the original "image of the result". In the case of a mismatch, the psychic activity continues until the necessary result is acquired. At the same time, the internal organs are maintained by the relatively autonomous vegetative nervous system. The sensations from internal organs do not quite reach unit II, while unit III is regulated by higher vegetative centers of unit I according to the programs of action. In normal conditions the person feels only somatic well-being. At the physical level they feel energy, strength, health and high spirits, which are represented by positive images – holograms – in the mind. Usually it is a tree, fruit, a bird, a rock, mythical heroes. On this base, the work of units II and III with good feedback gives the feelings “I exist”, “I can”, “I am fine”, endowing the person with self-assurance and internal freedom. The symbols of this level are also positive: an eagle, wings, a fountain, a creek, etc. Such a person is able to make a choice to reveal himself; he is ready for creative work, he faces the future with confidence, he is able to develop his relations with other people on the basis of respect and understanding. Attention is directed outside because the internal medium functions well. The person avoids addictions and can keep his identity while staying in a team due to his sufficient energy and feeling of internal comfort. These qualities are necessary for team work; they promote co-creativity, leading to additional positive symbols in the mind. The personality with this equipment aspires to unlock their creative potential. According to the wave dynamics of the Universe, this personality attracts positive people and situations. Such a personality is sustainable and successful [31, 32].

The neurologist Natalia Davydovskaya (2012) studied the role of the dominance of Ukhtomsky on a structural-functional model of Luria. She established that most often the dominance forms in unit I of the brain at the level of upper stem (associated with emotions and structures of the long-term memory). So, unit I contains pathological dominance. It is characterized by: 1) elevated excitation; 2) stability of excitation; 3) ability to accumulate excitation; 4) inertness and inhibition of other nervous centers of the first unit. Only the information relative to the dominance is transferred from this area of unit I to unit II. In other words, while unit I provides for mostly modal non-specific processes, and unit II for modal specific processes, the pathological dominance sends “pseudo-modal specific” information (the author’s term) to unit II. Thus, the dominance spreads to the brain cortex, developing the unpleasant holographic image, “shadow image”: dragon, snake, spider, mythical monster, etc. In months or years (depending on the exact situation and characteristic features of a person) the image enhances and takes more room, feeding on the energy of unit I.

Under these conditions, the information is sent to unit I from unit II in a partially distorted way; analysis and synthesis in unit II is inaccurate and unit III issues distorted programs of action relying on distorted data. Consequently, the result and the “image of the result” do not coincide. This leads to unpleasant emotions forming new unpleasant images – holodynes. Under such conditions the person has to spend more efforts and energy on the control of their actions and development of extra programs of the type “action program – realization – comparison – incorrect”, “control program – realization – comparison – correct – hesitation – estimation program – comparison – correct”. Hence, unit III starts to stimulate the vegetative centers of unit I for additional energy. The strain of unit I increases and influences the function of internal organs negatively. Moreover, the nervous centers of unit I are suppressed by pathological dominance that works “for itself”. The energy deficit increases and the vegetative centers are overworked. The organism is in stress fulfilling its routine work. Sometimes secondary pathological dominances develop, thus deteriorating the situation in unit I. The homeostasis is disordered and adaptation reduces; that is, the compensatory capacities of the organism decrease [18].

Neurophysiological and neuropsychological approaches to brain studies are still topical for the understanding of the mechanisms of the brain's operation. Strangman, Heindel, Anderson and Sutton, the researchers from the Department of Psychiatry at the Massachusetts General Hospital, Harvard Medical School, studied the behavioral and neural effects of knowledge that was based on the rules of motor sequences training [33]. The authors developed a novel 2-dimensional variant of the serial reaction time (SRT) task to test the effect of prior, verbalizable rule knowledge on motor learning behavior. To examine the neurophysiological effects, they also performed functional magnetic resonance imaging on a small cohort of subjects while performing the same task. Their results on behavioral data demonstrated that instruction on sequence-governing rules enhanced behavioral performance in both learning magnitudes and rates. The MRI data revealed substantially different, but partially overlapping, learning-related activation patterns with and without prior rule instruction. Direct comparison of these two conditions revealed the significantly different involvement of the bilateral superior and anterior prefrontal cortex (Brodmann areas 8 and 10, respectively), right superior temporal cortex (BA 38/21), and left cerebellum. These behavioral findings demonstrate an advantage of teaching governing rules prior to 2D-SRT task performance. While these neuroimaging findings remain to be replicated in a larger cohort of subjects, results suggest that substantially different - though partially overlapping - brain regions subserve learning in these 2 rehabilitation-relevant conditions. Thus, an appropriate choice of pretraining may benefit, for example, rehabilitation populations, at least in the acquisition of motor skills that require sequencing.

The supporters of the oscillatory theory of the brain (E. Basar, C. Basar-Eroglu, S. Karakas, M. Schurmann, 1999) were extremely skeptical of the works in the sphere of the structural-functional brain model [34]. They presumed that in the previous fifty years the false notion of the 19th century prevailed that the neurons were the carriers of nervous energy either in chemical or electrical forms. The populations of neurons interacted with each other across extended regions of the brain via large bundles and tracts of axons. Each part of the cortex and basal ganglia maintained its own "soap bubble" dynamics, with the specializations based on its history and input, and it was forced by these interactions into creating new patterns within itself that reflected and contributed to an ever-shifting global pattern involving the entire forebrain. These patterns were not re-entrant "mappings" that corresponded to the transfers of the information in computational neural networks. Rather, they were dynamical flows with continuous distributions and trajectories, comparable to hurricanes and tornadoes. The mathematics needed to describe these flows had undergone striking developments in recent years with the aid of computer graphics and digital computers. The founders of the oscillatory theory of the brain, E. Basar and the team, proposed the "integrative neurophysiology" which described the activity of several regions of the brain and their functions globally. It relies on voluminous experimental research: the EEG oscillations permit the evaluation of the sensor and cognitive functions together – both in independently behaving animals and humans in thinking and feeling. The processing of the sensor function and that of the cognitive function are closely interconnected; the approach used in the theory allegedly permits the analysis of the integrative functions of the brain. Integrative neurophysiology should also include physiologically important and cognitive functions. The integration of both types of functions is possible only in a common approach. Oscillations of the brain seem basic events to establish such integrative discipline. As far as the natural frequencies of the brain manifest in the EEG oscillations, then such an approach seems the most promising for the development of integrative neuroscience in the future. The supporters of the oscillatory brain theory presume that the analysis of natural frequencies opens up new opportunities in the combined analysis of sensor and cognitive functions at the level of separate neurons and field potentials (EEG or MEG).

Growing interest in gamma oscillations, now regarded as functionally relevant signals of the brain, underlines the importance of the concept of the event-related oscillations for bridging the gap between single neurons and neural assemblies. Elaborating on this concept, researchers from Germany (Prof. Erol Başar and the team.) reviewed the experiments, showing that such oscillatory phenomena as alpha, theta, and delta responses to the events were strongly interwoven with the sensory and cognitive functions [35]. Their review argued that selectively distributed delta, theta, alpha and gamma oscillatory systems act as resonant communication networks through the large populations of neurons. Thus, the oscillatory processes might play a major role in the functional communication in the brain in relation to memory and integrative functions.

For the past decade the founders of the oscillatory brain theory have participated in the development of theoretical approaches to non-linear dynamics of the brain and oscillatory processes of neural formations. Recently, three volumes have been issued, describing the oscillatory theory as a new evolution in neurosciences. The authors came to the conclusion that new integrative neurophysiology and a new theory of the brain are necessary to counter problems that were claimed essential for the decade of the brain in the 21st century. They say that the last revolution in terms of ideas about the brain happened in the middle of the 20th century, when the development in the sphere abruptly changed direction.

Mari Jibu and Kunio Yasue proposed the theory of the dynamics of the quantum brain and quantum consciousness. The authors, a brain researcher and a theoretical physicist, offered a new quantum structure to study such advanced functions of the brain as memory and consciousness. They were the first to provide a systematic description of the brain functioning as an integral system based on the fundamental principles of quantum physics. The quantum field theory was originated in the 1960s by the great theoretical physicist, Hiroomi Umezawa, to whom the book is dedicated. Both quantum physics, for sub-microscopic constituents of brain cells and tissues, and classical physics, for the microscopic and macroscopic constituents, were simultaneously justified by this theory. It posed an alternative to the dominant conceptions in the neuro- and cognitive sciences, which take neurons organized into networks as the basic constituents of the brain. Certain physical substrates in the brain were shown to support quantum field phenomena, and the resulting strange quantum properties were used to explain consciousness and memory. The whole of memory was stored in such a state of macroscopic order, and consciousness was realized by the creation and annihilation dynamics of energy quanta of the electromagnetic field and molecular fields of water and protein. This change of perspective resulted in a radically new vision of how the brain functions [36].

Beck and Eccles, in their research in the early 1990s, also discussed the quantum aspects of the brain's activity and their role in the formation of consciousness. The relationship between the brain's activity and conscious intentions was considered regarding the functional microstructure of the cerebral cortex. Every incoming nerve impulse caused the emission of transmitter molecules via the process of exocytosis. Since the exocytosis was a quantal phenomenon of the presynaptic vesicular grid with a probability of much less than 1, the authors presented a quantum mechanical model of it based on a tunneling process of the trigger mechanism. Consciousness manifested itself in mental intentions. The consequent voluntary actions were effective by momentary increases of the probability of vesicular emission in the thousands of synapses on each pyramidal cell by quantal selection [32].

Ruth Czarnecki, in her review, fully supports the quantum concept of the brain's organization and its scientific ideology [38]. The author notes that the studies of neurobiology have long been reduced to research into the actions between neurons and their synapses. Change in the concentration of different ions permits conductance both to and from the central nervous system and is responsible for all information processed in the nervous system as a whole. So, the quantum theory seems to the author to be the main alternative to theoretical views in neurobiology and theoretical neurology, and this view is supported by many researchers. In their work Globus and O'Carroll (2010) turn from quantum brain theory to the terms of non-local neurology, proposing to go beyond the localization of the functions in the brain to holonomy. According to the authors, the concept of local pathology has long served neurology admirably. Relevant models include self-organizing nonlinear brain dynamics, global workspace and dynamic core theories. However, such models are inconsistent with certain clinical phenomena found in Charles Bonnet syndrome, disjunctive agnosia and schizophrenia, where there is disunity of content within the unity of consciousness. This is contrasted with the split-brain case, where there is disunity of content and disunity of consciousnesses. The development of quantum brain theory with its nonlocal mechanisms under the law of the whole ("holonomy") offers new possibilities for explaining disintegration within unity. Dissipative quantum brain dynamics and its approach to the binding problem, memory and consciousness are presented. A non-local neurology armed with a holonomic understanding might look more deeply into what clinical neurology has always aspired to: the patient as a whole [39].

Joachim Keppler (2013) in his recent work also advocated fundamental quantum principles of brain functioning and their role in human consciousness, and offers new perspective views on the brain functioning and mechanisms that underlie conscious processes. In his article he presented an approach that in his opinion "sheds new light on these mechanisms". The approach was based on the stochastic electrodynamics (SED), a promising theoretical framework that provides a deeper understanding of quantum systems and reveals the origin of quantum phenomena. The author described the most important concepts and findings of SED and interpreted the neurophysiological body of evidence in the context of these findings, indicating that the functioning of the brain rested upon exactly the same principles that were characteristic of quantum systems. On this basis, Keppler constructed a new hypothesis on the mechanisms behind conscious processes and discussed the new perspectives this hypothesis opened up for consciousness research. In his opinion, it offered the possibility of elucidating the relationship between the brain and consciousness, of specifying the connection between consciousness and information, and of answering the question of what distinguishes conscious processes from unconscious processes [40].

The main trend of contemporary research in neurosciences lies in the development of a large unified theory of brain functioning that in this century has not been developed by the doctors, surprisingly, but by the physicists, mathematicians, programmers and specialists in robotics: those who have never seen the brain and have quite a vague understanding of its structure. To my mind, this is the main methodological mistake of our time. One cannot develop unified theories apart from the already known anatomy of the brain. The anatomy of the brain and surrounding structures offer many prompts that are on the surface and the researchers have to notice them, stepping over conventional ideas. Undoubtedly, the notions of the information and communication must become the basic foundation in the development of a new theory of the brain, which as yet has not been achieved.

As the physicists say, the aspiration to understand the most complex object in the investigated Universe is a long and complex process. By now we know much about the way the brain works, how our senses transform into electric signals, how different parts of the brain process these signals, how the memories are formed and the muscles are controlled. We know what parts of the brain are active when we listen to speech, look at pictures or buy something. We are even beginning to understand the neural processes that stand behind learning and decision making.

What we still lack is the method to gather all of these pieces together into an all-embracing theory of the brain. Despite decades of research, the neuroscientists have not developed their own equivalent of the Schrödinger equation in quantum mechanics or Einstein's $E = mc^2$; that is, a strong and exact mathematical law that would describe the work of the brain, just as we do not have a convincing roadmap in the sphere of "theory of everything", similarly to the string theory in physics. If we are able to approach an explanation of the Universe, the brain cannot be too hard a nut to crack. However, the human brain seems to be a more intricate construction than a physical system. It is the product of half a billion years of evolution, and we have studied it only for the past 200 years. It fulfills billions of functions: thinking, memory, perception, learning and emotions – and these are only a few of them – and it uses an unstable number of cell types, connections and receptors. Consequently, it is not susceptible to the descriptions in simple mathematical and physical laws. However, that does not discourage the neuro-researchers from their attempts to explain the higher psychic functions of the brain.

A physicist from Donetsk (Ukraine), Valeriy Andrus, displayed his viewpoint on the brain's setup and its principles of organization relying on physics, chemistry and astrophysics on the Internet [41]. Using a physical approach to the analysis of the fluids that wash and feed the brain, he tries to explain its information setup. According to Andrus, fluid is the main carrier of information; it stores and transfers it. In the immediate contact of a human body with water, its gases and fluid evaporations - that is, gas-vapor components - dissolve in it and this is a chemical aspect of information. The information component, in the author's opinion, is only possible if it has an electrical basis. Everybody knows that humans have electrostatic charges on their skin. It is also known that in fright the hairs of human and animal skin stand on end. Such a reaction of the hair is possible in the case of an acute increase of electrostatic stress. The researcher asks whether the electromagnetic wave in the brain can manifest in an electrostatic charge. Andrus claims that the electrostatic surface of a human body emits TV and radio signals, and these are not electromagnetic waves but electrostatic charges. All powerful TV and radio antennas work on high-voltage electrostatic charges. An electrostatic charge consists of a direct chain of electrical current with the South Pole in front and the magnetic field line (MFL) coiled around it with the North Pole in front. An electrostatic charge is negative; that is, its south pole is put forward along a whole construction. The "engines" of electric current push the charge in a straight line, and the "engines" of MFL, located along a helical line, curl it clockwise if we look in its end. These two facts, the existence of the waves and electrostatic charges result in electromagnetic carriers, represented as waves. Finally, a mythical electromagnetic wave receives a clear and precise electromagnetic carrier, i.e., an electrostatic charge (ESC). It is considered that the light is also an electromagnetic wave. The light needle has no α-particle – electric particle, and a magnetic component is based on neutrino, while the MFL based on a neutron is needed. Thus, there is observed some similarity of the light with electromagnetic wave based on ESC, but it is not true.

Two ESCs, moving toward each other at an angle and contacting as two rotating bodies with bulges, partially disintegrate into light needles with different frequencies. So it is obvious that crossing electromagnetic waves (interference) can yield a faint hologram observed by a personal viewer, such as a computer, but almost unobservable to others. This is the birth of images in reading, thinking, etc. The electromagnetic holograms emerge at the moment when we see true light images and hear sounds: this is our reference base to identify images or sounds. If we accept the point that high-voltage electrostatic charges emit their end parts, it becomes clear that high-voltage ESCs are fed with the charges too, and the sequence "transmitter→antenna→signal" is logical. The author examines the basics of the reception of electrostatic charges by a human body. How is a "TV-radio-receiver" of the human brain organized? As a true physicist, Andrus starts from afar; namely, from submarines. In salty sea water the stable radio-signal of extra-long waves reaches the antenna of a submarine at 28 meters' depth and no more, and then disperses. Meanwhile, the radio-signal can be captured by a current and reemitted in several minutes, hours or days, many miles away from the submarine. Hence, the conclusion is the following: the radio-signals can be captured by water and carried at large distances; the radio-signals can penetrate water. The capture and transfer of the signals under the water is the storage of information. The repeated emission of a signal at a large distance away from the submarine is retranslation. Andrus pays special attention to the fact that any special devices in the sea water are absent but the information can be registered and repeatedly translated without distortion. The scientist studies the mechanism of this phenomenon. The distributed radio-signal becomes more condensed when it approaches the submarine with the antenna, because the antenna is a capacitor. At the same time, it slows down in a denser medium. If the depth capability of a submarine, which is close to maximal, and the lower border of a flowing water current coincide, then the maximally inhibited row of the signals of ESCs begins the ionization of the molecules of dissolved salts, primarily NaCl. This ionized lower layer of salt ions is carried away by the current, and then the next layer follows, etc. So, we receive the film of saline ions in the total layer of flowing fluid which recorded all radio-transfer. To switch to the mode of the retranslator, this film should rise to the surface at some elevation of the bottom, where the motility of an ion will abruptly increase and lead to the loss of ESCs with their emission into the air in the same sequence. Andrus thinks that the main principle of radio-signal transfer and transmission in the brain lies in the ionization of the salts in fluids and their deionization - that is, the emission of the signal – and, due to this, all connections in the human body function, and the most stable is in fluids. Having stated that the fluids of a human body can receive TV- and radio-signals and emit them, the author figures out how the images appear in the organism. He thinks that everything begins from the radiation of a human with the signal, i.e., it comes through the body with a specific frequency. Different organs sort an input signal with the help of their specific saline solutions and specific crystalline materials of the organs that are responsible for input and output frequencies. When the frequencies of a signal and an organ coincide, the sorting implies the ionization; this means that it has accepted the signal; partial chaotic ionization is the warming up of an organ with further emission and passage through the organs without the ionization but with the general short-term excitation. Supposedly, the signal brought some image with it and a certain part of the brain tuned to the same frequency was ionized; that is, the signal was recorded. The ionization of this part of the brain is also its heating, which abruptly enhances the blood supply to cool it. Thus, we receive a rapid flow of blood/fluid (0.2 m/s), and the part of the brain re-ionizes blood with a preset sequence as a magnetic strip on a film. Andrus accentuates that blood becomes a temporary recording track. The part of the brain is connected to the visual and auditory organs with the help of this tape-blood through ion connection. When blood gets to the ears and eyes of a human, it discharges ions in other saline solution and does not ionize it further; this is radiation of a signal to the surface of an organ which changes its electrostatic charge, the oscillations of which cause sounds and images. Normally, the light/images initiate the oscillations of cones and rods in the eye with their further transformation into electric signals, while in the case of the brain it is the opposite process.

Andrus questions, why do we need this double address if humans can "watch" with the brain? As he says, "The funniest thing is that humankind thinks so because the scientists said so. Ask yourself a question, what is the mechanism of this sight? Does the brain have "eyes" of its own and a "TV-set" to record the information for long-term storage?" Then the researcher analyzes: every educated person knows that we perceive images at a speed of 24 frames per second, i.e., approximately every 40 milliseconds every picture stops in an unknown place accompanied by continuous light signals; and how is the rhythm of the frames counted? (In silent films the standard speed was 16 frames per second. When sound was introduced, the speed was standardized to 24 frames per second, as the previous speed could not be adequately coupled with the sound.) Imagine that a human eye receives continuous light with a specific frequency. The cones and rods vibrate under the mechanical pressure of the light, and one frame of 24 is registered as a steady image. How can it be, that the continuous vibration of cones and rods yields the flow of electric impulses, and the image of a frame is steady?

Andrus analyzes the memory as a function of the brain and as an example describes an artist who paints the portrait of a girl from memory. According to him, the memory is the record of the girl's image stored as ions, but it should be remembered that at multiple recollections we do not extract all of the stored abundance, but record it again to extract it again. He thinks that here we again observe a double process, i.e., we recall the image and automatically record it again. So, the artist recalls the electrical package of the girl's image from his memories; that is, the flow of released electrostatic charges that attack the part of the brain which is responsible for visual perception as an antenna that divides electrostatic charges into magnetic and electric, and which in turn transfers electrical signals by nervous connections to the cones and rods projecting the image through the eye's cornea to the space even if the eyes are closed. The image consists of the light flows issued by the cones and rods that vibrate, compress and thus break electrical signals into α-particles and γ-packages of light.

The Swiss scientists of the Blue Brain Project, Reimann et al. (2013), offer a detailed biophysical model of the neocortical potentials of the local fields which promises an important role to the active membrane currents of neurons. Brain activity generates fluctuations of extracellular tension, registered as the local field potentials (LFP). It is known that the relevant microvariables, the ionic currents across membranes, jointly generate the macrovariables, the extracellular voltage, but neither the detailed biophysical knowledge nor the required computational power have been available to model these processes. The researchers simulated the LFP in a model of the rodent neocortical column composed of >12,000 reconstructed, multicompartmental, and spiking cortical layer 4 and 5 pyramidal neurons and basket cells, including five million dendritic and somatic compartments with voltage- and ion-dependent currents, realistic connectivity, and probabilistic AMPA, NMDA, and GABA synapses. They found that, depending on a number of factors, the LFP reflects local and cross-layer processing. Active currents dominate the generation of LFPs, not synaptic ones. Spike-related currents impact the LFP not only at higher frequencies but below 50 Hz. This work calls for re-evaluating the genesis of LFPs [42].

Canadian engineers and mathematicians from the Department of Computer Science, University of Toronto, Natarajan, Huys, Dayan, and Zemel (2008), consider the fundamental organization of the brain to be based on the principles of coding and decoding of the spikes for dynamic stimuli and established that spiking neural populations might transfer the information about continuous dynamic stimulus variables. The combination of simple encoders and temporal stimulus correlations leads to a code in which the information is not readily available to downstream neurons. The authors explored a complex encoder that was paired with a simple decoder which allowed for the representation and manipulation of the dynamic information in neural systems. The encoder that they presented took the form of a biologically plausible recurrent spiking neural network where the output population recoded its inputs to produce spikes that were independently decodable. The researchers showed that this network could be learned in a supervised manner by a simple local learning rule [43].

Engineers from the University of California, San Diego, Sarajedini, Hecht-Nielsen and Chau (1999), also seriously treated the opportunities to train neural networks and their use as brain models. They developed methods of conditional probability density function estimation that can be helpful in solving real-world problems (pattern recognition, signal detection, and financial prediction) and should certainly improve understanding of the human brain's functioning. Previous developments in this direction used neural networks to estimate statistics of the distribution or the marginal or joint distributions of the input-output variables. The scientists modified the joint distribution estimating the sigmoidal neural network to evaluate the conditional distribution. Thus, the probability density of the output conditioned on the inputs was estimated using a neural network. They derived and implemented the learning laws to train the network and showed that this network had computational advantages over a ratio of joint and marginal distributions. They also compared its performance to a kernel conditional density estimator in a larger scale (higher dimensional) problem simulating more realistic conditions [44].

Prof. Walter Freeman from the Department of Molecular and Cell Biology, University of California, Berkeley, thinks that the key problem for cognitive scientists is in the calculation and explanation of the neural mechanisms of the rapid transposition between stimulus energy and recalled memory – between the specific (sensation) and the generic (perception) – in both material and mental aspects. The researchers are attempting three explanations in terms of neural codes. The microscopic code: cellular neurobiologists correlate stimulus properties with the rates and frequencies of trains of action potentials induced by stimuli and carried by topologically organized axons. The mesoscopic code: cognitive scientists formulate symbolic codes in trains of action potentials from feature-detector neurons of phonemes, lines, odorants, vibrations, faces, etc., which object-detector neurons bind into representations of stimuli. The macroscopic code: neurodynamicists extract neural correlates of stimuli and associated behaviors in spatial patterns of oscillatory fields of dendritic activity, which self-organize and evolve on trajectories through high-dimensional brain state space. This multivariate code is expressed in landscapes of chaotic attractors. Unlike other scientific codes, such as DNA and the periodic table, these neural codes have no alphabet or syntax. They are epistemological metaphors that experimentalists need to measure neural activity and engineers need to model brain functions. The author's aim is to describe the main properties of the macroscopic code and the grand challenge it poses: how do very large patterns of textured synchronized oscillations form in the cortex so quickly? Transactions between the levels happen in all areas of the cortex – upwards by integration (abstraction, generalization), and downwards by differentiation (specification). The levels are united by a cyclic causal connection: microscopic activity upwards sets the mesoscopic parameters that limit transaction downwards [45, 46].

Capolupo, Freeman and Vitiello, neuroscientists from Italy, developed (2013) a thermodynamic model of cortical neurodynamics expressed at the classical level by neural networks and at the quantum level by dissipative quantum field theory. Their model is based on features in the spatial images of cortical activity newly revealed by high-density electrode arrays. The researchers incorporated the mechanism and necessity for so-called dark energy in knowledge retrieval. They extended the model first using the Carnot cycle to define their measures for energy, entropy and temperature, and then using the Rankine cycle to incorporate criticality and phase transitions. They also described the dynamics of two interactive fields of neural activity that express knowledge, one at high and the other at low-energy density, and the two operators that create and annihilate the fields. The authors postulated that the extremely high density of energy sequestered briefly in cortical activity patterns could account for the vividness, richness of associations, and emotional intensity of memories recalled by stimuli [47].

Lawrence J. Cauller, the distinguished American scientist of the Department of Neurosciences of the Texas University at Dallas (2000), claimed the main principles of cortical neuroactivity of the brain [48]. According to Cauller, the conceptual framework of this neurointeractive explanation of emerging higher functions must be based on the functional architecture of the cortex, whose damage directly affects higher activity. Apart from the enormous associative capacity of these extensively connected neural networks, at least five relatively underestimated characteristics of the cortex are essential for dynamic neurointeractivity; these are subordinated to the emergence of a higher function:

1. All areas of the cortex are always active. Although the states of the cortex can be associated with fundamentally different activity modes (i.e., slow-wave sleep versus alert desynchronization), the neurons of the cortex are always active.
2. The majority of inputs to cortical neurons originate within the cortex itself. Almost all of the remaining inputs come from the thalamus, but the cortex is the major source of the inputs to the thalamus. Therefore, taking into account the cerebral cortical system, which should be considered the network of interacting cortico-thalamic circuits, almost all connections in the cortex provide cortical feedback.
3. Output signals from a wide cortex area, including motor areas and primary and higher order areas, project directly to the subcortical structures responsible for the directed movements of the head, ear, finger, that generate sensory input signals.
4. All cortical connections are reciprocal. These reciprocal connections provide the anatomical basis for cortical neurointeractivity. For example, the primary sensory

areas send "bottom-up" projections to the secondary sensory areas. These "bottom-up" projections are reciprocated by "top-down" projections from the secondary areas to the primary areas. This directionality of the sensory path defines the cortical hierarchy from the primary areas, which are the direct targets of sensory inputs, to the higher order areas which receive indirect sensory inputs through the primary areas. In both directions these cortical projections are always excitatory and it is likely that all areas may be activated by either bottom-up or top-down inputs. However, this top-down influence over cortical activity has not been properly studied, because the conventional transfer function approach would require careful manipulation of the top-down inputs, which are nearly inaccessible. The potential significance of this top-down activation of primary sensory areas is indicated by the finding that the primary visual areas may be activated in humans during mental imagery when the eyes are closed [49]. It is not useful to refer to either bottom-up or top-down projections as "the feedback" pathway because they are both sources of feedback with respect to the other. The dynamical complexity of cortical neurointeractivity is generated by this pervasive reciprocity, which extends across all areas of the cortex, creating a richly embedded system of multiple time-scales and interwoven levels of organization; that is, interactivity between reciprocally connected primary sensory and motor areas is embedded into the interactivity between primary and secondary shells. The complexity of this collective neurointeractivity rises above the sum of all of the embedded activities.

5. Reciprocal connections between cortical areas are structurally and functionally asymmetric with respect to the spatial distribution of the axon projections, and to the synaptic physiology of the connections.

Cauller described a dynamic neurointeractive paradigm according to which the dynamic mechanics of interactive processes in the brain lead to higher cortical function. The theory is based on the recently established biological principles of neural connectivism and promotes a neurointeractive paradigm of the brain and behavior, and accentuates interactivity between the neurons in cortical areas, between the regions of the cortex, and between the cortex and environment. This paradigm admits the closed architecture of the organism with respect to motor/sensory integration within the dynamic environment, where the major part of sensory activity is the direct consequence of self-oriented movements. The input signals of the cortex that predict the discriminating behavior in monkeys selectively activate cortical-bulbar neurons that function as the mediators in targeted movements [50]. As distinct from the widely distributed axons and long-term excitatory synaptic effector projections top-down, which generate the associative context for motor/sensory interactivity, the bottom-up sensor projections are spatially exact and activate short excitation followed by long-term inhibition [51]. Accordingly, the sensor consequences of motor actions are the main source of negative feedback, which completes an interactive cycle of associative hypothesis testing: a winner-takes-all motor/sensory pattern initiates a behavioral action within a top-down associative context; the bottom-up sensory consequences of that action interfere with the top-down sensory predictions and strengthen or refine the associative hypothesis; then the testing cycle repeats as the sensory negative feedback inhibits the motor/sensory pattern and releases the next winner-takes-all action.

Taking into account this neurointeractivity, the perception is a proactive behavior rather than information processing, so there is no need to impose representationalism: neurons simply respond to their inputs rather than encoding sensory properties; neural activity patterns are self-organized dynamical attractors rather than sensory driven transformations; action is based upon a purely subjective model of the environment rather than a reconstruction. The associative hypothesis is the neurointeractive equivalent to awareness and hypothesis testing is the basis for attention. This neurointeractive process of action/prediction association explains early development: from self-organized cortical attractors in utero; to the emergence of self-identity in the newborn, who learns to predict the immediate effects of self-action (i.e., listening to his own speech sounds); to the discovery of ecological contingencies; to the emergence of speech through the prediction of the mother's responses to infant speech. Ultimately, our scientific paradigm likewise emerges through neurointeractivity as we learn to see the world in a way that explains more of the effects of our actions.

In this way, Larry Cauller (2003) supports the dynamic approach to the cortical functions. As other brain models and constructs, Cauller's theory was tested on a computer and demonstrated many interesting and relevant features. Particularly, he comes to the conclusion that the dynamic attractors of neural networks are fundamental, repeated, basic elements of information storage and processing. Such ideas as the neurons that function as "the detectors of characteristics" are rejected. Hence, we are offered an unconventional and fresh concept of the functioning of the brain's cortex.

The viewpoint of John G. Taylor, the British mathematician (2007), who proposed the theory of neurodynamics of consciousness, is close to that of Cauller. Supposedly, consciousness has specific temporal dynamics. The model of Corollary Discharge of Attention Movement (CODAM) developed out of an engineering approach to attention and motor attention. Briefly, the model can be explained as the support arising from brain dynamics, especially that for the attentional blink. The understanding of known temporal dynamics in the brain associated with the emergence of consciousness is then developed from CODAM, and specifically related to the N2 ERP brain signal. How the pre-reflective self, as content-free, interacts with the content of experience is discussed in terms of the possibility that such experience arises from some proto-self generated by body signals; experiments are described which indicate that no pre-reflective self based on body signals is observable. Only a content-free pre-reflective self is consistent with this data, as CODAM suggests. How such a pre-reflective self can be further fused to give temporal continuity of a sense of self is considered in terms of various mechanisms which could be present for preserving the sense of self. The observation of the N2 signal in hippocampal encoding is proposed as providing a justification for the encoding of the N2-P3 sequence of brain signals. This would correspond to episodic encoding of the sequence of experiences of the pre-reflective self; this will thereby provide the necessary control signals in time so that 'I' is experienced as part of the retrieval of such memories [52].

Oleg Favorov and his colleagues (2003) share a radically different point of view. They think that Frank Rosenblatt was right and the brain consists of the multilayered networks of neurons similar to perception, trained by backward distribution. Favorov's theory is backed by sound arguments, and the main one is that their concept agrees with many known properties of cerebral information processing and behavior. The fact that "connectivistic" cognitive science achieved amazing success in the development of phenomenological models of multiple operations in cortical information processing is another strong argument in favor of this theory [53].

Walter Freeman's (2003) theory of the brain coincides with that of Larry Cauller philosophically, but it goes further by considering chaos, the key ingredient of the brain's dynamics. According to Freeman, every neuron participates in multiple interrelated dynamic interactions with other neurons. Going further than Cauller, Freeman perceives the trajectories of the transfer from one neuron to the other as information representations. The processes of training and behavior depend on the distribution of these transfers, and not on the consequent acquisition of margin cycles of stable attractors. The appropriate (target-satisfying) transfers enhance, while the neutral or target-negating transfers suppress. Freeman's idea has serious grounds, as its major issues rely on behavior that, possibly, can be reached by neurons, and because it helps understand why conventional concepts are not very successful in the explanation of information processing by the brain [54].

Robert Hecht-Nielsen (2003) presents an almost new, detailed and complete theory of processing thalamic-cortical information. According to the theory, all processing of thalamic-cortical information can be explained by two types of neural networks of associative memory, and each of them is actively used. The first of these networks is a fast-acting two-step system of attractors (implemented by two reciprocal connections between cortex and thalamus), which transmits all information in one of many thousands of disseminated neuronal codes (representative signs) designed for life. It is considered that the brain cortex is paved with tens of thousands of similar but weaker interacting networks. The second network learns to connect certain pairs of these signs in different regions. The power of connection is a new unclear information quantity named "the support of preceding"; that is, the only information learned, stored and used in the thalamocortex. The idea of the fundamentally symbolical cortex can attract the old-school supporters of artificial intelligence. The fans of the "Computational mind" may like the theory, because learning relations between the couples of solid symbols are informational-theoretical in essence and actually present software. The neuroscientists may like the theory because on the whole it seems to coincide with the known anatomy and physiology of the thalamocortex and related structures [55].

The theory of the brain brought forward by Henry Markram, the head of the Blue Brain Project, is the manifestation of proficiency in advanced understanding of the most critical elements of the brain, i.e., synapses. Markram's synthesis of an enormous scope of sophisticated literature on the subject is maintained by his personal findings, which are ahead of the entire world. Particularly, in resonance with other theories of the brain, he accentuates the dynamics of synaptic transmission: the post-synaptic effect of emerging potential to the action is critically dependent on the recent history of other action potentials. Going considerably further than a mere retelling of the facts, Markram identifies and characterizes the main categories of synaptic dynamic behavior. This theory provides broad and valuable expertise to all interested in the theory of the cortex [56].

Thomas McKenna's (2003) theoretical views on the brain are a sound commentary of various cortical theories and their interrelations. In particular, McKenna studies existing gaps between cortical theories and biology. These gaps are then used as the indicators for promising directions of theory construction. A valuable feature of McKenna's theory is the characteristics and comparisons of the theories that easily operate at different levels of abstraction. Going far beyond the "top-down" and "bottom-up" taxonomy, the theories are discussed from the standpoint of their ability to achieve success at the individual level of abstraction. Hopefully, in two hundred years, any college student will be able to provide a simple explanation of how the brain presents objects, learns, stores facts and then employs these facts to process information. The key point is that a good theory can function without gaps at any level of elaboration. The other issue considered here is the applicability of the cortex theories. The theories that are complete and correct must support practical implementation that is able to provide solutions to the vitally important problems of humans [57].

Jeffrey Sutton and Gary Strangman (2003) think that the cerebral cortex can be viewed as consisting of hierarchical groups of neural networks or, as they call it, the network of networks. The main point of this theory is that the modeling of the networks of individual associative memory on itself cannot explain the function of the brain's cortex. The main missing ingredient is that the groups of such networks are employed, controlled and trained as an ensemble, not individually. The theory of Sutton and Strangman explains how it can be implemented and why this viewpoint can be so important in understanding the obvious hierarchy of processing that we know so well (our cortex can deal with "throwing the ball" as with a conceptual unit just as with "a slight contraction of the biceps") [58].

John Taylor (2003) presents a theory for the processing of cerebral information concentrated on the way in which consciousness can emerge from the combined activity of the ensembles of cortical-subcortical control stimulus-driven structures adjusted to the behavior's goals and needs. The analysis of Taylor is free from the details targeted at the high-level information properties of the brain. Examining the discoveries of different theoretical perspectives, Taylor integrates them into a whole that manifests as a vision of how gatherings of relatively straightforward "thermostatic" functions of the brain that can support high-level processes become self-conscious due to powerful causative connections between their activating stimuli. Distinct from "toy-like systemic" studies of "emerging" features, the theory of Taylor comes close to explaining how and why the consciousness emerged phylogenetically. This theory illustrates the meaning and shows an excellent example of theory development at the highest conceptual level [59].

Neil Taylor and John Taylor (2003, 2004, 2005) address other key elements of the theory of the cortex: language. They performed a fundamental research of how neural architecture can be developed to implement the Language Acquisitional Device (LAD) of Noam Chomsky. The structures of division and uniting of word sequences (for example, hierarchical networks) are central to their theory. Using them, the authors developed a range of neutrally valid language data proceeding from the components and procedures for LAD. The resulting theory is not a final theory of language learning and understanding, but it gives a good basis for further research [60].

Richard Zemel (2003) describes a theory of population codes that, in the opinion of many researchers, can underlie the processing of cortical information. In the past almost all researchers of population codes thought that the group of neurons involved in the code was a group of turn-on neurons (while the other neighboring neurons are off-neurons). If we accept this binary theory, many interesting properties of these codes can be established. R. Zemel in his theory expands this proposal: according to him, the population codes can have variable non-negative levels of activity ascribed to them. Then he shows that these levels of activity can be interpreted from the point of view of the conjugated distribution of probability. Zemel says that the process of the activation of the population code is the calculation of probability. Moreover, he shows that the groups of associated population codes can interact and form a network of suppositions that looks easily compatible with cortical neuronal anatomy, physiology and function. The result is the basis for a new and very promising direction of research in the sphere of neural networks [61].

Canadian researchers Zemel and Mozer (2001) reached these conclusions due to their studies of attractor networks, in which they mapped the space of input into the discrete space of output, used to complete patterns: to clean up noisy or missing input features. However, designing a net to have a given set of attractors is complicated; training procedures are calculation-intensive and often produce spurious attractors and ill-conditioned attractor basins. These difficulties occur because each connection in the network participates in the encoding of multiple attractors. The researchers described an alternative formulation of attractor networks in which the encoding of knowledge was local, not distributed. Although localist attractor networks had similar dynamics to their distributed counterparts, they were much easier to work with and interpret. They proposed a statistical formulation of localist attractor net dynamics, which yielded a convergence proof and a mathematical interpretation of model parameters. Zemel and Mozer presented simulation experiments that explored the behavior of localist attractor networks, showing that they yielded few spurious attractors, and readily exhibited two desirable properties of psychological and neurobiological models: priming (faster convergence to an attractor if the attractor has been recently visited) and gang effects (in which the presence of an attractor enhances the attractor basins of neighboring attractors) [62].

In the past, scientists worked on unifying the ideas on information processing so that they would be applicable to the development of intellectual computers. Up to now their ideas have been general and testable to excite neuroscience. But a group from the University College, London, has probably got the ball rolling. Karl Friston and his colleagues (2012) proposed a mathematical law that seems close to a big universal theory of the brain [63]. This law permits Karl Friston to provide an explanation for almost everything about the brain's nerve tissue. This statement is disputable but it draws attention. The work of Karl Friston made the neuroscientist and psychologist Stanislas Dehaene change his mind about the opportunity to develop the Schrödinger equation for the brain. Like most neuroscientists, Dehaene was pessimistic, but then he claimed that for the first time in neuroscience we had a theory that was strong, broad and deep. I would like to dwell on the research of Karl Friston in more detail, as it is acknowledged to be outstanding work in the sphere of scientific theories of the brain's functioning and organization.

The ideas of Karl Friston are based on the theory known as the Bayesian brain, which conceptualized the brain as a probability machine that constantly makes predictions and revises them on the basis of what it feels. The idea was born in 1983 when Geoffrey Hinton of the University of Toronto in Canada and Terry Sejnowski, then at Johns Hopkins University in Baltimore, Maryland, suggested that the brain could be viewed as a machine that made decisions based on the uncertainties of the outside world. In the 1990s, other researchers proposed that the brain represented knowledge of the world in terms of probabilities. Instead of estimating the distance to an object as a number, for instance, the brain would treat it as a range of possible values, some more likely than others.

A crucial element of the approach is that the probabilities are based on experience, but they change when relevant new information, such as visual information about the object's location, becomes available. Karl Friston said that the brain was an inferential agent, optimizing its models of what is going on at this moment and in the future. In other words, the brain runs on Bayesian probability. Named after the 18th-century mathematician Thomas Bayes, this is a systematic way of calculating how the likelihood of an event changes as new information comes to light (see New Scientist, 10 May, p 44, for more on Bayesian theory).

The work of Karl Friston and his team describes a free energy principle that explains the ability of biological systems to resist a natural tendency to disorder. The work appeals to circular causality, found in synergetic formulations of self-organization (e.g., the slaving principle) and models of coupled dynamical systems, using nonlinear Fokker Planck equations. Here, circular causality is induced by separating the states of a random dynamical system into *external* and *internal* states, where external states are subject to random fluctuations and internal states are not. This reduces the problem of finding some (deterministic) dynamics of the internal states that ensure the system visits a limited number of external states; in other words, the measure of its (random) attracting set, or the Shannon entropy of the external states is small. The researchers motivate a solution using a principle of least action based on variational free energy (from statistical physics) and establish the conditions under which it is formally equivalent to the information bottleneck method. This approach proved useful in understanding the functional architecture of the brain. The generality of variational free energy minimization and corresponding information theoretical formulations may speak to interesting applications beyond the neurosciences; e.g., in molecular or evolutionary biology.

Over the past decade, neuroscientists have found that the brain seemed to work in this way. In perception and learning experiments, for example, people tend to make estimates – of the location or speed of a moving object, say – in a way that fits with Bayesian probability theory. There is also evidence that the brain makes internal predictions and updates them in a Bayesian manner. When one listens to someone, for example, the brain is not simply receiving information, it also predicts what it expects to hear and constantly revises its predictions based on what information comes next. These predictions strongly influence what we hear, allowing us, for instance, to make sense of distorted or partially obscured speech.

In fact, making predictions and re-evaluating them seems to be a universal feature of the brain. At all times your brain is weighing all input information and comparing it with internal predictions in order to make sense of the world. "It's a general computational principle that can explain how the brain handles problems ranging from low-level perception to high-level cognition," says Alex Pouget, a computational neuroscientist at the University of Rochester in New York [64].

However, the Bayesian brain is not quite a general law. It is a collection of related approaches that each use Bayesian probability theory to understand one aspect of brain function, such as speech analysis, recognizing objects or learning words. No one has been able to integrate these disparate approaches together, nor explain why the brain works like this in the first place. An overarching law, if one exists, should attempt to do this [65].

In the 1990s Karl Friston was working next door to Geoffrey Hinton at UCL. At that time Hinton explored the concept of "free energy" as it applied to artificial neural networks. Free energy originates from thermodynamics and statistical mechanics, where it is defined as the amount of useful work that can be extracted from a system, such as a steam engine. It is roughly equivalent to the difference between the total energy in the system and its "useless energy", or entropy.

Geoffrey Hinton realized that free energy was mathematically equivalent to a well-known problem: the difference between the predictions made by an artificial neural network and what it actually senses. He showed that you could solve some complicated problems in machine learning by treating this "prediction error" as free energy, and then minimizing it. In the next few years Friston investigated whether the same concept could underlie the functioning of a real brain. His idea was that the constant updating of the brain's probabilities could also be expressed in terms of minimizing free energy. Around 2005 he proposed that a "free energy principle" explained at least one aspect of brain function – sensory perception.

To illustrate this, Karl Friston used the example of peripheral vision. First, there was a big error between the prediction of the brain and what it really senses. According to Friston, to reduce this prediction error, one of two things can happen: the brain can either change its prediction or change the way it gathers data from the environment (Journal of Physiology-Paris, vol 100, p 70). If the brain takes the second option, you will instinctively turn your head and center the object in your field of view. "It's about minimizing surprise," he explains. "Mathematically, free energy is always bigger than surprise; therefore, if you can minimize free energy you can avoid surprising encounters with the world."

Karl Friston developed the free-energy principle to explain perception, but then he generalized it to other kinds of brain processes. He claims that everything the brain does is designed to minimize free energy or prediction error (Synthese, vol 159, p 417). "In short, everything that can change in the brain will change to suppress prediction errors, from the firing of neurons to the wiring between them, and from the movements of our eyes to the choices we make in daily life," he says.

Let us consider neural plasticity, the well-established idea that the brain alters its internal pathways and connections with experience. First proposed by Canadian psychologist Donald Hebb in the 1940s, it is thought to be the basic mechanism behind learning and memory.

Friston's principle accounts for the process by describing how individual neurons interact after encountering a novel stimulus. Neuron A "predicts" that neuron B will respond to the stimulus in a certain way. If the prediction is wrong, neuron A changes the strength of its connection to neuron B to decrease the prediction error. In this case the brain changes its internal predictions until it minimizes its error, and learning or memory forming is the result.

It sounds nice in theory, but how can we know whether real brains actually work this way? To answer this question, Friston and others have focused on the cortex, the 3-millimetere-thick mass of convoluted folds that forms the brain's outer surface. This is the seat of "higher" functions such as cognition, learning, perception and language. It has a distinctive anatomy: a hierarchy of neuronal layers, each of which has connections to neurons in the other levels.

Friston created a computer simulation of the cortex with layers of "neurons" passing signals back and forth. Signals going from higher to lower levels represent the brain's internal predictions, while signals going the other way represent sensory input. As new information comes in, the higher neurons adjust their predictions according to Bayesian theory. This seems abstract, but there is a concrete reason for doing it: it indicates what patterns of activity to look for in a real brain.

Last year Friston's group used functional magnetic resonance imaging to examine what is going on in the cortex during a visual task (NeuroImage, vol 34, p 1199). Volunteers watched two sets of moving dots, which sometimes moved in synchrony and at other times more randomly, to change the predictability of the stimulus. The patterns of brain activity matched Friston's model of the visual cortex reasonably well. He argues that this supports the idea that top-down signals are indeed sent downstream to reduce prediction errors.

More recently, Friston's team has shown that signals from higher levels of the auditory cortex are responsible for modifying brain activity in lower levels as people listen to repeated and predictable sounds (Proceedings of the National Academy of Sciences, vol 104, p 20961). This also complies with Friston's model of the top-down minimization of prediction error.

Despite these successes, not everyone in the Bayesian brain camp agrees with the theory. They say it is hard to know whether Friston's results are ground-breaking or just repackaged old concepts. However, nobody says he is wrong. Others say the free-energy principle is not falsifiable. "I do not think it is testable, and I am pretty sure it does not tell you how to build a machine which emulates some aspect of intelligence," says theoretical neuroscientist Tomaso Poggio of the Massachusetts Institute of Technology.

Friston disagrees, pointing out that there are experiments that would definitively test whether or not a given population of neurons is minimizing prediction error. He proposes knocking out a higher region of the cortex – using transcranial magnetic stimulation, for example – and seeing whether free-energy models can predict how the activity of a lower region of neurons would change in response.

Several groups are planning such experiments, but they need to work out exactly which neurons to target. "This would, I think, be an aspect of the theory that could be proved or falsified," says Thomas Wennekers, a computational neuroscientist at the University of Plymouth in the UK.

Meanwhile, Friston claims that the free-energy principle also gives plausible explanations for other important features of the cortex. These include "adaptation" effects, in which neurons stop firing after prolonged exposure to a stimulus such as a rattling fan, so that after a while you do not hear it. It also explains other phenomena: patterns of mirror-neuron activation that reflect the brain's responses to watching someone else make a movement; basic communication patterns between neurons that might underlie how we think; and even the hierarchical anatomy of the cortex itself.

Friston's results have earned praise for bringing together so many disparate strands of neuroscience. "It is quite certainly the most advanced conceptual framework regarding an application of these ideas to brain function in general," says Wennekers. Marsel Mesulam, a cognitive neurologist from Northwestern University in Chicago, adds: "Friston's work is pivotal. It resonates entirely with the sort of model that I would like to see emerge."

Friston's free-energy principle clearly is not the ultimate theory; yet, it remains to be tested fully and needs to produce more predictions of how real brains behave. If all goes well, though, the outcome will be a concise mathematical law of brain function, perhaps something as brief and iconic as E = mc2. "The final equation you write on a T-shirt will be quite simple," Friston predicts.

On a more practical level, he says the approach will change our concepts of how the brain works and could help us understand the deeper mechanisms of psychological disorders, especially those thought to be caused by faulty connections in the cortex, such as schizophrenia. It could also shine a light on bigger questions such as the nature of human consciousness.

There is much work still to be done, but for now Friston's is the most promising approach of all available. "It will take time to spin off all of the consequences of the theory – but I take that property as a sure sign that this is a very important theory," says Dehaene. "Most other models, including mine, are just models of one small aspect of the brain, very limited in their scope. This one falls much closer to a grand theory" [65].

Neill R. Taylor and John G. Taylor, the British mathematicians from the Department of Mathematics, King's College London, developed hard-wired simulations of temporal sequence storage and generation by multi-modular networks based on the frontal lobe system (cortex, basal ganglia and thalamus). Single cell activity was shown to have been constructed so as to mimic results measured in monkeys on a similar task, indicating that a suitable form of chunking had been achieved in the models. The mathematical nature of these processes was discussed, from the viewpoint of bifurcation theory [66].

In other work (2006), they studied the microstructure of attention in the brain profoundly and accurately. They investigated three possible methods for specifying the microstructure of attention feedback: contrast gain, additive and output gain, and using simple single node and 3-layer cortical models composed of graded or spiking neurons. Contrast gain and additive attention were also tested in a spiking network which was simplified by mean field methods. The simulation task used two stimuli, probe and reference, presented singly or together within the neuronal receptive fields, while attention was directed toward or away from the receptive field. Model neurons were differentially activated in the different stimuli and attention and equilibrium potentials or average firing rates, depending on neuron type, were recorded. The scientists compared results for the different modes of attention and architectures with experimental single cell recordings which showed how neuronal firing rates changed in response to attention, with a bias toward neurons that responded more effectively to the attended stimulus, to investigate which attentional method best fitted the experimental data. The simulation results were also mathematically analyzed. Their conclusion was that there was most experimental support for contrast gain, although some additional feedback gain would be possible. As a result of their study, the authors proposed a tentative method by which attention as a contrast gain might occur in the primate brain using acetylcholine and nicotinic receptors [67].

The press release of Carnegie Mellon University informs us about a novel theory of brain flexibility that explains how the brain compensates for damage caused in such disorders as stroke and others [68]. The neuroscientist Marcel Just and Stanford postdoctoral fellow Sashank Varma put forward a new computational theory of brain function that provided answers to one of the central questions of modern science: How does the human brain organize itself to give rise to complex cognitive tasks such as reading, problem solving and spatial reasoning? Just and Varma's theory, called 4CAPS, was described in the Cognitive, Affective, and Behavioral Neuroscience journal.

More than a decade of research involving functional Magnetic Resonance Imaging brain scans in hundreds of laboratories has yielded a tremendous amount of information about what parts of the brain are activated when a person performs various tasks. Some researchers were tempted to conclude that a simple one-to-one relationship existed between high-level mental tasks and brain areas. For example, some believed that a specific brain area was responsible for a specific cognitive task, such as identifying a face.

However, Marcel Just and Sashank Varma (2007) proposed that the evidence revealed a more complex picture in which thinking was a network function — a collaboration of several brain areas that was constantly adapting itself, based on the task at hand and the brain's own resources and biological limitations. The collaborating parts of the brain, according to Just, were like members of a sports team whose players substitute in and out of the action. 4CAPS (an acronym for Capacity Constrained Concurrent Cortical Activation-based Production System) proposed a decentralized process by which members of the cortical team volunteer themselves when their strengths are called for, but also permit less efficient but capable members to step forward when the primary player is injured or disabled, as might occur as a result of a stroke. Just and Varma constructed a number of computational models to demonstrate this process, such as a model that understands English sentences.

A unique characteristic of the theory was that it could accurately predict the change in brain activation that resulted from some types of brain damage or disease. For example, if a stroke damages the part of the brain known as Broca's area — which is located in the left prefrontal cortex and is involved in language processing — then the corresponding site on the right side of the brain often becomes activated during language processing, even within hours after a stroke. According to 4CAPS, the same dynamic allocation mechanism that allows brain areas to volunteer themselves on a moment-by-moment basis would also come into play if Broca's area were damaged, and would allow any excess computational load to spill over to the right hemisphere mirror site on a more permanent basis. Another example occurs with Alzheimer's disease, where the damage to some brain areas causes additional "helper" areas to be recruited to perform a task – additional areas that were not typically used by control subjects who did not have the disease. "Many brain-imaging studies have shown as the nature of the task changes, so does the set of activating brain areas," said Just, the D.O. Hebb Professor of Psychology. "It is as though substitutions of team players are being made dynamically in response to changes in the game."

4CAPS provided a framework for scientists and medical researchers to better understand nascent topics in neuroscience, such as how brain areas communicate and collaborate with one another during the thought process and how this can go wrong. For example, Just and his colleagues proposed an influential theory of autism, called the underconnectivity theory, which attributes the disorder to poor connectivity and hence communication between frontal areas of the brain and more posterior areas. The individual areas still have their specializations, according to the theory, but they cannot communicate as well with each other, and may develop a tendency to operate more independently of each. The theory also provides an account of what limits our ability to perform multitasking [69].

As the researchers consider, thousands of facts acquired due to visualization techniques of the brain demand organization and coordination, some agreement that would result in an understanding of the brain. Theory provides a new framework for understanding how a flow of thoughts emerges from the brain's activity dynamics. As far as neurological issues come up in education, aging, development, and as the basis for knowledge-based economics, it becomes more and more important that brain function is made clear to students, parents, education workers, patients and doctors, trainers and managers, citizens and politicians [68].

For decades neuroscientists have been convinced that they had a clear understanding of how the signals move through the brain cortex. Studies of the anatomy of axons took them to the conclusion that information was transferred through the column of six layers of specialized nervous cells in the series of automated signals originating from the midlayer of the cortex and then moving to other layers till the behavior response is triggered. However, new research from Dr. Randy Bruno (2013) demonstrates that the concept is incorrect. Bruno studied the processing of sensory information in rats and discovered that the signals are processed in two parts of the cortex simultaneously, and not in a series – as if there were two brains. "Our findings challenge dogma," says Bruno, Assistant Professor of Neuroscience and a faculty member at Columbia's new Mortimer B. Zuckerman Mind Brain Behavior Institute and the Kavli Institute for Brain Science. "The upper and lower layers form separate circuits that do separate things." The discovery, he says, "opens up a different way of thinking about how the cerebral cortex does what it does, which includes not only processing sight, sound and touch but higher functions such as speech, decision-making and abstract thought" [70]. The research was done with Christine Constantinople, as co-author, who now is a post-doctoral researcher at the Princeton Neuroscience Institute and the results were published in the *Science*, 2013 [71]. They studied a well-known sensory system of rat whiskers, which functions similarly to that of human fingers, providing tactile information about shape and texture. This information follows from nervous fibers at the base of the whiskers to the thalamus in the midbrain and is then processed in the cerebral cortex. Previous research has mapped each whisker to a specific barrel-shaped cluster of neurons in the brain. The new study relies on a sensitive technique that allows researchers to record how signals move across synapses from one neuron to the next in a live animal by using micropipettes, whose tips are just 1 micron wide—one-thousandth of a millimeter. The records showed that signals were relayed from the thalamus to the mid- and deeper layers of the cortex simultaneously, with surprisingly robust signaling to the deeper layer.

To confirm that the deeper layer receives sensory information directly from the thalamus, the researchers blocked all signals from the mid-layer using a local anesthetic. Activity in the deeper layer remained unchanged.

"This was very surprising," says Constantinople. "We expected activity in the lower layers to be turned off or very much diminished." The study suggests that the upper and lower layers of the cerebral cortex form separate circuits that play separate roles in processing sensory information. Researchers believe that the deeper layers are evolutionarily older—they are found in reptiles, for example, while the upper and middle layers appear in more evolved species and are thickest in humans.

One of the versions is that basic sensory processing occurs in the lower layers; for example, visually tracking a tennis ball. Processing that involves integrating context or experience might be done in the upper layers – for example, watching where an opponent is hitting the ball and planning where to return the shot.

Bert Sakmann, the German neurobiologist, who won a 1991 Nobel Prize for developing the micropipette system of mapping nerve impulses, describes the study as a game-changer. "Dr. Bruno has produced a technical masterpiece that now firmly establishes two separate input streams to the cortex," he says [69].

Konstantin Baev (2007) from St. Joseph's Hospital and Medical Center (USA) offered a basically different conceptual understanding of the brain functioning and basic mechanisms of normal and pathological behavior conditioned by the brain. His work of 2007 shows why the classical conceptual views of the brain that can be found in any neuroscience textbook are not capable of providing an adequate explanation of brain-initiated normal and pathological behaviors and why the classical view should therefore be replaced with a new concept of the brain. The major reason for the inadequacy of the classical model is its explanation of the relationship between the structure and the function in the brain. This article introduces a new brain concept based on two discoveries: the discovery of the neural network computational principle and the discovery of the generic functional organization of hierarchical neural optimal control systems. A neural optimal control system is a learning system that possesses a model of the behavior of its controlled object. A hierarchy of neural optimal control systems is functionally organized in such a way that a higher level neural optimal control system treats a lower one as its controlled object and creates a model of its behavior. The ability of the new conceptual brain model to explain the brain mechanisms of normal and pathological behaviors is demonstrated through the examples of spinal reflexes and central pattern generators, the cerebellum, skeletomotor cortico-basal ganglia-thalamocortical loop, and Parkinson's disease and some other brain disorders. In this article, a new understanding of the relationship between structure and function in the brain is introduced [72].

The idea of controllers, proposed by Baev to explain the mechanisms of brain functioning in the neurosciences, is not new. An article by Lisa Zyga describes the theory of brain controllers that explains brain functioning from the standpoint of information theory and systems of artificial intelligence (AI) [73]. It was found by Asim Roy, the professor of information systems, who in the 1990s started writing his work on the new theory of the brain. According to this theory, special controllers for the brain functions of a higher level are absent, and all control is local and distributed evenly throughout all areas. In his work, Asim Roy describes the theory of brain controllers, according to which there exist parts of the brain controlling other parts, organizing them into a hierarchical system [74]. According to the theory of controllers that agrees with the so-called computational theory, the brain learns a lot of rules and uses them in a hierarchically organized top-down method. To illustrate the efficiency of the theory, the researchers offer the example of its use in chess. In 1997, IBM's *Deep Blue* computer, which is famous for its victory over Garry Kasparov, the world chess champion, operated by relying on countless rules that were programmed by its programmers. Despite the success of the rule-based AI system in chess, no AI system has come close to learning and interacting with the world at the human level, using either the connectionist approach or the computational approach.

Roy's theory undermines the roots of connectionism, and that is why his ideas have experienced resistance from the cognitive science community. For the past 15 years, Roy has engaged researchers in public debates, in which he had to argue with a dozen or so connectionist researchers.

One reason why it was so difficult for researchers to accept his theory was that, in cognitive science, terms are not always defined in a very strict way, as they are in other sciences, he explained. He said that he ran into many circular arguments with reviewers regarding his paper, and that was why much of the paper was dedicated to defining what a controller was.

Psychology Professor James McClelland at Stanford University, whose early work Roy cites in his paper, thinks that modern connectionist thought allows for some controlling parts of the brain, though not to the extent shown in Roy's model [73].

Meanwhile, neuroscientist Walter J. Freeman of the University of California at Berkeley also said that he agreed with the notion that there were controllers or guidance systems within the brain. Freeman, who had taught brain sciences at Berkeley since 1959, developed a model of the brain's intentional system. The model involved a control loop that predicted future states, future sensory input and future plans of action. The spatiotemporal pattern that implemented this plan was transmitted by cortical neurons into the brain stem and spinal cord, using feedback from various parts of the brain. So the guidance, control and monitoring of actions played an important part in Freeman's model.

No matter exactly where or what the brain controllers are, Roy hopes that his theory will enable research on new kinds of learning algorithms. Currently, restrictions such as local and memoryless learning have limited AI designers, but these concepts are derived directly from the idea that control is local, not high-level. Possibly, a controller-based theory could lead to the development of truly autonomous learning systems, and a next generation of intelligent robots. "The controller theory gives us much more freedom in creating brain-like learning systems," he said. "The science is currently stuck, and we have not made any significant progress toward creating robots that can learn on their own like humans."

Ten years later and after several rejections and resubmissions, the paper "Connectionism, Controllers, and a Brain Theory" has finally been published in the November issue of *IEEE Transactions on Systems, Man, and Cybernetics – Part A: Systems and Humans* [74]. However, Roy's controversial ideas on how the brain works and learns probably will not immediately win over many of his colleagues, who have spent decades teaching robots and AI systems how to think using the classic connectionist theory of the brain. Connectionists propose that the brain consists of an interacting network of neurons and cells, and that it solves problems based on how these components are connected.

In his research using logical arguments and neurological data, Asim Roy shows that connectivism theory is actually based on a controller. He explains that some of the simplest connectivity systems use controllers to accomplish the operations, and, as more complicated connectivity systems are based on simpler ones, they also involve controllers. If Roy's logic correctly describes how the brain functions, it could help AI researchers to overcome some of the inherent limitations in connectionist algorithms. The criticism of this theory argues that connectivism demands a human babysitter for its learning algorithms, and that is not like human brain at all.

Roy acknowledges that only neuroscience, and not information science, can determine whether connectionist algorithms such as the back-propagation algorithm actually exist in the brain. But if they do, he says that they must rely on controllers. He highlights evidence from a variety of neuroscience studies that support the existence of controllers in the brain. For example, past research has proposed the existence of control centers of the brain, such as the prefrontal portion of the cerebral cortex. Studies of dopamine and other neural transmitters, as well as the presence of "neurogenesis" in adults, are also compatible with a controller-based brain theory.

Roy clarifies that there is not necessarily a single executive controller in the brain, but rather that multiple distributed controllers could be responsible for different subsystems of the brain. After all, he says, if the connectionist theory is correct and the brain is a network of changing connections, there must be some control mechanism to determine how all of those connections are made.

Finally, if the theory of connectivity is right and the brain is network of changing connections, there must be the mechanisms to specify how to establish these connections. But the controller theory can form and train neural networks in a different way from that of connectivity so that, actually, a new science emerges and we look forward to new algorithms of human-like learning [73].

The Northwestern University public release dated January 2005 describes another theory about the memory challenging conventional concept of long-term memory storage in the brain [75]. The current view of memory is that, at the molecular level, new proteins are manufactured, in a process known as translation, and it is these newly synthesized proteins that subsequently stabilize the changes underlying the memory. Thus, every new memory results in a permanent representation in the brain.

The Northwestern University neuroscientist Aryeh Routtenberg presented a provocative new theory that took issue with that view [76]. Routtenberg and his doctoral student Jerome

L. Rekart outlined their new theory on memory storage in the January issue of the journal Trends in Neuroscience. According to the authors, rather than permanent storage, there is a "dynamic, meta-stable" process. Our subjective experience of permanence is a result of the re-duplication of memories across many different brain networks.

For example, one's name is represented in innumerable neural circuits; thus, it is extremely difficult to forget. But each individual component is malleable and transient, and as no particular neural network lasts a lifetime, it is theoretically possible to forget one's own name.

This is observed in the most advanced stages of Alzheimer's disease, the researchers stated. The advantage of such a precarious storage mechanism is that it is a highly flexible system, enabling the rapid retrieval of even infrequent elements, with great advantages over models of permanent storage, said Routtenberg, Professor in the Department of Psychology and in the Department of Neurobiology and Physiology, Judd A. and Marjorie Weinberg College of Arts and Sciences and a leading researcher in the Institute for Neuroscience, Northwestern University.

To achieve this high degree of flexibility, Routtenberg's new theory goes on to propose that the brain stores long-term memory by rapidly changing the shape of proteins already present at those synapses activated by learning. While it is universally agreed that brain proteins are critical for memory storage, Routtenberg's hypothesis challenges the widely accepted, 40-year-old model that long-term memories are stabilized only once newly synthesized proteins are transported to recently activated synapses.

Indeed, this view is central to the theory of Eric Kandel, who in his Nobel Prize address reinforced the central position of this model in forming long-term memory. So does memory form because you make more protein, as most neuroscientists believe, or because you change the shape of existing proteins, which are known to be strategically located to effect change within milliseconds of activation?

Part of the answer to this question lies in the fact that there are critical weaknesses in the prevailing view. "There are enough instances of memory storage in the virtual absence of protein synthesis to compel consideration of alternative models," said Routtenberg. The authors noted that most of the evidence supporting the current view had been obtained by studying the effects of certain drugs, called protein synthesis inhibitors, on memory, leading to the conclusion that synthesis was necessary. The authors outline specific evidence that calls those results into question.

For example, synthesis inhibitors that block the production of new proteins by more than 90 percent often cause no discernible memory impairments. Additionally, protein synthesis inhibitors cause a number of side effects that could lead to memory loss caused by something other than protein synthesis inhibition.

Routtenberg agrees with the view that it is the synapse that is modified in response to learning-associated activity, a position first articulated by Nobel Prize winner Ramon y Cajal a century ago. But the difference with the current theory is that he and Rekart do not believe that synaptic modification is brought about by recently synthesized proteins.

Routtenberg's theory, derived from a consideration of extensive, fundamental biochemical information, advocates that learning leads to a post-synthesis (or, post-translational) synaptic protein modification that results in changes to the shape, activity and/or location of existing synaptic proteins. In the Routtenberg-Rekart proposal, this is the only mechanism required for long-term memory.

To maintain some residue of this modification, Routtenberg proposes that the "spontaneous activity" of the brain actually acts to "cryptically rehearse" past events. So, long-term memory storage relies on a positive-feedback rehearsal system that continually updates or fine-tunes post-translational modification of previously modified synaptic proteins. It is in this manner that this model allows for the continual modifications of memories.

In the Routtenberg-Rekart model, post-translational modifications within cells and synaptic dialog and endogenous activity between cells and networks work in concert to perpetuate and update memory representations.

A group of post-translational protein modifications that affect neuronal plasticity – present in activated pre-synaptic and post-synaptic elements and regulated by proteases, kinases and phosphatases – regulates the efficacy of the synapse in response to a learning event.

These modifications are, in turn, maintained via positive feedback between cells (dialog), which are regulated by synaptic excitation (e.g., via the neurotransmitter glutamate) or inhibition (e.g., via the neurotransmitter GABA).

Thus, the self-sustaining positive feedback system also carries built-in control mechanisms that would prevent runaway feedback leading to the detonation of one massive memory or "thermonuclear" engram. Although Routtenberg's model seems different from the current view of how long-term memories are stored, he believes that scientists need to articulate alternative models other than the prevailing one.

A more accurate description will help address issues of memory loss in mental retardation, aging and Alzheimer's disease. Indeed, new hypotheses can lead to the development of new chemical agents that would successfully target the chemical reactions that require appropriate correction. "We would assert that there is enough substance both in the concerns raised and in the post-translational modification/positive feedback model proposed to energize the search for yet more plausible models of long-term memory storage, and to redirect and reinvigorate the quest to understand the brain substrates of information storage," Routtenberg said [75].

Steve Ramirez, Xu Liu, Pei-Ann Lin et al. (2013) from the Massachusetts Institute of Technology (USA) claim that the hippocampus is the sought substrate of the brain [77]. The researchers created a false memory in mice by optogenetically manipulating memory engram-bearing cells in the hippocampus. Dentate gyrus (DG) or CA1 neurons activated by exposure to a particular context were labeled with channelrhodopsin-2. These neurons were later optically reactivated during fear conditioning in a different context. The DG experimental group showed increased freezing in the original context, in which a foot shock was never delivered. The recall of this false memory was context-specific, activated similar downstream regions engaged during natural fear memory recall, and was also capable of driving an active fear response. These data demonstrate that it is possible to generate an internally represented and behaviorally expressed fear memory via artificial means. The idea of the memory cells located in the hippocampus was pronounced by Karl Pribram in the 1950s, though no evidence had been received. The data of American researchers on the photo-stimulation of neurons do not prove that the neural structures of the hippocampal area of the brain are the neurons of the memory [77].

There is another quite unusual spatiotemporal concept of the brain's functioning, which was developed by Andrew A. Fingelkurts, Alexander A. Fingelkurts and Carlos F. H. Neves (2010) from the Brain and Mind Technologies Research Centre (Espoo, Finland) [78]. The concepts of space and time are widely developed in physics. However, there is a considerable lack of biologically plausible theoretical frameworks that can demonstrate how space and time dimensions are implemented in the activity of the most complex life-system – the brain with a mind. Brain activity is organized both temporally and spatially, thus representing space-time in the brain. Critical analysis of recent research on the space-time organization of the brain's activity pointed to the existence of so-called operational space-time in the brain. This space-time is limited to the execution of brain operations of differing complexity. During each such brain operation a particular short-term spatio-temporal pattern of integrated activity of different brain areas emerges within related operational space-time. At the same time, to have a fully functional human brain one needs to have a subjective mental experience. Current research on the subjective mental experience offers a detailed analysis of the space-time organization of the mind. According to this research, subjective mental experience (subjective virtual world) has definitive spatial and temporal properties similar to many physical phenomena. Based on a systematic review of the propositions and tenets of brain and mind space-time descriptions, the aim of the researchers is to explore the relationships between the two. They proposed the hypothesis that via the brain operational space-time the mind subjective space-time is connected to otherwise distant physical space-time reality [78].

To support their space-time concept of the brain A. A. Fingelkurts and A. A. Fingelkurts explored the operational architectonics of alpha activity in different normal and pathological brain states. An aggregated analysis of a set of diverse previously conducted EEG/MEG experimental studies was performed within the same methodological and conceptual framework. It was shown that the characteristics of short alpha activity periods (segments), as well as the spatial structural synchrony of alpha activity, changed considerably in accordance with the type of brain functional state, stimulation, cognitive task, pharmacological influence, and the type of pathology. The results of this study suggest that particular neurophysiological pattern(s) of cortex alpha activity indicate a resting state network, which is characterized by well-defined structure in both the temporal as well as the spatial domain. The optimal functional state of the brain depends upon a delicate metastable balance between local specialized processes and their global integration. An excess or lack of either component would be a deviation from the optimal condition and could lead to pathology. The fact that all observed results were significantly different from surrogate EEG data reflects a non-occasional nature of spatio-temporal dynamics in the operational architectonics of alpha activity. A better understanding of the specific ways in which the disrupted dynamics of different characteristics of alpha-generating neuronal assemblies (and their functional connectivity) may underlie neuro/psychopathology might suggest new targets for therapeutic agents [79].

The novel neuro-technological approach of Emre Neftci and the team (2013) throws light onto general issues of the organization of neural circuits in the brain and future neuromorphic (brain-like) technologies capable of cognitive behavior. They performed neuromorphic emulations that expressed the dynamics of neural circuits in analogous electronic circuits offering distributed low-energy technology for the development of intellectual systems. However, neuromorphic circuits are characterized by noise and inaccuracy, and currently there is no method to change the configuration of safe behavior dynamics on these substrates. Emre Neftci et al. (2013) describe a new method able to install simple cognitive behavior on neuromorphic substrate. To answer how neural circuits of the brain work, Neftci et al. (2013) attempted intellectual processing in electronic neuromorphic systems, which, however, lack the methods of achievements of safe behavior dynamics in the originally inaccurate and noise neuron substrates. They reported a solution to this problem that involved first mapping an unreliable hardware layer of spiking silicon neurons into an abstract computational layer composed of generic reliable subnetworks of model neurons and then composing the target behavioral dynamics as a "soft state machine" running on these reliable subnets. In the first step, the neural networks of the abstract layer were realized on the hardware substrate by mapping the neuron circuit bias voltages to the model parameters. This mapping was obtained by an automatic method in which the electronic circuit biases were calibrated against the model parameters by a series of population activity measurements. The abstract computational layer was formed by configuring neural networks as generic soft winner-takes-all subnetworks that provided reliable processing by virtue of their active gain, signal restoration, and multistability. The necessary states and transitions of the desired high-level behavior were then easily embedded in the computational layer by introducing only sparse connections between some neurons of the various subnets. They demonstrated this synthesis method for a neuromorphic sensory agent that performs the real-time context-dependent classification of motion patterns observed by a silicon retina [80].

There is another methodological approach to biotechnological studies of the human brain developed by the Allen Institute for Brain Science [81]. Paul Allen, a co-founder of Microsoft, established the Allen Institute for Brain Science, a medical Manhattan Project. The institute focused on creating tools, such as the mouse laser, which is technically a new type of microscope. "As an ex-programmer I'm still just curious about how the brain functions, how that flow of information really happens," said Allen in a rare interview. "The thing you realize when you get into studying neuroscience, even a little bit, is that everything is connected to everything else. So it's as if the brain is trying to use everything at its disposal– what it is seeing, what it is hearing, what is the temperature, past experience. It's using all of this to try to compute what the animal should do next, whether that animal is a mouse or human being."

In the Allen Institute for Brain Science Paul Allen developed a huge computer genome model of a mouse brain to demonstrate how genes work. Allen initiated the development of a similar model to the human brain that would help to develop new theories of the brain's functioning. Allen and his team want to know how the visual cortex of the brain works, as a way to understand how nerve cells work in brains in general. Other projects aim to isolate all of the kinds of cells in the brain and use stem cells to learn how they develop. Scientists think there may be 1,000 of these basic building blocks, but they do not even know that. The sequencing of the human genome, an example of the power of industrial-scale science, inspired Paul Allen, and he wanted to fund something similar, such as an atlas of brain genes work or a computer map of genes working in a mouse brain.

Every cell in a mouse has the same 20,000 genes. What makes a heart cell different from a brain cell is how those genes are used. "It appealed to me because it was something that hadn't been done, something that could be scaled, something that created a database that could be accessible worldwide and would lift all boats in the area of neuroscience," Allen said. It was also similar to the role he'd played at Microsoft, where he had created emulators that allowed others to write software; again, he was creating developer tools, but this time for neuroscientists.

Today the research in the Allen Institute for Brain Science is done at a neurobiological level. Mice brains were frozen and sliced by automated machines; each slice fit on a single microscope slide. Technicians dipped each slice in an RNA solution that stained cells containing a single sequence of RNA in a particular color. Only one gene can be captured per slice and six per brain, meaning it took 4,000 mice to create the Allen Brain Atlas, made available free on the Web in December 2004 and largely finished in 2006. The completed atlas involved 85 million images on 250,000 slides, or 600 terabytes of data–half as big as the entire Internet in 2003.

The Mouse Brain Atlas fast became a standard tool for neuroscientists in both industry and academia worldwide. In 2006 the scientists outside Allen's institute had used the atlas to find genes that might influence susceptibility to multiple sclerosis in humans, as well as eating disorders and memory. With the success of the mouse atlas, Allen put another $100 million toward a tougher proposition; an atlas of the human brain, which is 3,000 times as big, with 1,000 times as many cells.

All of the equipment used for slicing and staining the brains had to be refitted. And, more critically, the brains themselves were hard to acquire. Rather than 1,000 human brains, the map would have to be built with fewer than 10, which needed to come from people who had died in the prime of life without the brain being damaged by injury or illness.

Four years later, six brains have been donated and four analyzed to some degree. The project is due to be finished this year, but the first brain images, put online in 2010, are already yielding scientific results.

Understanding the brain, Allen argued, was much like being a medieval blacksmith trying to reverse engineer a jet plane. It was not just that you did not understand how the wing attached to the fuselage or what made the engine go. You did not even know the basic theory of how air going over a wing creates lift. "Moore's Law-based technology is so much easier than neuroscience," Allen said. "The brain works in such a different way from the way a computer does. The computer is a very regular structure. It's very uniform. It's got a bunch of memory, and it's got a little element that computes bits of memory and combines them with each other and puts them back somewhere. It is a very simple thing. You can start programming. I did it in high school. Me and Bill Gates and our friends did that. Probably in a few months we were programming and probably understood what there was to understand about computing within a few years of diving into it. In the human brain, designed by evolution, every tiny part is very different from every other tiny part. It's hideously complex," Allen said. "And it's going to take "decades and decades" of more research to understand. We are talking about dozens and dozens of Nobel Prizes that have yet to be won to understand how the brain works." [81].

Colombian neuroscientist Ricardo Dolmetsch, on leave from Stanford, is heading up another challenge: using stem cells to figure out what the brain is made of. "If a mechanic didn't know how many parts were in a car, would you trust that mechanic?" queried Koch, who likens the current drugs for depression and schizophrenia to fixing that car by pouring oil over the top and hoping some gets into the motor. Science, like the early days of software, has generally been practiced by hundreds or thousands of individual scientists working independently, competing to scoop one another – even large-scale research labs such as Salk and Rockefeller work this way. Allen's industrialized approach is known by researchers as "big science," a worrisome trend to some. "The state of funding in neuroscience is worse than it's ever been in my career," says NYU neuroscientist Tony Movshon. "I think small, investigator-initiated science is the best way to get creative ideas" [82].

The French-German-Canadian team of scientists of the Institut de Neurosciences des Systèmes, Aix Marseille Université (Marseille, France), Charité University of Medicine (Berlin, Germany) and Rotman Research Institute at Baycrest, (Toronto, ON, Canada) attempted to understand the principles of the brain's workings through the development of a virtual brain presented as the model of the primate brain network dynamics (P. S. Leon, A. Knock, Woodman et al., 2013) [83]. The researchers presented The Virtual Brain (TVB), a neuroinformatics platform for full brain network simulations using biologically realistic connectivity. This simulation environment enables the model-based inference of neurophysiological mechanisms across different brain scales that underlie the generation of macroscopic neuroimaging signals including functional MRI (fMRI), EEG and MEG. Researchers from different backgrounds can benefit from an integrative software platform including a supporting framework for data management (generation, organization, storage, integration and sharing) and a simulation core written in Python. TVB allows the reproduction and evaluation of personalized configurations of the brain by using individual subject data. This personalization facilitates an exploration of the consequences of pathological changes in the system, permitting investigation of the potential ways of counteracting such unfavorable processes. The architecture of TVB supports interaction with MATLAB packages, for example, the well-known Brain Connectivity Toolbox. TVB can be used in a client-server configuration, such that it can be remotely accessed through the Internet thanks to its web-based HTML5, JS, and WebGL graphical user interface. TVB is also accessible as a standalone cross-platform Python library and application, and users can interact with the scientific core through the scripting interface IDLE, enabling the easy modeling, development and debugging of the scientific kernel. This second interface makes TVB extensible by combining it with other libraries and modules developed by the Python scientific community. In this article, we describe the theoretical background and foundations that led to the development of TVB, the architecture and features of its major software components as well as its potential neuroscience applications [83].

Therefore, until now there has been no clear understanding or any integral ubiquitously acknowledged theory of brain structure and organization. All previously mentioned informational, biophysical and biochemical aspects of the theory are acceptable and all of them have an important rational kernel taken by the authors as the main and system-forming basis for their theoretical construct. In some works, it is entropy; in others, it is connectivity, and in yet another it is protein memory, etc. These theories correctly reflect the hierarchical connections in the brain that control the informational relations. But they do not provide a full explanation for all biophysical (magnetic-field and magnetic-wave) and biochemical (genome, transcriptome, proteome, metabolome and secretome) relations observed in the human and mammal nerve tissue. How are they connected? Where is the borderline when biochemistry replaces biophysics and then the biophysical component emerges again? These theories cannot answer the simple, primitive questions of an ordinary neurologist or a first year medical student: 1) Why does the brain look so strange; why does it have the gyri that are not found in any other organs of mammals? 2) Why is the area of spinal cord washed by CSF intensively, while in the areas of the brain and the neocortex the CSF space is suddenly divided into two sectors by the arachnoid mater? 3) Why does the pia mater of the brain differ so much from an external capsule of any other mammalian organ? 4) Why cannot we imitate the thoughts and cognitive functions when we develop a complete simulator of neuron networks of the brain? 5) Why do the conducting fibers, vessels, glial cells, and synapses constitute the major part of the brain (75%) and the neurons comprise only 25%? 6) Where and how in the brain do the holographic processes, acknowledged to be central in the brain's functioning, occur? The questions seem stupid, but the answers that we want to receive must be smart and clear even for a schoolchild. However, none of the current concepts of the brain's structure and organization can give answers to these questions that would be clear even to a professor of neurology. Obviously, there is no complete clarity in the sphere. One can speak a lot about the shape of mobile communication towers, the distance between them, the brands of mobile phones and their characteristics, but it will not drive you closer to an understanding of mobile communication. One still does not understand the main laws of the information transfer between the subscribers and the role of the mobile operator. This situation is similar to the understanding of the brain setup and its functions. The visual methodological approach observed in neuro-research yields very nice pictures of the brain (MRI, CT, MEG, PET, FMRI, EEG), but does not allow an understanding of their information identity. Looking at the nice images of the MRI of the brain, we forget that the physical principle of the magnetic resonance of the nerve tissue reflects the magnetization or fundamental parameters of the nerve tissue magnetic field, and the magnetoencephalography of the brain presents magnetic-wave processes in large areas of the nerve tissue. We forget that the PET of the brain can help us to describe the metabolism of the nerve cells of the brain, depending on the level of radioactive glucose distribution in them, while biochemical tests of the brain tissue can tell us what every part of the brain secretes. The genome, transcriptome and proteome of nerve cells seem very distant from the sphere of contemporary multidimensional biology and laboratory tests, and not data that could be of use to clinicians and neuroscientists. We have not achieved a complete information image of the events, and still speak of the shape and geometry of the nerve cells, gathering gene networks of them, protein networks, and floundering in them. We color the fibers (or wires) connecting different parts and enjoy the images of the brain's connectivity. And this is the main philosophical and methodological mistake. One should go deeply into the nature of the phenomena and the relations between them.

In conclusion, we would like to dwell on an important summary made by the Russian neuroscientist Evgheny Vityaev. He asked how one can make sense of a huge number of the brain theories and what the methodology of the brain theory should be. In terms of the work of the brain being multifaceted, it is described at different standpoints in different theories and in different terms; thus, these theories are hardly compatible. The situation is similarly complicated in the theories of perception that were described by Alexander Logvinenko in the preface to the translation of James Gibson's book (1988): "The first introduction into the theories of perception embarrasses. The abundance of theories, their eclectic diversity and occasionally complete incompatibility knock you down. Those who have enough patience to make out this extremely confusing bulk of ideas, approaches, trends and the rest will be surprised once more. It appeared that the theory of perception had never ever existed. There were more or less successful ideas, but there never was a well-developed theory". This picture is equally applicable to the theories of the brain, its functions, structure and setup. One should have a clear idea of what is meant under the development of such a theory of the brain and what can be considered an integral theory of the brain.

Evgheny Vityaev thinks that the theories are diverse for natural reasons: they have different conceptual frameworks (ontologies) that condition the angle at which the object of the studies (brain and its organization) is perceived; they have different a priori guesses and supportive theories and methods. Altogether, this constitutes the reference basis of the natural-scientific theory (paradigm) that determines the subject of studies, baseline natural-scientific theory and the further direction of research. The natural-scientific theory is developed within this paradigm and consists in the specification and clarification of this basis: new hypotheses formulated within the conceptual framework are forwarded and studied; the theory develops when new confirmed hypotheses are added; new consequences of the theory are examined, etc. When a sufficient number of facts is accumulated, they are summarized as new postulates, principles, axioms, equations, etc. These summaries are usually done simultaneously with the introduction of new and rather abstract terms (theoretical notions). The process of summarizing evolves to quite abstract and usually simple postulates, principles, axioms or equations that provide the basis for the main assertions of the theory. Such assertions are called the principles by Vityaev; that is, the *principles* of the theories are the general assertions of the theory from which follow the most important statements of the theory. In other words, the principle must be an assertion (postulate, axiom, equation) from which almost a whole theory is drawn. If the theory follows out of some principle, we call it the *theory-principle*. Traditionally it is considered that the theory developed within a certain paradigm gives the "picture" of the subjects of study that agree with its basis. However, it is not so. Usually, the exact analysis of the principle (including mathematical) comes into conflict with the basis of the theory. In the principles the theory can rise over the details of the suppositions, research methods and involved machinery that were done and used in the process of the development of the theory and, hence, we approach the truth. It is well known that in psychology the perception follows from the whole to the particular. Perception of the details and the particulars is guided and corrected by the perception of the whole. The same happens with the theories. If the theory evolves to the theory-principle, the latter is closer to the "truth". Theoretical notions are introduced into the theory to deepen the "image", the "standpoint" of the subject of the study and to penetrate it to the core. If in this case the basis of the theory contradicts the theory-principle, then the basis should be changed and not the principles. However, with rare exception, nobody thinks that the principles are more important than the basis, so the detected contradiction is not accepted by the academic community as it demands a revision of the basis and, respectively, the available paradigm. As far as the paradigm is more important than the principles and its revision signifies a scientific "revolution", the contradiction of the basis to the theory-principle is viewed as the *paradox* and is underrated. However, there are many examples proving the opposite – that the basis of the theory requires revision. Such revision is considered revolutionary. The method of theory development when the principles are detected, then the theory-principle is derived, and then there is a "scientific revolution" due to the revision of the basis, would be a regular method for the development of theories, including both development of the theory within one paradigm and the change of paradigms. Now a *method of research* can be formulated that will permit finding the principle of brain functioning and its formal model. The theories-principles exhibit an important feature: they permit the establishment of *conceptual bridges*. If the principle of the theory-principle can be interpreted within the conceptual framework of another theory-principle, then a whole theory-principle derived from this principle can be interpreted within the conceptual framework of this theory. Therefore, these theories become conceptually bridged. If the principles of two theories-principles express some general key notion or principle, then the principles as well as the theories are mutually interpretable or one of the theories is embedded in the other. This permits the *synthesis of different theories through their principles*, which is impossible if only baseline theories are used.

To come to an understanding of the brain seems possible only due to the synthesis of various theories through their principles. First, the appropriate principles should be specified in the studied theories. Then these theories should be brought to the theories-principles with mutually interpretable principles. In the case that some principles appear interpretable in a suitable mathematical theory, then we formalize the corresponding theory. In this case, not only the principle is formalized, but a whole theory-principle, by means of acquisition of all consequences from the principle. Reverse interpretation of the formalization to baseline theory can be tested for adequacy by experiments, thus raising higher demands to formalization. As the available examples show, the development of a mathematical theory-principal is an unconventional thing. This method of research has not been acknowledged and current work is attempting to demonstrate its efficiency [84, 85].

The work of Vityaev showed that the synthesis of several theories-principles could be performed along with their formalizations as mathematical theories-principles. Baseline theories are sub-theories in the synthesized formal theory. Not only the baseline theories, but also other theories-principles can be embedded into the synthesized formal theory, together with their formal theories, the principles of which are interpreted in this theory. The synthesis of principles gives us a fuller principle of the work of the brain. This method of research is attempted in this work to detect the principles of brain functioning.

Chapter 3

Current Global Research of the Brain: Theoretical, Methodological and Technological Bases for Discoveries, Inventions and Innovations in Contemporary Neuroscience

Abstract

The chapter begins with the analytical statement that in the 21st century the research innovations and breakthroughs were achieved by the "collective mind" of the international researchers, which can be illustrated by the Internet, Large Hadron Collider, space flights or missile defense. The Human Genome Project demonstrated an amazing capacity to integrate scientists around the world for research into the DNA structure of the eukaryotic genome. The 21st century was claimed to be the century of brain understanding. As the development of this trend, the chapter describes almost all of the current international research on the human brain, as well as its goals and objectives. During the past decade over 11 large-scale international neuro-research studies have been launched, initiated by the leaders of the unions (the EU, the USA) and countries with highly developed (Canada, the UK, Switzerland, etc.) and developing (China) economies. The Blue Brain (2005, Switzerland), the Human Connectome Project (2009, the USA), the Human Brain Project (2012, the EU), BRAIN Initiative (2013, the USA) and other projects have been financed by both public and private grants. In the next decade, various public organizations will spend about 20 billion USD on brain research, while private companies and specialized funds will invest about 5 billion USD. The Human Brain Project (HBP) is analyzed in this chapter as an example, and its main scientific and methodological errors are discussed. The HBP should lay the foundation for a new model (simulation) of the human brain on the bases of the information-communication platforms (ICPs) of the brain research, management of the integration of the data and knowledge from different spheres and development of new brain-like computing technologies. The author expresses his criticism and doubts about the efficiency of the proposed methodology of the system approach as a universal tool of analysis, synthesis and processing of the data about the brain. Several discrepancies between the claimed objectives and expected results have been found along with the practical impossibility of reaching the set goals due to the outdated morphological and functional system understanding of the brain. The author proposes a new project, Brainstorming of the

Brain, which can be implemented by relying on the information approach and the development of new information-commutation technologies but will be cheaper, more energy saving and science-driven.

Keywords: international projects of brain research, the Human Brain Project, BRAIN Initiative, the Human Brain Connectome, the Blue Brain, the BigBrain, dual-use technologies, neuro-technologies, military neuro-technologies

Until the middle of the 20th century all of the scientific breakthroughs and grand discoveries had been the results of the insights of the brightest scientists and advanced specialists. By now, the scope of knowledge is so great and multidisciplinary that it can hardly be covered and stored in one supercomputer, not to mention the human mind, even that of an extremely intelligent person. We live in an amazing era of the integration of scientific speculation and intellect, when the cooperation and joint efforts of all of the scientists and experts of the world brainstorm the academic challenges of humanity. The collective intelligence of scientists from all over the world develops innovations and inventions of global strategic meaning. We are the witnesses of the milestone events, discoveries and breakthrough technologies that lead to the realization of bold science-driven projects, which for centuries seemed only dreams and delusory hopes for the people of the world. What yesterday seemed fantastic and incredible today appears real and even commonplace. This can be illustrated by numerous examples: global mobile telephony, the Internet, international space flights, systems of collective security to prevent natural disasters and wars of aggression, Large Hadron Collider, etc.

Generally, the implemented multi-scale research projects were conditioned by the scientific theoretical developments and technological breakthroughs of 20th century scientists. Humankind brought several multi-scale research projects and initiatives from the 20th century to the 21st. These projects were to overthrow the basic notions of the biological identity of humankind and to outline its potential in the reorganization of the world.

The first project of this type was the ambitious Human Genome Project, with its 3 billion USD funding from the National Institute of Health and the Department of Energy. The project was launched in 1988 and James Watson was appointed to head the Office of Human Genome research [86]. That was one of the most sophisticated, labor-consuming and expensive projects in the history of science. After the completion of the project in 2005, it became obvious that the received bulk of fundamental scientific evidence neither helped to answer the main challenges of contemporary healthcare, nor offered efficient novel therapeutic strategies to treat the main diseases of civilization (cancer and malignant tumors, AIDS, obesity, degenerative nervous diseases, etc.). However, the biotechnological leap in research into the fundamentals of life biology on Earth that was performed by the USA and their partners during the project, along with social and political preferences, military-economic and technological advantages over other countries, provided a breakthrough in the field of biology of living systems and the global scientific and technical superiority of the participating countries. Meanwhile, a large part of the obtained results remains classified and was not provided to the global scientific community. Still, by now the volume of the global market of genome production exceeds 1 billion USD, and it has not yet achieved its limit.

The project displayed the amazing opportunities that can be achieved due to pioneer research and the development of innovations when the leading experts of the world unite their efforts to answer global challenges of the modern age; the project permitted the establishment of new working places in the US and EU and the re-equipment of the leading scientific centers and laboratories according to the latest scientific needs. The US Administration highly appreciated the mobilizing, organizing, political and economic advantages that resulted from the implementation of such global projects. The US began to introduce new national ideas for the development of real sectors of the economy and business, as well as to initiate new incentives for novel solutions to national challenges. According to the opinions of the leading US analysts, one of the possible solutions to the problems that the country faces can be in the new ambitious national projects that aim to integrate frontier scientific thinking and to organize the international experts' brainstorms on the available challenges of healthcare and the needs of the biotechnological industry.

The advanced scientific and socially active communities turned their eyes to the innovative technologies of multidimensional biology: proteomics, metabolomics, RNomics, secretomics and others. The coming era was called post-genomic and no less ambitious a project than that known as the Human Proteome has been initiated to map, catalogue and examine the functions of all proteins found in eukaryotic cells [87]. The USA and their partners in the project have already distributed the scope of work in the planned research. However, the practical goals for the use of this new "proteomic" data in medicine and biotechnologies are not clear so far, and it seems extremely important to impart not only fundamental, but primarily clear practical healthcare meaning to this generation of new knowledge. It must be remembered that the new generation of knowledge in the area of life sciences on the one hand should neither give groundless and unreasonable hopes to specialists nor create an illusion of a cure-all to the patients. On the other hand, from the new methodological, biotechnological and informational positions, only novel biotechnological research can provide unique evidence about the structure and pathogenetic mechanisms of most of the incurable diseases of civilization and help to find efficient therapies. Humankind should not repeat the mistakes of genomics and genetic engineering; everything must be foreseen at the very start of new projects. While the Human Proteome Project is still under discussion, other global research projects have been put into action.

In 2008 Barak Obama, the US President, lifted the ban on stem cell research, and declared a revolutionary initiative of public funding for them (while the previous administration of George Bush banned their public funding), and establishing the national biotechnological base of regenerative medicine and the formation of a market of cell products [88]. In 2008 the US Congress allocated 300 million USD to this and within the next three years under the Department of Defense the Armed Forces Institute of Regenerative Medicine (AFIRM) was established, comprising of two scientific consortia and uniting about 30 leading American universities, several private funds and large biotechnological companies [89]. Over 250 public and private companies and institutes of regenerative medicine have been found in the US and other countries within two years. The patronage of the US Department of Defense conditioned the military priorities and main directions of the project development. Although the politicians accentuate humanitarian reasons for the project, dressing it in the "white clothes" of great goals to assist diseased and injured people, it is obvious that the key commercial goal of the project was to develop a global market for cell products, which, by a modest computation, will exceed the market of genomic production twofold or threefold. The other goal of the project is to develop the national basis of the military healthcare of the USA and to establish a new sector of the world's biotechnological industry. It is supposed that the market for the cell products will considerably exceed all existing world markets of the pharmaceutical industry.

The United Nations organization named the 21st century the century of brain understanding. The efficiency and validity of global research strategy in the production of new knowledge and advanced technologies of brain research, as well as the research intensity of academic policy, led to the initiation of the Human Connectome, another global research project, in 2009 [90]. The term *connectome* is used by neurologists to denote the network of all synapses; that is, contacts between the neurons in the human brain. Accordingly, over 30 million dollars per year have been allocated to researchers from Harvard, Washington University in St. Louis and the University of Minnesota, who were to construct a map of the network activity of the brain with the help of diffuse-tensor MRI. However, the reality appeared to be more complicated than expected. Images of unreal beauty showing the complete connectome of the brain have been received (Figure 1) and the presentation of a multifunctional device as a quick realization of the project's results was predicted. Also, the images of the connectomes of different brain regions (Figure 2) have been received and for future reference considered the analogues of military technology samples. Gary Marcus, a Professor of Cognitive Science at New York University, said "In principle, data of this sort might contribute to understanding how the brain works, and might have important implications for treating neurological disease—especially when the project is complete, and the researchers have scanned all one thousand two hundred subjects. But, for now, we know how much data has been collected, but not what it all means" [91]. Although formally the project is not completed, Professor Botstein has claimed the magnetic resonance imaging to be morally outdated, just like the current cytoarchitectonic research of the brain.

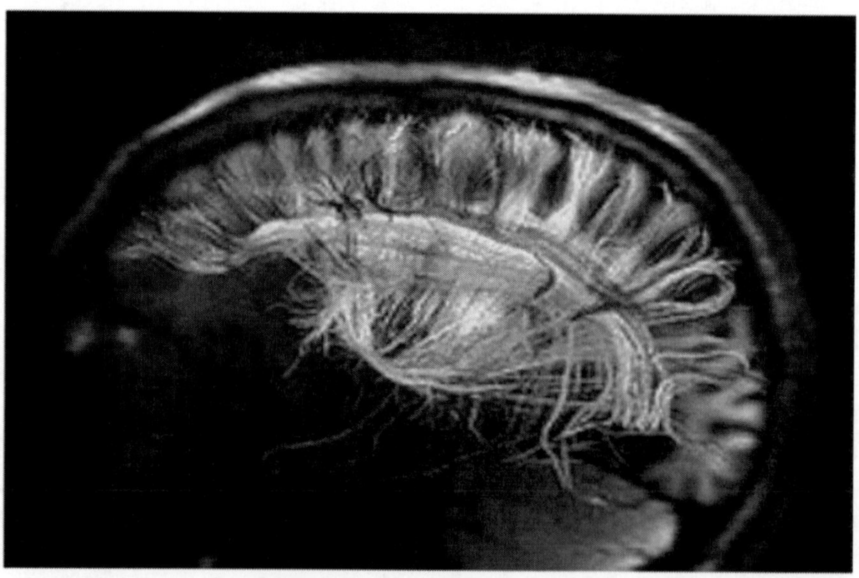

Figure 1. Three-dimensional connectome model of the neural networks in the human brain received by the diffuse-tensor MRI of the brain in the Human Connectome Project (Photo of MGH-UCLA Human Connectome Project).

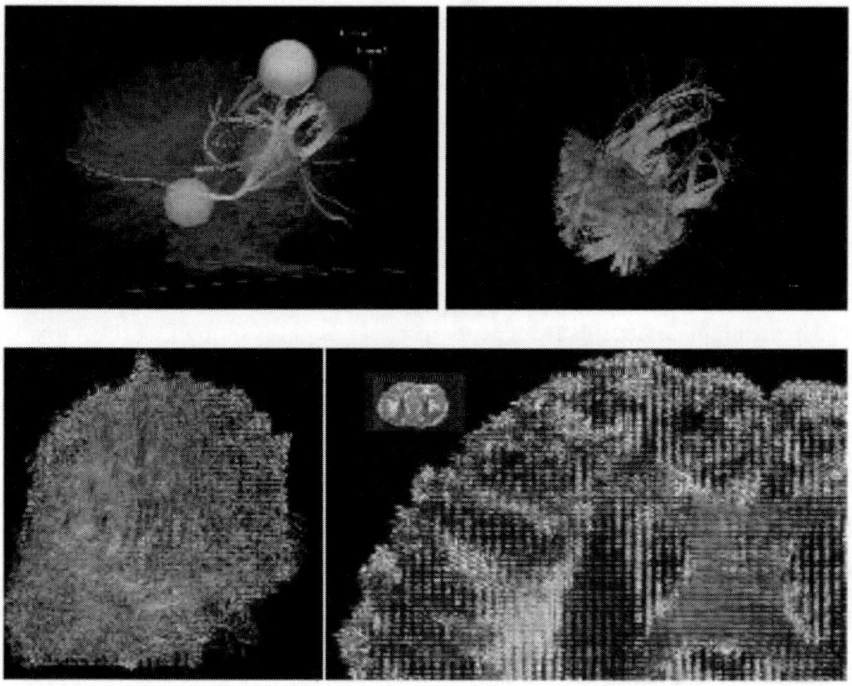

Figure 2. Images of the connectome of different parts of the human brain (a, b, c) and the map of network activity (d) (Photo by: MGH-UCLA Human Connectome Project).

Without waiting for the accomplishment of the Human Connectome Project, in April 2013 the US government launched another large-scale brain research under the working title BRAIN (Brain Research through Advancing Innovative Neuro-technologies) Initiative (Figure 3). The research and its funding began in 2014 [7].

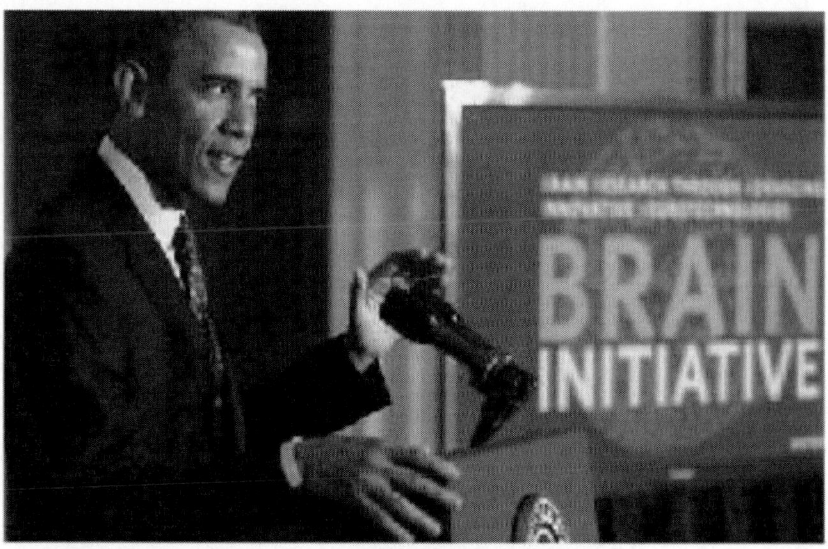

Figure 3. Presentation of the Brain Initiative project by the US President Barack Obama in 2013.

The appropriate funding of 100 million dollars is planned for the project with the prospect of its rising to 3 billion USD; that is, 300 million dollars a year for a decade. The project will involve the National Institutes of Health, the Defense Advanced Research Projects Agency, the National Science Foundation, the Allen Institute of Brain Science (which will invest 60 million into the Brain Initiative projects) and others [92]. The funds will be allocated to the development of new technologies that will show the interaction of separate cells of the brain and functional ensembles of neurons presented as neural networks.

Also, the scientists plan to focus on the way in which the brain processes, records, stores and reproduces information and on the relationship between the brain's operation and its behavior. The available materials from academic and popular sources showed that the goal of the project is not only the mapping of the brain, as claimed in the President's speech, but also a fundamental biotechnological study of the framework and operational principles of the human brain as well as the principles of program functioning of different brain regions. New biotechnologies of control, maintenance and regulation of the human brain will be based on these system principles and models. The tasks of the BRAIN Initiative include the development of innovative military neuro-technologies for the remote control of the brain with the help of brain-implantable micro and nano-systems of electronic chips and, conversely, the control of robotics by brain-implanted microchips. Preparing for the implementation of the BRAIN Initiative, the University of Pittsburgh finished a unique research in this area on monkeys and even humans with severe spinal injury. It is intended to attract super-neurocomputing training technologies and databases to analyze the received information "at the speed of thought" and search for the technologies to enter into human consciousness and sub-consciousness. The new BRAIN Initiative can be compared to the Human Genome Project in its size and scale, but should have greater significant political resonance and military and economic meaning. Both private and public institutions will be involved in the research.

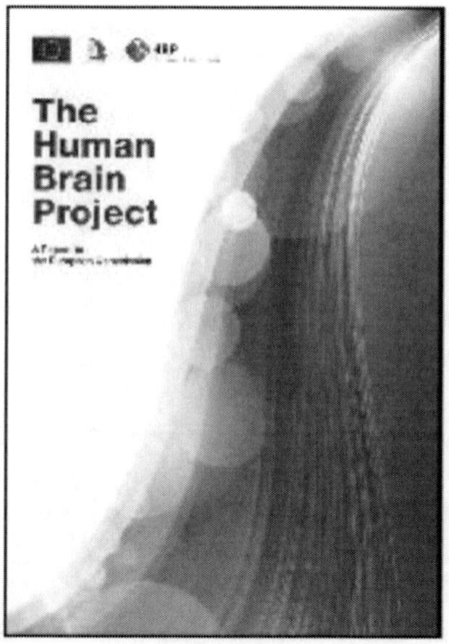

Figure 4. The 2012 Human Brain Project flagship report to the European Commission to validate the project launch and funding.

It is important to note that the US project was announced a year after a flagship report to the European Commission on the similar Human Brain Project (HBP) was published in April 2012 (Figure 4). We would like to discuss the HBP in detail, insofar as it is the most advanced research project observed in neuroscience. About 80 European institutes as well as organizations from outside the EU are uniting their efforts in the project. As we have already noted, the project was expected to cost 1 billion 190 million Euros. The scientists are using contemporary computer models and simulations to construct a virtual brain and develop new pharmaceuticals.

According to the HBP authors, the goal of the project is the following: *The Human Brain Project should lay the technical foundations for a new model of Information and Communication Technologies (ICT)-based brain research, driving integration between data and knowledge from different disciplines, and catalysing a community effort to achieve a new understanding of the brain, new treatments for brain disease and new brain-like computing technologies* [1].

We have several questions to ask the authors of the project. Why should the priority be given to the development of the ICTs in the research of the brain? And generally, what is it, if applied to the existing methodology of the brain studies and contemporary neurology? Why has the EU allocated these enormous funds to fundamental science now, rather than earlier or later? Why do these goals demand an initiative that can be only realized as a flagship financial and economic transnational research project? Why have pragmatic and rational officials and neuroscientists of the EU become so ambitious and somewhat megalomaniacal, which is not typical of them at all? Their project is now positioned as the flagship of global neuroscience, rather than one of many studies being undertaken.

The experts of the Human Brain Project studied the scientific and technical feasibility of the project, described its specific goals and the main methods of the applicable sciences, and determined the challenges and possible solutions, having concluded that there is every reason to launch such a project and to meet the target date. However, we do not think that it is clear what the European Commission can expect in terms of data gathering and processing, the development of a new theory of the brain, and the development and use of the ICT platforms and appendixes of the project. According to the managers of the HBP, it should be regulated by know-how and technical resources, expenses, and the possible risks and potential advantages that it can gain for the European industry and population. Moreover, the executives of the project suppose that the developed ICTs will become beneficial five years after the launch [1].

What are the strategic goals set by this innovative project? As claimed by the project analysts, HBP has four main goals, each of which is based on the current work and catalyzes new ideas and research.

1. *Data: generate strategically selected data essential to seed brain atlases, build brain models and catalyze contributions from other groups.*
2. *Theory: identify mathematical principles underlying the relationships between different levels of brain organization and their role in the brain's ability to acquire, represent and store information.*
3. *ICT platforms: provide an integrated system of ICT platforms offering services to neuroscientists, clinical researchers and technology developers that accelerate the pace of their research.*

4. *Applications: develop first draft models and prototype technologies, demonstrating how the platforms can be used to produce results with immediate value for basic neuroscience, medicine and computing technology[1].*

The consortium of top European neuroscientists answered the question of why the brain research should start now, saying that the *similarity of the ICT and advances of contemporary biology had achieved a point at which the dream of brain understanding could be turned into reality*. The opportunity to realize the dream inspired the launch of the preparatory study of the HBP for a year, financed by the EU as a coordination program, which united three hundred experts in neurosciences, neurology and cybernetics to develop a new "ICT-accelerated" vision of brain research and to work out new software for it. The scientists of the project think that "the major obstacle that hinders our understanding of the brain is the fragmentation of brain research and the data it produces. Modern neuroscience has been enormously productive but unsystematic. The data it produces describes different levels of biological organization, in different areas of the brain in different species, at different stages of development. Today we urgently need to integrate this data – to show how the parts fit together in a single multilevel system" [1].

The main goal of the project is the development of a multilevel systemic model of the human brain on the basis of the integration and synthesis of all recent (morphological, histological, genomic, post-genomic, visual, ultrastructural, etc.) methods of acquisition of data about the human brain, generating a structure of strategically selected data as a catalyst for the future joint research and further modeling of the structure and functions of the virtual brain that will be used to generate new knowledge about the brain, to solve theoretical and practical problems in the neurosciences, to develop novel strategies in the therapy of neurological disorders, to develop military neuro-technologies for the remote control of the brain through a brain-computer interface and innovative computers inspired by the discovered mechanisms and patterns of the brain operation and capable of efficiently working at minimal energy consumption and demanding no additional reprogramming.

The designers of the Human Brain Project presume that to understand the role of different levels of biological organization of the function of the human brain, we should understand their joint action in mammals. For that we need system data that describe different levels of the brain's organization in different species and analysis of the correlation of the variability of the structure with genetic variability. The available evidence in genetics, molecular and cell biology as well as experimental techniques is largely based on research in rodents. Therefore, the authors propose that the Human Brain Project generates system data complexes on rodent genomes, molecules, cells and schemes and use the results to fill the gaps in our knowledge and to detect general patterns planning to engage them in their multilevel simulations of the human brain.

Particularly, we would like to dwell on the development of the innovative ICTs in the project that will be actualized in a range of information and communication technologies on the basis of the scientific platforms (ICT-scientific platforms).

As the experts from the coordination board of the HBP believe, the *Neuroinformatics Platform* should provide technical capabilities making it easier for neuroscientists to analyze structural and functional brain data and to build and navigate multilevel brain atlases. The platform should also include tools for *predictive neuroinformatics*, making it possible to detect statistical regularities in the relationships between data representing different levels of brain organization and to estimate the values of parameters that are difficult or impossible to measure experimentally. These tools will provide a new way of filling the gaps in the data and knowledge that currently prevent us from achieving an integrated understanding of the brain.

The *Brain Simulation* platform is meant to make it possible to build and simulate multi-scale brain models at different levels of detail appropriate to different scientific questions. The platform, which would play a central role in the whole project, should provide researchers with modeling tools, workflows and simulators allowing them to integrate large volumes of heterogeneous data in multi-scale models of mouse and human brains, and to simulate their dynamics. This possibility would allow them to perform silico experiments that are impossible in the lab.

The HBP *High Performance Computing Platform* is expected to provide the project and the community with the computing power needed to build and simulate models of the brain. This should include both the latest, most powerful supercomputing technology, and the exascale and completely new capabilities for interactive computing and visualization.

The HBP *Medical Informatics Platform* should federate clinical data from hospital archives and proprietary databases, while providing strong protection for patient data. Such capabilities would allow researchers to identify "biological signatures" for specific disease processes – a fundamental breakthrough.

The HBP *Neuromorphic Computing Platform* should provide researchers and application developers with the hardware and design tools they need to develop systems and devices modeled on the architecture of the brain and prototype applications. The new platform would allow researchers to develop a completely new category of compact, low-power devices and systems approaching brain-like intelligence.

The HBP *Neurorobotics Platform* should provide researchers with tools and workflows allowing them to interface detailed brain models to a simulated body in a simulated environment, comparing the behavior they can learn against results from human and animal experiments. These capabilities would offer neuroscientists new strategies for studying the multilevel mechanisms' underlying behavior.

However, there is another financial and industrial side of the project. I would like to quote the ambitious specialists who wrote the HBP Flagship report: "European groups are already world leaders in many of the relevant areas of science and technology" [1].

The coordination board presumes that "a European-led Human Brain Project in the FET Flagship Programme would reinforce this leadership and help the transfer of basic research knowledge to industry. However, there is a limited window of opportunity. Neuroscience and ICT are progressing rapidly. If Europe does not take the lead, others will. In the world economy of the 2020s and the 2030s, the pharmacological treatment for brain disease and brain-inspired computing will be key drivers of economic growth. If Europe wants to establish a strong competitive position in these sectors, the time to act is now [1].

To prevent and cure brain disease, researchers need to understand their underlying causes. Studies have shown that conditions classified as a single disease can have completely different genetic causes and that diseases with different causes can produce very similar symptoms. This means we need to move beyond isolated studies of individual disorders and investigate brain diseases systematically, identifying key similarities and distinctions, creating new biologically grounded classifications, and understanding the complex disease processes leading from changes at lower levels of brain organization to clinical symptoms. Only then will it be possible to intervene effectively. Today, the knowledge we need is lacking.

Less obviously, poor understanding of the brain is also an obstacle for ICT. The computing technologies that have driven world economic growth since the 1950s are rapidly approaching fundamental limits on processing speed, power consumption, reliability and programmability. This creates an urgent need for new architectures – perhaps also for completely new computing paradigms. According to the experts responsible for the International Technology Roadmap for Semiconductors, the most effective strategy for moving forward is to complement current information technology with compact, low-power computing systems inspired by the architecture of the brain, with human-like intelligence. But to actually implement such systems, we first have to reach a deep understanding of the brain's cognitive architectures: the way in which the different levels of organization work together to acquire, represent, and store information. In summary, neuroscience, medicine, and ICT all require an integrated multilevel understanding of the brain" [1].

All of this is reminiscent of the words of Barak Obama. Still, the methodology of the system approach as the methodology of choice can be seen in every sentence of the quote from the HBP report. Why are the governments and parliaments of the EU and the USA ready to spend billions on such global biotechnological research projects? I have already mentioned that in the Introduction and I would like to repeat it here. These projects will provide strategic economic and biotechnological advantage over the partners and possible enemies of the USA and the EU and, most importantly, they will also provide a fundamental national and international technological basis for scientific and technical progress in these countries and unrestricted superiority in the newly developed markets of highly technological innovative products.

A significant delay in the generation of new knowledge, the accumulation of new fundamental scientific achievements and the absence of breakthrough biotechnologies can become critical for the sovereignty and independence of even the well-developed and successful states. We can say that *those who own the information, innovations and technologies own the world*. Hence, the initiation of global research is not due to a presidential obsession with megalomaniacal projects but a forced measure to provide the biotechnological safety balance, social and political priority, technological deterrence and strategic parity. Therefore, the principle "a day late, and a dollar short" is meaningful and relevant for the race of the states for biotechnologies and innovations.

What is left for the countries that are not involved in these great national and international projects? How can they secure their technological parity and strategic balance and reduce the scientific and technological gap? The way out is to unite and develop breakthrough cross-border clusters of strategic scientific development, to develop alternative global research projects of technological deterrence together and to form their own international integral technological base of innovative data of biotechnological safety within the framework of existing political preferences and state alliances. An alliance could include all interested participants from the developed and developing countries of Asia, Africa, the Middle East and Latin America. The already existing geopolitical and economic alliances can also be used to realize such a project.

Today the International Association of Neurorestoratology (IANR), a public non-commercial organization that unites the leading neuroscientists from 35 countries, is taking the opportunity to address the governments and parliaments of the interested states with an appeal for participation in an alternative global neurobiotechnological project under the working title *Brainstorming of the Brain* ***(Brain Research by Advanced Innovative Neurobioinformative Systems and Technologies & Onward Restoration of the Brain by Molecular-Induced Neurobioengineering Grafts and Brain Function Reprogramming by Artificial Interface between Microchips and Neurotissue)***. The Project *Brainstorming of the Brain* can become an opportunity for the developing countries to make their contribution to global scientific research, to become the developers and partners in the innovative solutions of collective biotechnological safety and the co-owners of new competitive bioneuro-technologies and innovations that would be able to enter the global market of biotechnological and medical services.

Provisionally, the required volume of funding will be significantly smaller when compared to similar projects in the US and the EU. The expected costs of the planned volume of work are about 300 million USD. The IANR plans to propose participation in the project to the governments of the BRICS (Brazil, Russia, India, China, South-Africa) countries, some of the Middle East countries (the OAE, Egypt, etc.) and the Far East countries (Japan, South Korea, Thailand, Singapore, etc.).

The IANR specialists believe that they should not copy the projects of the world leaders of biotechnological industry from the economically developed countries and follow the way chosen by the US and the EU. Their method of a system approach to large-scale fundamental research and brain mapping methodology is valid, academic and methodologically appropriate and, undoubtedly, from a long-term perspective can provide significant advantages and benefits in the generation of new knowledge about the brain and development of the technologies of its regulation. The methodology of the system approach to brain research demands considerable financial assets and, being developed at the end of the 20th century, is now methodologically outdated. The IANR specialists understand that our competitors have been working on the object of the research for a long time and have accumulated considerable experience in the research in this field: Europe for the past two years and the USA for the past 5-6 years have been very active in the research in the area. For the past several years the researchers have attempted to thoroughly systemize the entire scope of the acquired and yet-to-be acquired knowledge and employ it in the development of the so-called *image of the human brain* that provides the interaction of different brain structures, all previously existing, currently existing and predicted relations and interrelations of the elements and structures of the brain at different levels (neurophysiological, biochemical, histological, etc.) of the research through their integration in one database. Viewed from the viewpoint of classical science, everything seems academic and fundamental, but extremely bulky, ineffective and low-informative. What do the adepts of the system approach to brain research want to receive from the BRAIN Initiative and the Human Brain Project? They plan to map and catalogue morphofunctional changes and the integration of different brain regions in norm and to detect system-forming patterns by means of the accumulation and integration of the acquired knowledge in order to use them in the maintenance of the brain in health and in disease, and, possibly, to develop new technologies to treat brain pathology. We will discuss these approaches in the next chapter.

Chapter 4

A System Approach as the Basic Methodology of Contemporary Neuro-Research: Its Advantages and Disadvantages

Abstract

In this chapter the author discusses the methodology and opportunities of the system approach as the main toolkit for neuro-research of the HBP in detail, as well as analyzing the expectations that are placed on this methodology. The author concentrates on the advantages that the system approach has provided to neuroscientists in setting the goals and objectives of large-scale projects. At the end of the chapter the author proves an important fact that the methodology of the system approach was the engine for the scientific progress in all spheres of science and engineering in the 20th century. In the 21st century this methodological tool slows the progress due to the rigidness of its rules, the bulkiness of graphs and the low-informative capacity of its technologies. In the 21st century the masses of data received by contemporary diagnostic and research equipment are so large that they demand new toolkits for their gathering, processing, storage and analysis as well as for systemic work with already available databases in the adjacent and competing fields.

Keywords: benefits and shortcomings of the system approach in the 21st century, the methodology of the system approach, masses of biological data, multilevel research of the brain, genome, transcriptome, proteome, metabolome, cell, synapse, a whole brain

The methodology of the system approach is not new in the science and is widely used by the global medical community generally and in brain research particularly. As with any methodology or, in other words, theoretical foundation of fundamental research, it has certain advantages over other methodological approaches and some drawbacks, which to a certain extent cancel out the positive aspects of using the methodology in research. In this chapter I would like to discuss the advantages as well as the disadvantages of the methodology of the system approach in the neurosciences and to talk about its limitations in neuro-research. Also, using the example of the *Methodology* section of the Human Brain Project, I would like to show how the methodology of the system approach to the brain research helped European neuroscientists to propose a novel strategy of brain research and to define an innovative conceptual approach to the available discrepant evidence. Undoubtedly, the methodology of the system approach allowed the authors their own theory of how to develop information and communication technologies that would integrate in one information field anatomy, histology, histochemistry and pathomorphology of the brain with neurology, neuromathematics and advanced cybernetics represented as superneurocomputers and robots integrated in one object of research on the basis of newly developed platforms. The methodology of the system approach of the HBP permitted the clear definition of the key issues of contemporary neurosciences and neurology today and the outlining of possible solutions.

In the 20th century the system approach led to the greatest achievements in science, as it was the most advanced and revolutionary methodology of scientific experience that permitted the integration of different methodological approaches and description of the brain functions' organization, viewed from the standpoint of the contemporary theory of systems. The system approach has been applied to research of the brain in health and in disease, and in many respects it has radically changed the views of the researchers on the mechanism of the functioning of the brain and spinal cord, established systemic patterns of cerebral connections in the brain at the morphological and functional levels, and identified systemic solutions in the diagnostics of a range of the nervous diseases.

Apparently, for decades the fundamental research of the brain and brain diseases relied on traditional morphofunctional principles of neuro-research: anatomic-topographic, neuro-morphological, neuro-physiological, system-functional and neuropsychological. The introduction of a large number of innovative genome and post-genome biotechnologies (genomics, transcriptomics, proteomics, metabolomics, etc.), of up-do-date computerized diagnostic equipment to study the brain in neuro-morphological tests (confocal microscopy, electronic microscopy, tunnel microscopy, atomic force microscopy, CT and MRI), specialized neuro-visualization of the brain (neuro-endoscopy, neuro-navigation and stereotaxic systems), computerized diagnostic neuro-functional equipment (EEG cerebral mapping, magnetic encephalography and others) into neurosciences along with clinical neurology led to the accumulation of a bulk of unique, but discrepant and irregular evidence. It resulted in a situation where the obtained results do not correlate with conventional evidence of the biological organization of the brain, entailing even more confusion and mismatch with our concepts of the brain's operation and functions. This led to new research goals and the necessity to search for novel systemic solutions. Obviously, the absence of a theoretical foundation for the development of neurosciences renders further progress that relies on the trial-and-error approach unpromising and practically impossible. We need a new system of concepts about the brain's operation where all fragmentary evidence will be systemized and arranged in a system accurately. Traditional views on the brain should be reconciled with the innovations in the sphere of notions and concepts. We should work out a new ideology, methodology and terminology for neurosciences that would be clear to neurologists, neurosurgeons, basic scientists, physicists, mathematicians and even engineers who work far from the field of medicine. This "trans-scientific" interface and new scientific Esperanto between absolutely different liberal arts and exact sciences must be worked out in the near future without delay.

The next stage of the work in the area seems to be the development of a multilevel hierarchical system in which these data and knowledge take an appropriate position and functional significance in the hierarchical system of dominating signs and dominated subsystems. Moreover, it is necessary to learn to predict the characteristics of the features and the structure of composing system elements in this hierarchical system. A biotechnological system-forming structure, similar to the Element Periodic Table, is necessary. Only then will we be able to understand how changes in the genome of nervous cells influence the cognitive sphere, or how changes in the proteome of a nervous cell manifest in its phenotype. It is clear to many neuroscientists that the newly received evidence about the brain is the evidence from different levels of a biological organization and their relations and interactions must be the object of thorough research. The systematization and cataloging of rapidly growing results of experimental research in clinical and theoretical neurology demand large memory resources and computing capacities. To date the memory resources of the superneurocomputers are unable to cope with the volume of the information to be processed and analyzed. The system approach to the neuro-physiological (electroencephalographic, neuromyographic and somatosensory biopotentials of the brain) data processing led to the definition of the concept of bioelectrical activity of the brain, systematization of the available evidence of EEG and development of the EEG cerebral mapping. Due to the system approach to the analysis of neuropsychological and experimental psychological research, the available evidence about the localization of higher psychic functions in the brain was structured and correlated with the morphological structure of the brain and specific personal features.

The European neuroscientists who described the methodology of the planned research in the HBP mostly relied on the theoretical systemic scientific views and notions. The system approach in this project permitted step-by-step structurization of the sequence of main stages of the research by means of the isolation of the levels of biological organization of the brain. As the experts conclude, to understand the role of different levels of biological organization of the human brain's functions in its structure, it is necessary to understand their cooperative systemic work in other mammals. For that they need system data that describe different levels of organization of the brain in some species of mammal, and analysis of the correlation of structural variability with genetic variability. The available evidence of the genetics, molecular and cell biology and behavior of the brain, as well as their experimental techniques, is mostly based on the studies of rodents; hence, in the project the research into rat brains will be accentuated. The authors of the project proposed the methodology of the system approach, according to which the HBP will generate system complexes of the data on genomes and molecules, cells and schemes in rodents, using these results to fill the gaps in our knowledge and detect general patterns that are planned to be used for multilevel simulations of the human brain.

According to the classical system approach, the methodology of European research of the brain seems a very accurate system that includes investigations from the level of genome to the level of higher cognitive functions (Figure 5). This is an attempt to construct a logical and interdependent system of the levels that influence each other and to manipulate them. Multilevel data about the specific morphological structures of the brain received in various diagnostic testing (genome sequencing, complete transcriptome analysis of gene expression, proteomic research, microdissection and immunochemistry, MRI, psychophysiological and neuropsychological testing) are to be organized in a multi-scale model of the brain, the European scientists believe.

Furthermore, the structure of strategically selected data and systemic data complexes is planned to be used as a catalyst for new joint research between neuroscientists and experts in cybernetics and computation. In the HBP the methodology of the system approach is demonstrably represented in the schemes of formation and evaluation of the multilevel structure of brain research and in the schemes of space continuum of the structures of the functional organization of the neurobiological system of the brain.

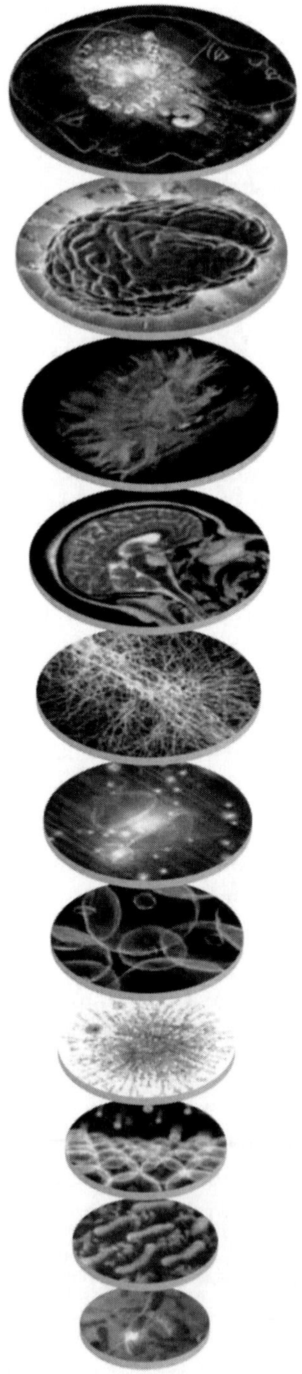

Multi-level data required for multiscale brain models

Cognition. Structured cognitive tests, combined with fMRI and MEG, constrain brain circuit models for visual perception-action, decision and reward, memory encoding and retrieval, space, time, number and language. Changes in circuits during development and aging and differences between adults constrain network models of cognition at different ages and provide benchmark data to validate detailed cellular brain models.

Whole brain. Multi-modal sensory physiology and anatomy map how different brain regions come together to shape perception-action and our sense of body ownership, awareness and consciousness, and can help validate human brain models. Whole brain synchrotron scans reveal the vasculature supporting cognition, and provide constraints for models of blood flow and brain metabolism.

Connectivity. Whole brain fibre tract tracing and DTI yield paths and fibre densities for connectivity within and between brain regions and provide global fibre projection parameters constraining connectivity in brain models. Whole brain ultramicroscopy yields constraints for single neuron projections and provides high-resolution validation of DTI tracts. EM provides high-resolution images of the synapses formed on individual neurons, principles of fibre selection, and structural features of synapses.

Brain regions. Structural and functional MRI yield dimensions of brain regions which can be used to build models. Region-specific cellular architecture and densities constrain the cellular composition of model regions. Receptor, ion channel, signalling and other protein distributions further constrain neurochemical organisation within and across brain regions. Correlations between protein distributions, cognitive circuits and genomic variability point to neural mechanisms of cognition, provide global constraints for detailed brain models and generate data for model validation.

Microcircuits. The cellular and molecular composition of microcircuits supports their role in cognition. Single-cell gene expression yields sets of genes that form different types of neurons and glia and determine their morphological and electrical properties. Global brain maps of gene and protein distributions constrain the cellular composition of microcircuit models. Cell geometry and synaptic selection rules constrain local synaptic connectivity in microcircuit models. Electrophysiology, multi-electrode recordings, voltage sensitive dye mapping and optogenetic studies provide data to validate microcircuit models.

Cells. 3D reconstruction of the anatomy of single cells yields the structural geometry needed to establish the morphological properties of different cell types. Correlations between gene expression and the geometric properties of cells constrain the artificial synthesis of cellular morphologies from gene expression patterns, as well as models of morphological plasticity. Single-cell gene expression, combined with general rules for the production and distribution of proteins and for protein interactions, constrain molecularly detailed models of neurons and glia.

Synapses. Physiological, biophysical and imaging studies of synaptic transmission, plasticity and neuromodulation constrain synaptic models. Pair-wise single cell gene expression constrains the repertoire of synaptic proteins at the synapses between pairs of neurons of known type, making it possible to model synapse diversity. The dynamics of single cell gene expression constrain long-term molecular changes in synapses in response to environmental stimuli. Comparing synaptic proteins across species constrains species-specific synaptic models.

Metabolome. The intricate biochemical network linking neurons, synapses and glia constrains molecular brain models, in which activity, plasticity, neuromodulation, homeostasis and nutrition depend on metabolic processes. Coupling neurotransmitter receptors and their signalling pathways to the biochemical pathways that supply energy to cells and synapses, constrains activity-driven changes in blood flow, and the resulting fMRI signals.

Proteome. The number and different types of proteins cells produce, the different parts of the cell where they are located, and their respective life cycles all constrain how many and which proteins can come together in a single cell. The set of proteins, other biochemicals, and ions that each protein binds to and reacts with forms the protein's interactome. Results on protein-protein interactions from biochemical studies, molecular dynamic simulations, and predictive informatics constrain reaction-diffusion models of cells.

Transcriptome. Combined with data on the genes expressed in single cells, 3D maps of gene expression constrain the total number of neurons in the brain and the types of genetically identifiable cells the brain can produce. Single cell gene expression changes in response to stimulation, determining how cells can change with experience. Single cell gene expression, combined with predictions of which proteins the cell can produce and basic principles of proteomics, constrains detailed molecular-level cell models.

Genome. The state of the chromosome reflects when genes are active or inactive and constrains gene network models. It is likely that the genome constrains the number of genetic cell types in the brain, the size of brain regions, connectivity between brain regions, and total brain size. It may also predict cognitive functions, behavioural traits, epigenetic vulnerability, and brain disorders.

Figure 5. Multilevel data for multi-scale models of the Human Brain Project.

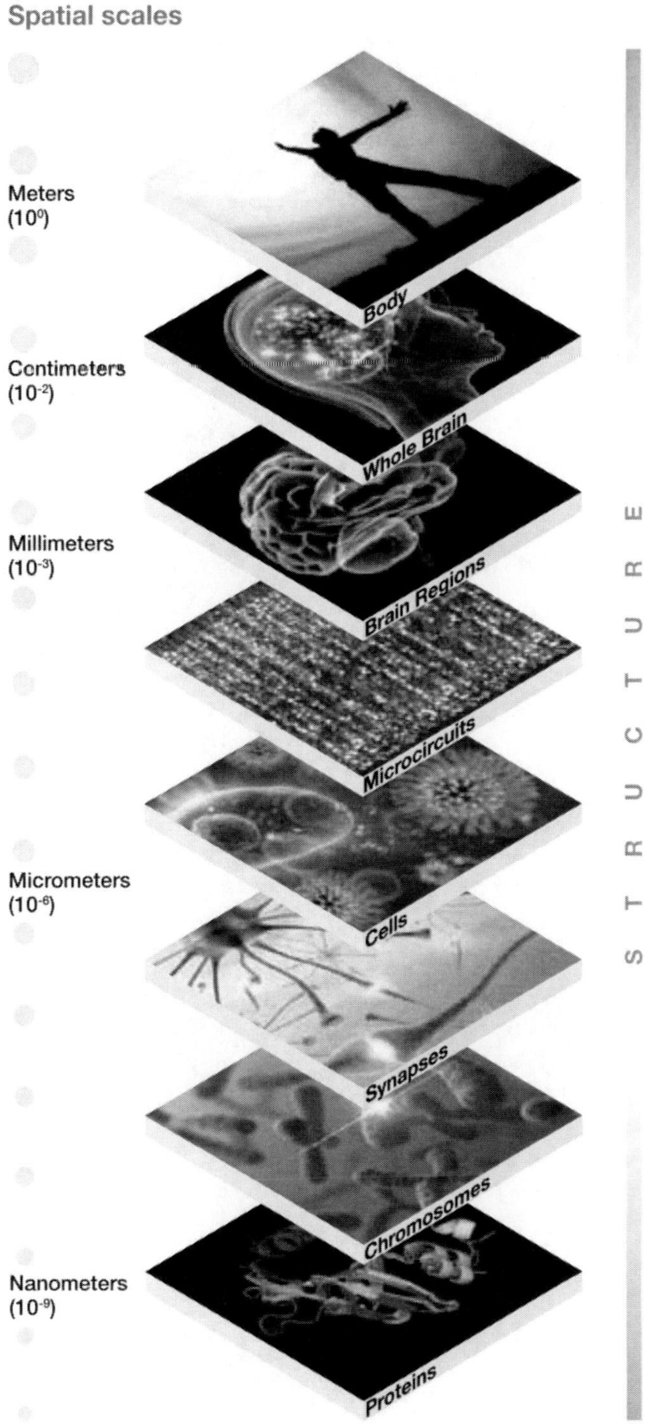

Figure 6. The scheme of spatial continuum of the functional organization of the neurobiological system of the brain (the Human Brain Project).

They define several levels of the space continuum of the structure of the operation of the brain's biological substrate (Figure 6) from the level of proteins (10^9 – nanometers) to the level of cells' and synapses' functioning (10^6 – micrometers) and the level of cellular microcircuits and tissue level of various regions of the brain (10^3 – millimeters) and further to the level of a whole brain (10^2 – centimeters) and finally to the level of a whole body (meters).

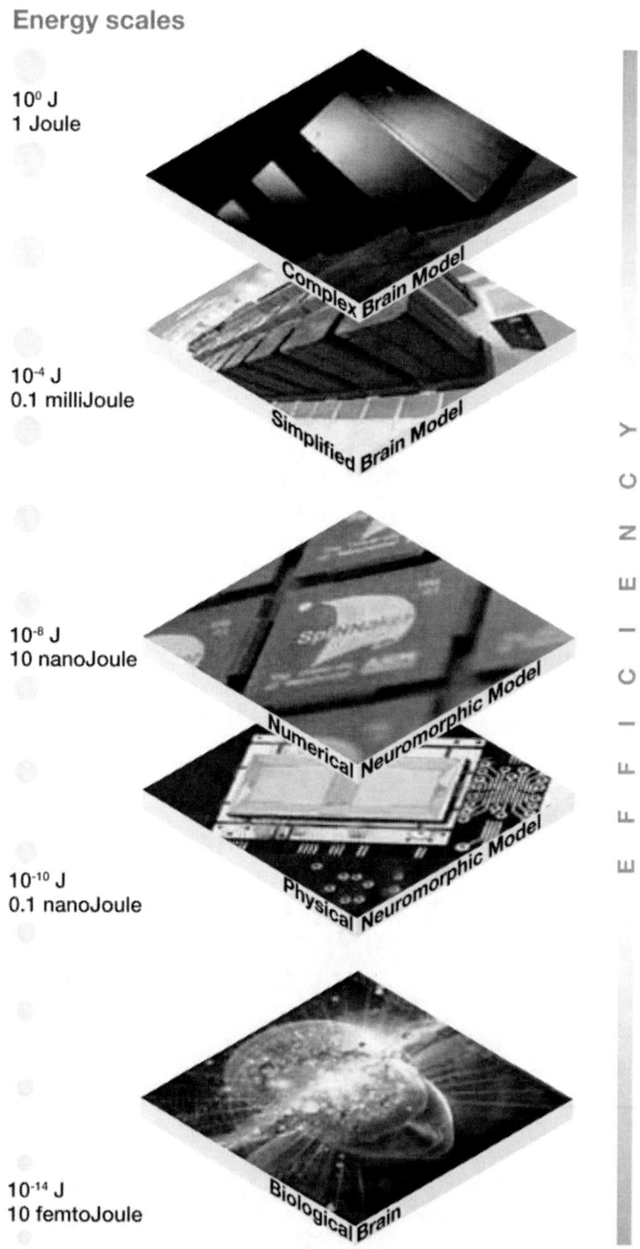

Figure 7. Systemic representation of energy consumption of computing systems in efficient work located at different levels of systemic functioning in the Human Brain Project: from biological brain to supercomputer stimulator.

As we have already noted, one of the key goals of the HBP is the development of brain-like structures for the intellectual processing of various data. The developers presume that these systems of artificial intelligence will copy the principles of brain operation and will be able to process volumes of data at minimal energy consumption, similar to those stored and analyzed only by the network of supercomputers.

The reduction of energy consumption is one of the most important tasks set to the designers and developers of the HBP, and in analyzing this parameter they too used the methodology of the system approach to illustrate the efficiency of the neuromorphic computation technologies that they develop in the project. The system-forming gradation of the energy-consuming processes of various sources of computation is shown in Figure 7, which illustrates the efficiency of energy consumption from a biological brain to the virtual brain simulation modeled by a supercomputer.

The energy that a biological brain spends on a synaptic transfer is minimal and does not exceed 10^{14} J, or 10 femtojoules, while a complex brain simulation on the basis of a superneurocomputer consumes about 10^{2} J of energy. The energy consumed by neuromorphic computing takes an intermediate position between a biological brain and a system of supercomputer modeling, so it promises huge energy saving.

The system approach to the analysis of the biochemical tests of the cells of the brain permits an understanding of the systems of interaction of different proteins at the level of a cell and nerve tissue. The system approach applied to the protein research resulted in the systems of protein networks in the cells of the nerve tissue and other somatic cells. The team of Prof. Terentyev from the Department of Biochemistry from the Pirogov State Medical University published their work in the journal *Uspekhi biologicheskoy khimii* (*The Achievements of Biological Chemistry*), giving a classical illustration of the use of the system approach in contemporary biochemical research [94]. This is a serious and fundamental work of national researchers that fully relies on classical biochemistry and systemic biology. It is methodologically precise and perfectly structured according to the system approach and it gives accurate and correct explanations to the systemic relations in the protein interactions from the position of the contemporary theory of systems. No accomplished, comprehensive concept can be seen in the description of protein relations in the proteome of a somatic cell and some of the provisions and systemized data require elaboration.

The evidence provided by classical biochemists in their serious analytical work is valuable and logical and must be used to confirm the correctness of methodological and scientific systemic structures in cell system research. As Terentyev and his team state (2009), the modeling, description and analysis of many existing processes, in biological as well as non-biological systems, require different types of networks formed by groups of interacting components. For studies of cell functioning, a special place among biological networks is taken by molecular networks that include gene, protein, metabolic and signal networks. All of these types of molecular networks refer to complex networks, according to their features and organizational principles. Reflecting the complexity of the organization of biological systems, they are the object of research for systemic biology [95].

A systemic analysis of molecular networks allows for the detection of functional modules in them and the definition of the role of every component of the network in the cell functioning. The groups of physically interacting proteins that function in a cell in a coordinated fashion and control interrelated processes that happen in the body organize the *protein networks* (Figure 8). The proteins, as the key biomacromolecules, are the main participants of almost all cell processes. Hence, it is not possible to model the information structure of a living cell without all complexes of the data of dynamic proteomics that studies the changes of concentrations and localization of the proteins and their interaction [95, 96, 97].

Disorder in the protein-protein interaction or their systemic relations can lead to various diseases including tumors, neurodegenerative, cardiovascular and autoimmune diseases and other diseases. Hence, the study of interacting partners and the analysis of protein networks formed by the protein-protein interactions is an important tool in the diagnostics of the disease and the mechanism of its development as well as the efficiency of certain therapeutic approaches [98, 99]. Moreover, the system approach at the level of protein research goes much further than their simple representation as the networks. Currently, it is acknowledged that most of the eukaryotic proteins are multi-module and multifunctional [100, 101]. Every module can fulfill an independent function and, as a result, the protein acquires the ability to fulfill a whole complex of different functions. Due to the multi-modality and multi-functionality of most of the eukaryotic proteins, their complex protein networks can fuse and overlap. Hence, the structural-functional mapping of the proteins is an important tool for modeling the proteomes of a living cell, permitting the localization of functionally important areas including those involved in protein-protein interactions or informational relations.

In my latest book (Bryukhovetskiy A.S. *Clinical oncoproteomics: personalized anti-tumor therapy*; 2013) I have shown the systemic relations of various proteins in the protein networks, as many of the proteins in a cell are dynamically related to each other and these interactions condition the functions and behavior of a living cell [12]. Reversible protein-protein interactions represent one of the types of dynamic processes that happen in a cell and permit judgment of its functioning. Intensive research in the area in recent years has contributed to the gradual accumulation of evidence about interaction pairs of proteins and the protein complexes that they form.

I would like to demonstrate the opportunities of the system approach methodology and its advantages and disadvantages using the example of the protein research in a neural cell. During the course of the past two decades a range of highly efficient and highly productive experimental methods to study the protein-protein interactions has been developed, all of which, however, have their flaws. This is why the experimental methods are supplemented with various theoretical approaches including mathematical and computing methods of research. Meanwhile, protein-protein interactions are studied separately depending on different biological species, and for higher eukaryotic organisms they are separate for different tissues and cell types. The whole complex of protein-protein interactions, which are characteristic of a specific organism, was named ***interactome***. The structural and systemic organization of interactomes and the total number of interactions in them is one of the most important factors determining the complexity of biological systems.

The number of copies of the cell proteins can vary from several tens (less than 50) to millions [102]. So, the interactomes of simple organisms can be formed by a rather large number of interactions. For example, the interactome of *S. cerevisiae* yeast can vary from 10 to 17 thousand, according to one source, and from 25 to 35 thousand interactions according to another source [103]. Statistics evaluates the possible size of a human interactome as 650 thousand interactions approximately. The human interactome appeared to be about 10 times larger than in the *D. melanogaster*, and can be three times larger than the *C. elegans* interactome [104]. The mapping of the human interactome is only at the initial phase of research. However, according to the evidence of Venkatesan K. et al., the human interactome presents 130 thousand interactions and the interacting partners have not been detected for the major part of them [105].

These data permitted a proposal that the size of the interactome of the neuron correlates with the level of complexity of the organization of the species. The detection of physically interacting protein pairs enables the mapping of the interactome, resulting in graphs consisting of the nodes where the proteins are located and links between them that show pair interactions. Interactome maps are viewed as the keys to new knowledge about protein functioning in cells [106].

Relying on the *in vitro* evidence, the statistic interactome maps are drawn and their analysis provides a description of dynamic protein-protein interactions *in vivo*. The interactome maps are useful for fundamental medicine too, and namely for determining the role of specific proteins and their relations in the onset and development of diseases, their diagnostics, as well as possible targets for different pharmaceuticals and control of the treatment efficiency. Currently, even the maps available for the protozoa are incomplete. Moreover, the data received by different authors are often contradictory. Interacting pairs and protein complexes that have been identified by one research team cannot be found by other researchers. Still, the development of new experimental and theoretical approaches leads to the gradual accumulation of data that are necessary to analyze the protein-protein interactions observed in the cell. The protein-protein interactions are fundamental elements of the information structure of a somatic cell and changes or transformations of it can be judged by them.

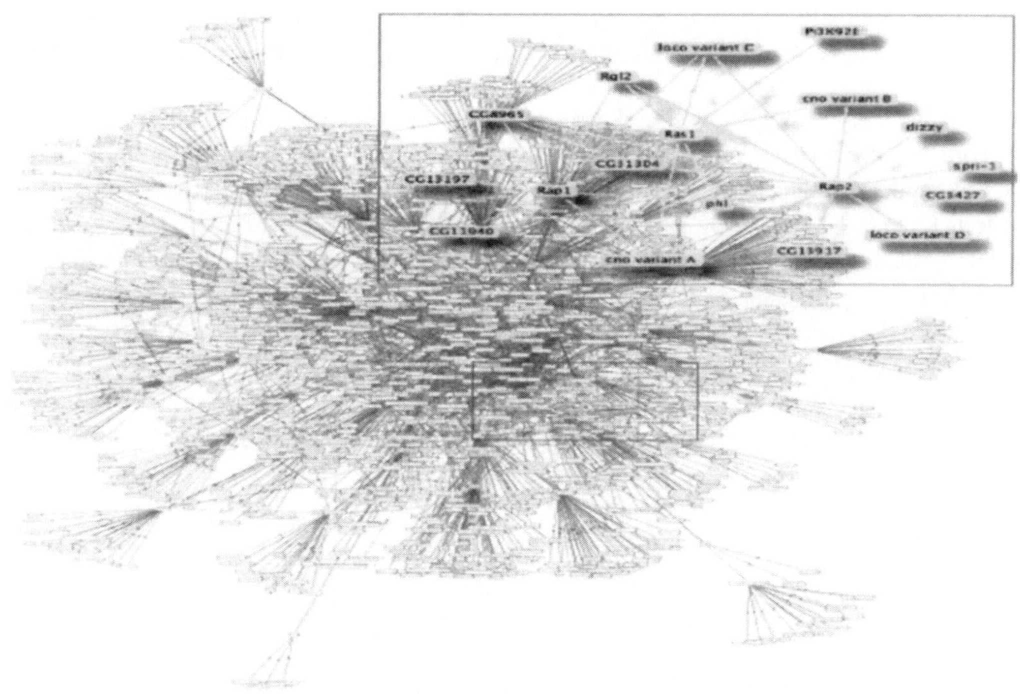

Figure 8. Systemic graphs of "protein networks" of a somatic cell describe and systemize obtained information and permit an understanding of the systemic relationship and interrelationship of the proteins in the networks.

The experimental methods can now determine interacting protein pairs and protein complexes mostly in prokaryotic or simple eukaryotic organisms. To detect protein-protein interactions in more complex organisms, such as mammals, the prediction method is used, which is based on the homology with the proteins, the interacting partners for which were detected in simpler organisms [107]. The approach is based on the homology between related proteins and comparison of the degree of conservation of the primary and spatial structure of the same protein in various species. For example, if it was shown experimentally that two proteins in yeasts interact, it is supposed that these proteins in humans interact too. Two pairs of proteins in different organisms that evolutionarily retained the ability for interaction were named *interologs*. The prediction of interacting pairs gives more or less reliable results only in the case of a high similarity of their primary consequences.

Initially, such biochemical methods as chemical cross-linking, co-fractionation during chromatography and immunoprecipitation have been used to study protein-protein interactions. However, later, to detect the interactomes of specific organisms the highly efficient and highly productive methods as Y2H – yeast two-hybrid assay, phage display, TAP-MS – tandem affinity purification-mass spectrometry were used [108, 109, 110, 111]. Different methods of microscopy, as well as mathematical and computing methods described by several research teams, offer broad opportunities, too [108, 112, 113]. We are not going to discuss laboratory issues here and will leave it to the experts in biochemistry. It is more important for us to consider the correlations of protein-protein interactions with the results of the proteome assays of the studied cell systems in the course of the informational processing.

Contemporary databases contain information about hundreds of thousands of interactions that are formed by several thousand proteins in tens of species [114, 115, 116]. For example, the BioGRID (Biological General Repository for Interaction Datasets) database currently boasts the data of about 198 thousand interactions for six species [117]. Such databases contain the information about interacting protein pairs that were received either through experimental methods, or by relying on the homology between amino acid sequences, or they were computer predicted. The goal of such databases as the DIP (Database of Interacting Proteins), the BIND (Biomolecular Interaction Network Database) and the INTERACT is to integrate a huge bulk of the data, to provide easy access to them and the opportunity to visualize them. The databases are also equipped with the tools to evaluate the accuracy of the experimentally obtained results. They are widely used to construct and analyze the protein networks that provide the basis of the functioning of a living cell.

The widely established databases not only contain information about the interacting partners, but also permit detailed structural analysis of the regions responsible for interaction [118, 119, 120]. For example, the SCOWLP (Structural Characterization of Water, Ligands and Proteins) database contains information about amino acid residues and atom groups that participate in the interactions. Due to this, it provides a detailed analysis of the interactions between the proteins, domains and peptide motives of different proteins, as well as their interactions with solvent [118, 119]. Another example is a global interactome map known as PSIMAP (Protein Structural Interactome Map); it is based on the data about domain-domain interactions of all proteins, for which a 3D structure that is represented in the PDB Protein Data Bank) database was experimentally established. The PSIMAP algorithm calculates the Euclidean distance to determine interactions between possible pairs of structural domains in proteins [121]. Two domains are considered interacting if at least five amino acid residues are located at a distance of less than 5Å (the 5-5 rule). Using this algorithm, it is possible to predict interacting partners on the basis of the homology of the primary amino acid sequences of the proteins and their structural domains. The database *PSIbase* contains the information about interacting partners.

I discussed the demonstration of protein networks in a nerve cell in such detail on purpose; they perfectly illustrate the methodological basis of the system approach. Similar "signal networks" are described in somatic cells as the main system-forming element of a whole system of signal transduction in a cell. In the literature one can find a description of gene networks in a cell, etc.

The application of the system approach to the analysis of the identity of the processes and phenomena in the biology and medicine of the 20th century provided novelty and future for the systemic scientific methodology. But in the 21st century the methodology of systemic analysis of the newly appeared masses of information cannot provide adequate processing of the data and plays the role of a dead-weight to the scientific progress. As the practice shows, the system approach to the research of the brain in health and in pathology has specific limitations and does not permit the correlation of such "non-materialistic" facts of the brain's functioning as its holographic nature, wave, field and trace interactions of the brain structures.

The system approach studies the brain as an object (system) as a whole, describes changes in the system depending on the changed environment, studies the structure (elements) of the object and system and does not permit the complete follow-up of the concealed relations of its structured elements. It demands compliance with the rigid framework within which the network graphs, the goal trees and complex analytical objective functions (models) must be developed, thus leading to ineffective and unreasonable expenses.

The system approach that lays in the basis of all fundamental medical and biological research describes only the evidence-based and objectively visualized part of the received results of the analysis of the studied living system, but does not disclose all deep processes and information relations inside it. The impossibility of disclosing the internal relations of the system elements inside the system as well as its relations with the environment or microenvironment imposes major limitations on its further use for analysis of the evidence received by contemporary neuroscience. Use of the methodology of the system approach and systemic analysis provides an opportunity to process and to study only the visible or visualized part of these relations inside the system, thus leading to the significant loss of matrix information. These aspects of the methodology prevent further use of the system approach as the basic scientific instrument for neuro-research. But the solution is available and it was proposed by the mathematicians over five decades ago, when they had to face a similar scientific problem in the research of the system theory.

This methodological approach can be efficiently realized to obtain the novel generation of knowledge with at least twice less financial and material expenses. Partially, it can be achieved by the methodology of "cloud computer solutions" at a more advanced methodological and technological level of scientific knowledge involving not only the systemic, but also, and mostly, the information approach. This means that the mapping and systematization of the functions of the human brain in health depending on the histology, morphology and neurophysiology of the brain activity is not the only basis for brain research. It is more reasonable to model specific pathology at the information virtual level of the normalized integrated data of post-genome (proteome, secretome, transcriptome, metabolome, etc.) research of specific cells and cell system of the brain and spinal cord and to attempt to bring it to norm not through systemic studies of material objects and phenomena in the brain, but through the restoration of the information structure of the damaged brain by means of the evaluation of the informational relations of healthy and disordered areas of the brain, the foundation of neuroregeneration and neuroplasticity within the framework of classical science about information and, namely, informationology. The elements of this ideology are used only partially by the European authors of the Human Brain Project.

In the next chapter we will discuss the concept of the information approach and will apply it to our goals and tasks.

Chapter 5

An Information Approach to the Fundamental and Theoretical Research of the Brain

Abstract

The history of the information approach is outlined in this chapter, beginning from the works of Claude Shannon, the founder of the mathematical theory of communication (1948), to the present day when the students of Anokhin-Sudakov neurophysiological school (1966-2013) realized the information approach in the theory of the functional systems of the brain and developed the information theory of emotions of Simonov PV. The chapter sums up the contemporary viewpoints on the scientific and mathematical perception of the methodology of the information approach in science and engineering. The author makes an attempt to adapt the information approach and the tools of informationology to the goals and objectives of neuroscience and to explain the results of the research of the brain, as seen from the information approach perspective. The HBP experts laid down the fundamentals of multilevel research of the brain for the first time in neuroscience, but did not develop it further. The author proposes taking a step further to evaluate the opportunities of another scientific methodology for brain research, which is termed informationology. It is obvious that only the information approach opens up new avenues in human brain modeling. The information approach permits a new viewpoint of the role and information meaning of the brain membranes, cerebrospinal fluid, and arachnoid granulations in the processing of the information received from brain regions. According to the information approach, the brain can be viewed as a switchboard and moderator of information, and the intermeningeal spaces (the space between the membranes) as the main neuroprocessor. The author considers the information levels of a neural cell, nerve tissue and a whole brain as the modules of organ structure. For the first time the movement and transformation of the information at different levels of the nerve tissue is considered. The role of the information structure of a whole brain in the information system of a body is presented.

Keywords: history of computer science and informationology, information approach in neuro-research, information neurobiology, information interrelationship, information structure of the human brain

By now the fundamentals of the information approach have been claimed and acknowledged in physical and mathematical research. The science concerned with receiving, using and processing information was named computer science, and the science related to using the information approach is informationology. It is well known that the ideology of computer science and informationology originates in the USA, and its history began in 1948 when the pioneers of informationology published cornerstone works about the basics of computer science. In that year Claude Shannon (1948) published his famous *A Mathematical Theory of Communication* in which he stated the fundamentals of computer science and introduced the terms of *information* and *entropy* in their contemporary understanding [122], and Norbert Wiener (1948) issued his theory of cybernetics under the title *Cybernetics: Or Control and Communication in the Animal and the Machine* [123]. Other famous mathematicians (Weaver, 1949; Turing, 1950; Miller, 1955) of the middle of the 20th century appreciated these theories and supported the research of Shannon and Wiener with their own theories, which became a new theoretical platform for global information science and a theoretical basis for the development of computing machines in the last century. The theories of communication, automata and control systems grew out of the communication theory of Claude Shannon and the cybernetic theory of Norbert Wiener.

In Russia Andrey Kolmogorov, the great mathematician (1903-1987), is considered a founder of the academic school of information theory, who focused greatly on the development of the framework of informationology. His works in the area of information theory became canonical both in Russia and abroad. From the mid-1990s a new direction of computer science was boosted due to the scientific research of the academic school of the mathematicians of the Russian Academy of Sciences [124]. To date the appropriateness of the information approach in exact sciences is not questioned; it is the main tool in the development of innovative approaches and technologies in science and technology.

Hence, all science about the information and methodology of the information approach to the research traces its roots to the works of outstanding American mathematicians of the previous century. We will not dwell on this exciting historical theme instead we will direct the reader to the appropriate literature on the issue. Here we will bridge the gap between mathematics and contemporary neuroscience and neurology.

Unfortunately, Russian neurologists did not have much interest in foreign and national works on computer science and informationology. However, several attempts to apply the information approach to the research of the brain were made in the works of neurophysiologists Piotr Anokhin (1974-1980) and Konstantin Sudakov (1978-2012), as well as their students. There is the information theory of emotions, by Pavel Simonov, which does not relate to the mathematical theory of information directly, but is an original hypothesis of information reasons for the emergence of emotions [125, 126]. The author considers emotions to be the consequence of a lack or excess of the information necessary to satisfy the demands. According to Simonov, the degree of emotional tension is determined by the strength of the demand and the value of the deficit of pragmatic information necessary to achieve the goal. He described it in the formula $E = D (In - Ia)$, where E stands for emotion, D is for demand, In is the information necessary to meet the demand and Ia is the information available at the moment of the demand. According to this formula, emotions arise only when demanded. If there is no demand, then there is no emotion, as the product of $E = 0 (In - Ia)$ also equals zero. There will be no emotion either, if the demand is present but $(In - Ia)$ equals zero; that is, if the person possesses the information necessary to meet their demand $(In = Ia)$. Simonov explains the significance of the remainder *(In – Ia)* by the fact that the probabilistic forecast of demand satisfaction is constructed on it. This formula permitted Simonov to state that due to the emotions the paradoxical initial evaluation of the lack of knowledge was provided [125].

Outside Russia the information approach to brain research is fundamental and accurate. It was profoundly studied by different neuroscientists at the end of the previous century [127, 128, 129]. In 2000 the Cambridge University Press published *Information Theory And The Brain* edited by Baddeley, Hancock and Foldiak; it is a fundamental summarizing work, in which the information approach to science in general and to the brain in particular, along with the brain's functions, is analyzed from the radically new information standpoint of theoretical neurology [130]. I strongly recommend this interesting and educational scientific work to the readers.

In 2003 I described my scientific concepts of the information approach to the research of the brain in the book *Cell Transplantation and Tissue Engineering in Nervous Diseases* and stated the theoretical framework of the approach as applied to general transplantology and the transplantation of neural cells in nervous diseases and injuries [131]. For the past decade a lot of new data and experimental evidence in the informationology of neuro-research have been accumulated and, accordingly, my views on the methodological and technological opportunities of the information approach, especially in the sphere of brain research, have changed. Hence, I decided to return to this complicated and extremely interesting theoretical topic and look at it from another, mostly methodological perspective or, to be exact, from the perspective of the development of a novel methodology for contemporary neural research. Also, I would like to state my new vision of the information approach in contemporary neuroscience as a new methodology of scientific cognition in neurobiology and medicine.

Therefore, to facilitate the process of sharing an understanding of the issue with my colleagues, neurologists, I would like to 'eradicate illiteracy' in the area of contemporary information theory and information processes, and in how they are understood in contemporary physics and mathematics. I will avoid the formulas and try to explain these complicated things in a simple language which is as understandable to me as to a practicing neurologist, and as clear to me as to a neuroscientist and professor of neurology. Hopefully, this means that I can explain it to my readers in a language clear enough for a doctor and a scientist. I would like to adapt the current information theoretical concepts and notions to our medical perception and humanitarian minds. Further, using these basic terms and notions, I want to explain the nature of the information approach and its place in theoretical neurology, which seems applicable to most contemporary neural research.

However, the concept of the information is significantly different for neurophysiologists, neuropsychologists and neurologists from the available concept of the information in exact science. For example, remember the information concept of Simonov in his theory of emotions, described previously. To my mind, as the novel methodology of the information approach gained a brilliant reputation in physics and mathematics, it can become the main tool of researchers aiming at understanding the mechanisms of the brain's organization and the basic issues of neurology that would allow the efficient therapy of nervous disorders. Moreover, the methodology of the information approach can change the general thinking pattern in a new generation of developers of computing equipment and lead them in a new direction of neuro-technological development. This novel direction of neuromorphic technologies is based on mimicking the principles of brain functioning and the development of a new model of information-communicative modules of nerve tissue, which relies on the information principles of organization and communication of the basic modules of nerve tissue and not on the biological morphofunctional principles of the neuron.

So, classical mathematical informationology (the science concerned with receiving, storing and processing the information) considers a process to be informational if it occurs due to research into the interaction and interrelationship of elementary particles, micro- and macro-bodies. The unit of an elementary relationship is known as an information bit, which is, in fact, a general physical elementary quantum of the relationship between micro and macro dynamic processes and the phenomena. Information interactions yield physical information fields, the constant intensity of which is supported by resonant-cellular, frequency-quantum and wave oscillation of molecules, atoms and elementary particles. All interactions between elementary particles, atoms, molecules, cells, tissues and body organs begin with field interaction, i.e., communication is carried out at the information level of fields of all types, their traces and all spin-spin, virtual, hypothetical, vacuum and other forms of micro- and macro-interactions.

Information therefore consists of principal links (e.g., between fields, spins and their traces) that can be revealed as fluctuations of (related) particles, frequencies, electrons, photons, resonances, oscillations and prompt emissions, which by virtue of their wave identity are massless. Information manifests as electromagnetic, gravitational and torsion (spin) fields. The torsion fields create relationships, interrelationships, interdependencies and interactions between massless and mass elementary, virtual and hypothetical particles which, according to the information code, determine their long existence or prompt decay. The interaction of *information bits* results in a cellular information space, which is wave, resonant, oscillating and fluctuating around an equilibrium state of electrons. The state represents a "standing" wave with its own resonant frequency, being a resonant oscillation of electrons, atoms and bodies. The identity of a standing wave of elementary particles lies in the interference when electromagnetic waves, being constantly reflected in space, interfere and create standing waves with a corresponding oscillation of electrons.

Having read this description, one understands that everything one knew and meant by the term "information" has nothing in common with the physical content of the term. Accordingly, the biblical "in the beginning was the Word" can be perceived in a different way; now it becomes obvious that "in the beginning was the information".

You might reasonably ask how these spins, electrons, standing waves and other information values relate to the brain and its information. Surprisingly, they have a direct relationship, which I will try to demonstrate.

It is well known that the information in biological fluids, cells and tissues is quantized with atoms and molecules of signal proteins, DNA, mRNA, microRNA, which are packed into micro vesicles and function as the main regulators of all sanogenetic processes in the body. But ***the information cannot be transferred by itself without material carriers***. This was proved by Claude Shannon in his mathematical theory of communication [122]. The biological information is not different from the physical and it is also transferred by various information carriers. Normally, the information is "loaded" or "packed" in the information carriers and it is received by the information channels in expressed microvesicles or exosomes on the molecules of regulatory proteins, DNA, transport RNA or microRNA secreted by a somatic cell in a dosed way. In other words, the information from every somatic cell is arranged in the information packages and isolated in microvesicles or exosomes that contain regulatory biologically active agents. Exosomes are the product of the proteome (protein structure) activity of these cells. Hence, the external information from the cell is transmitted by its secretome, which is produced or secreted by the proteome. This is an inherent part of cell proteomes functioning directed externally (into extracellular space) and capable of regulating and managing intercellular functions. Due to cell secretomes, the main relations between the cell proteomes are formed.

To date it is known that the main information relationships between the cells in a healthy tissue are achieved due to the fusion or intercellular exchange of the information through intercellular junctions. The intercellular junction, the means of the intercellular interactions, is a key structural-functional factor to support the metabolic homeostasis in the organs and tissues. This type of contact was first detected by electronic microscopy and looks like the spots of the close adherence of lateral membranes of neighboring cells with less than 0.2 nm gap between the membranes. This detail makes the intercellular junctions involved in all information processes of the organism's activity, and conditions their key role in tissue homeostasis support through an even distribution of molecular growth signals between neighboring cells. The information from one cell travels to the neighboring one through the intercellular junction; it is further transferred either by the lymphatic system or blood vessels and then through nervous fibers to executive organs and structures. The information between the neurons is exchanged by means of their secretome represented as the mediators, neurotrophines and trophic factors mostly through the synapses. The data inside the neurons are transferred by the packages of impulse current through the axons. Lymph, blood, cerebrospinal fluid and nervous fibers are the main *information channels* or *information buses* of interrelations between various information levels of eukaryotes. However, it should be noted that the bioinformation carriers (DNA, RNA, microRNA, proteins and somatic cells) differ from the information channels, information lines and information buses which are intercellular junctions, lymphatic vessels and nodes, arterial and venous vessels and sinuses, synapses, fibers of peripheral nerves and nervous ganglia, SCF system and others, and differ from the information. These things must not be confused. The information carriers are those biophysical and biochemical structures in the human/mammal body that provide storage, transport and different speeds of transmission and processing of different scopes of data, which is explained by their heterogeneous information capacity and genetically predetermined opportunities to use received information. They are always material. We would like to stress that the information is not able to move through the brain and human/mammal organism independently. To travel, the data need carriers. The data always locate on the carriers that fulfill the inter-level transfer. The speed of the data transfer depends on the characteristics of the carrier and on the characteristics of the information channel (information line, information bus). The slowest speed of the information transfer is observed in the tissue of solid organs and achieved through the intercellular junctions. In blood it is not high either, due to the high number of cells, each of which carries a volume of specific information. Consequently, these information channels are rather slow, although capacious. That is, blood is the best information line when a good quality of information exchange is necessary, and speed is not important. This information carrier unites all organs and tissues of humans and mammals. The speed of information transfer in the lymph is higher, due to the lower cell count and the protein count in this biological fluid. So the destinations (other organs and the brain) receive the data transmitted by the lymphatic track quicker than through the blood vascular systems.

Cerebrospinal fluid (CSF) is one of the best information carriers, and subarachnoid and subdural spaces are some of the best information channels of eukaryotic organisms. The speed of information transfer in CSF exceeds the speed of the information transfer by nervous fibers. The cell count in 1 μl of CSF varies from one to three; the protein count is about 0.33g/l and the electrolyte composition similar to that of sea water provides for excellent information properties of the human/mammal CSF. The information collapse in the nerve tissue in minimal traumatic hemorrhagic injuries of brain microvessels is extremely explicit, when the patient develops minor subarachnoid hemorrhage and the blood is found in the CSF. Even an insufficient number of blood cells in the CSF leads to severe disorders of consciousness in the patients, though morphological injury and suffusion are slight. Contemporary neurology is not able to explain the mechanism of consciousness disorder in this or other cases. Another example of the information failure in the brain cortex functioning is an increase of the CSF cell count in meningitis and meningoencephalitis. The direct correlation between the degree of the consciousness disorder, the value of the CSF cell count and protein-cellular dissociation in the CSF is observed. So, not only can the histology and cytology of the fluid be used to detect its cell composition, but also the mapping and profiling of the protein structure have huge diagnostic, prognostic and therapeutic potential. The biological fluids are the main reservoir of biological information about the tissues and organs they wash. The opportunities to decipher and use this information open up huge resources for the diagnostics and therapy of a range of diseases in civilization (diabetes, obesity, neurodegenerative diseases, etc.).

As already mentioned, the unit of information in contemporary scientific informationology is called an information bit. To specify the average scope of biological information in one information bit, we made a conditional assumption and equated the information capacity of an information bit to one unit of *normalized signal intensity* (NSI) of the protein, used in analytical biochemistry for the analysis of the proteome profile of the subject, i.e., a somatic cell of the brain (neuron) or biological fluid (blood, lymph, CSF, etc.). Presumably, the conditional juxtaposition that we made (1 information bit = 1 unit of protein NSI) permits the development of an integrating information system or the information "bridge" between contemporary information, biochemical, cell and proteome, metabolome, RN-ome and secretome technologies, along with discussions in a language that is clear to scientists of different specialties (mathematicians, biophysicists, biologists, biochemists, doctors, etc.).

From the standpoint of the information approach, all information is quantized and is distributed at different cell levels, each of which has specific features. The information characteristics of each level are described with the help of contemporary visualizing equipment: microscopy, electronic microscopy, mass-spectrometry, atomic force microscopy, MRI-spectroscopy, etc. These levels are obvious and cause no doubt for the major scientific skeptics. If we look at a somatic nerve cell on the whole, it becomes obvious that the information hierarchy of the cell is topped by the *cell information level* which can present visual microscopic data about the work and functioning of a cell as a living system. The cell level is characterized by the information from the cell in general; that is, its phenotype and function, as well as by information received from the cell membrane, organelles (mitochondrias, Goldgi complex, etc.) and cell cytoplasm. The protein level lies below the cell level; it is better characterized as the *molecular information level* that receives the information from protein molecules functioning and is determined by the functional significance of protein molecules, their precursors and metabolites in a cell. The molecules of DNA, RNA, microRNA, as well as various signaling molecules and the range of proteome molecular machinery that is described in every guidebook in biochemistry for medical students, belong to the molecular level. The molecules consist of atoms of the substance and obviously, the *atom information level* lies below the molecular information level. As we know from school, the atoms are composed of the nucleus and rotating around it are the elementary particles (electrons, protons, neutrons and other). Accordingly, the information sent from this level can be qualified as information from *the level of elementary particles*. Elementary particles that vigorously rotate around the nucleus develop an electromagnetic field characterized by specific frequency and intensity, by standing waves, oscillations, resonances and others. So, to describe its information identity, we propose naming this level a magnetic field level. This name of the level is clear to physicians and to scientists involved in brain research, as the MRI or MRI spectroscopy of the brain and some other methods rely on the principle of nuclear magnetic resonance. And the phenomena of field and magnetic resonance need not be explained to mathematicians and physicists.

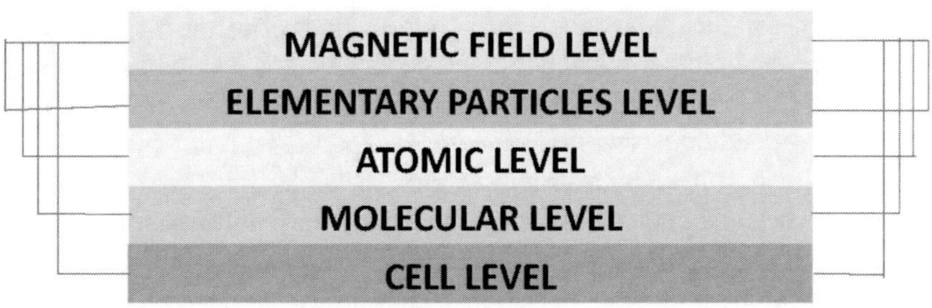

Figure 9. Information structure of a human/mammalian somatic cell.

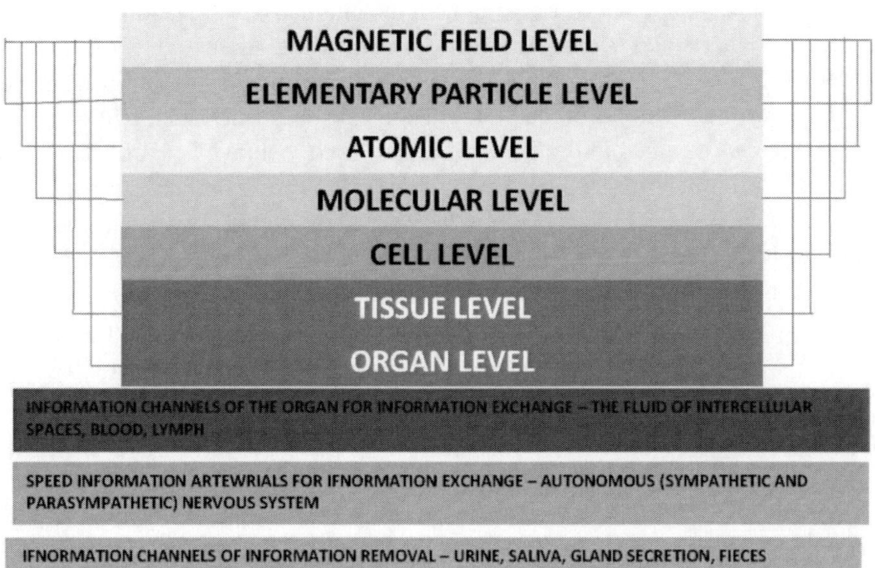

Figure 10. Information structure of human/mammalian somatic tissues and organs.

Therefore, we have constructed a specific and rather primitive information hierarchy of a somatic cell (neuron, neuroglia, vascular cell, etc.) in which every information level is quite obvious, exhibiting specific information relationships and interactions with all downstream and upstream information levels of the cell and certain information-cellular space (Figure 9). If the information structure of a tissue or an organ is studied from the same information standpoint, it would look quite similar; only appropriate tissue and organ information level should be added, along with appropriate information arterials that deliver necessary and remove unnecessary information and similar information structures of stroma cells. The information structure of an organ consists of the specific set of information structures of different parts of tissue united by one function. This organ structure has the elements of lymphatic supply and autonomous vegetative innervations (Figure 10).

According to the information approach, the human/mammal brain has the same information structure as any other organ. The brain and spinal cord are inseparable informationally, and represent an integral information structure, so we will further discuss the information structure of the brain implying their information integrity. However, the brain has certain features that make it different from any other somatic organ. One such difference is the technical aspect of the removal of extra information from the brain. As an actively functioning organ, the brain displays a high speed of data receiving and processing and, accordingly, excess information must be removed as rapidly as it was received. It is universally acknowledged that excess information is expressed directly into the CSF, where it is quickly removed and utilized by a strong current. The solid organ receives the information only through arterial and lymphatic systems, and the excess information is transferred by venous blood and is removed through the kidneys by urinary excretion.

The CSF system of the brain is a universal information bus typical only of the human/mammal brain. Long ago the neurologists used to call CSF “the urine of the brain”. There is a grain of truth in this name. Still, the brain, like any somatic organ, receives and removes some part of biological information with the blood and lymphatic systems, as well as with the vegetative nervous system. However, the CSF has a more significant function than just the removal of excess information. Obviously, the information should be removed from all organs, but only the brain has unique intermeningeal space filled with CSF around it. Due to the large scope of the information received and removed from the blood, the human/mammalian brain is one of the richest in blood vessels organs. And its systems of interconnections, collaterals and co-currents between the vascular pools and the systems of the information reset (venous sinuses and the CSF system) are the most perfect information systems created by nature. Another detail that makes the brain different from other organs is the absence of a fibrous capsule or a coat, which determines the size and geometry of other organs. Why do such “valuable” organs as the brain and spinal cord not have a sound protective fibrous capsule (as the kidneys, liver and other organs do), but instead are placed in the hard carcass of the skull and spine? Why does the brain have such a sophisticated system of membranes-meninges (the pia mater, the arachnoid mater and the dura mater)? Mechanical reasons such as making the brain float in a hard vessel do not seem satisfactory or physiologically grounded. We know that the brain is easily damaged even by light strokes to the skull and spine. The mechanisms of the coup injury of the brain against the skull, the hydraulic CSF stroke of the brain in trauma and the impossibility of expanding the volume of brain parenchyma in the hard carcass of the skull and spine lead to the loss of part of the brain or the whole organism. Consequently, we can say that the placement of the brain and spinal cord in a skull and spine was inspired by the complicated processing of the information received both from the environment and from the organism. Obviously, the brain is made to float in the skull for more significant reasons than mere physical protection. Further, we would explain the main reasons and aims of such localization of the brain and substantiate the main principles of its information organization. The information structure of the nerve tissue of the brain is presented in Figure11, and the information structure of the brain as of the organ of the human/mammalian organism is shown in Figure 12. The main difference between the information structure of the nerve tissue and the information structure of the brain as an organ lies in the information level of the field of consciousness, which is not observed in any other organ of humans/mammals. The information level of the field of consciousness characterizes the functioning of the system that consists of billions of various brain cells and distinguishes it from the functioning of the system consisting of billions of liver cells. We will discuss the tasks and mechanisms of its formation in the process of further structuring and systematization of our knowledge about the brain.

If it is not as complicated as it seems at first glance, then why can we not understand how the brain is organized and establish its main principles of work? What prevents us from answering these important questions? It seems that to answer them we have to revise all available scientific evidence about the brain, and understand its structure and significance for further research.

What is the main biological information about the brain that is analyzed by all neurologists and neuroscientists in their attempts to describe multilevel and multi-scale system of the brain? In current conventional neuroscience the scientists receive the main part of the evidence about the brain in clinical (neurological and psychopathological), neurophysiological, psychophysical, morphological, histological, cytological and immunohistochemical, MRI and CT) research of the brain substrate. There is another point of view on the information potential of contemporary neuro-research, mostly, of the experts in molecular neurobiology. They have their grounds to consider the main part of the information about the brain to be found at the molecular level of the nerve cells. Therefore, it seems rational to describe every brain cell with cellular, sub-cellular, genome, proteome, transcriptome, metabolome and secretome charts and protein profiles, their progenitors or metabolites, and compile a multilevel system of the cell of these most objective and personalized data, to transfer it to the level of the synapses and to the whole ensemble of the cell of the specific brain area (microcircuit) and then to follow the changes of the system at the level of different brain regions and the brain as a whole (the methodology of the Human Brain Project can be used as an example). Undoubtedly, the information about the brain as a complex multilevel system that was received using the main scientific and methodological techniques of the system approach is well-grounded and legitimate. But this information does not match itself as it is not scalable and cannot be formatted within the framework of this multilevel system. The main paradox of the system approach to the brain studies lies in the impossibility of connecting the interrelationships of different levels. It is unclear how changes in the genome correlate with the dynamics of psychophysiological and neuropsychological changes and how they influence the cognitive functions of the brain. Most probably, it can be explained by heterogeneity, the variety of levels and clusters of biological information received from the brain. Mostly, the information that was obtained using various clinical methods, questionnaires and tests and para-clinical methods of research reflects the morphofunctional state of the brain, while the information that was received using biochemical methods of brain tissues and cell research represents information of the fundamental genome/post-genome neurobiological properties of the substrate of the brain's nerve tissue. However, these two large volumes of information do not have an interface between them, through which we could observe their interaction and trace their information relationship. We know that the brain has a huge volume of biophysical (neurophysiological, bioelectric, etc.) information, which is correlated neither with the first, nor the second volumes. It is studied by biophysical institutions and scientific teams autonomously and independently, and is not associated with the first and second clusters of morphofunctional and genome/post-genome information data about the brain. Primitive understanding of the interaction between the structure and function of the brain elements seems basically incorrect. Biophysical information about the brain can and must become the buffer and interface for the integration of brain information of different levels and different scales, obtained through morphofunctional and fundamental genome/post-genome research.

I am convinced that the search for new theoretical constructs and a new methodology that would be able to provide the interface between the sets of morphofunctional, biophysical, genome and post-genome information can be realized only through the information approach to neuro-research. The information approach as a new methodology permits the answers to many fundamental questions of brain functioning. The information approach offers the possibility of structuring the information received from every level and of following its transformation from level to level and back.

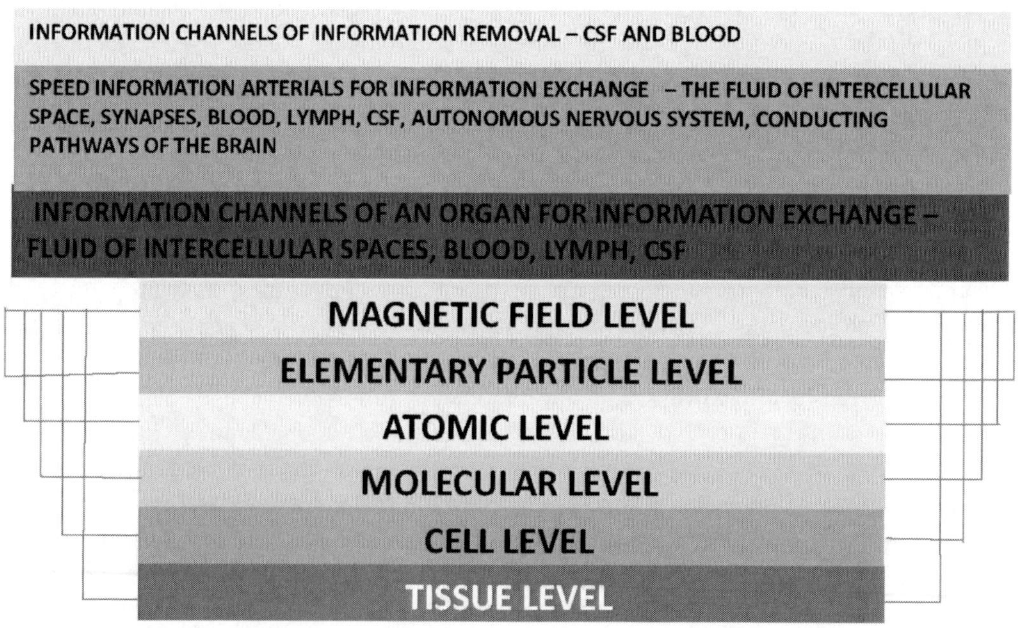

Figure 11. Information structure of nerve tissue of the human/mammalian brain and spinal cord.

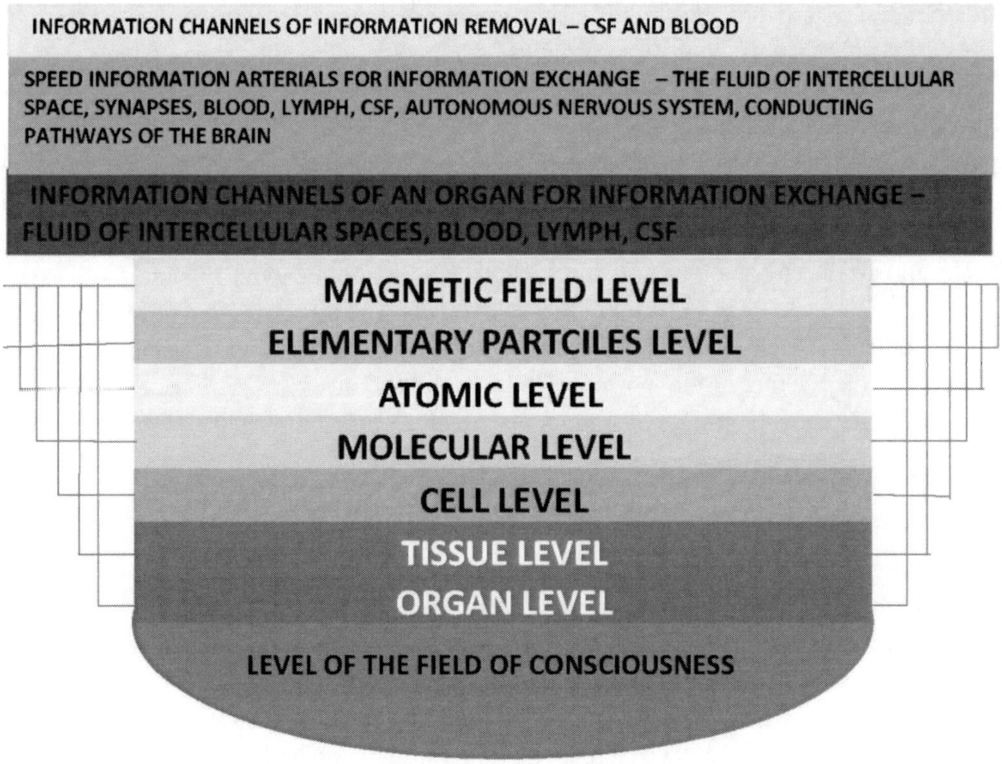

Figure 12. Information structure of the human/mammalian brain and spinal cord.

Let us look at the best studied molecular level of a cell and range it according to some of the basic characteristics of the proteins that are known in molecular biology and systemic biology. The first information characteristic is the molecular weight of the proteins. According to this, most of the proteins can be ranged from lower to upper molecular weight or *vice versa*. The second information characteristic is the protein localization in a cell. This characteristic helps to determine the amount of protein in the membrane, cytoplasm or cell organelles. The third information characteristic is the protein function in the cell. This allows for the description of all functional processes in which the studied protein is involved. All of these information characteristics, just like other informational characteristics, are important and necessary for the evaluation of a nerve cell, but carry little information if viewed from the standpoint of informationology. Using the methods of the system approach to studies of the protein structure of a cell, we can draw a systemic graph of their interactions, as shown in Figure 8. However, with the system approach one cannot distract oneself from details, but sticks to them in the attempt to present proteins, protein progenitors and their metabolites in a structured fashion, depending on the informational significance and the role in a cell.

What does the informational approach offer? It permits us to trace all inter-level relationships and to receive a clear answer to some of the most important questions, such as how the genome correlates with other information levels of the cell and to follow up their influence on the genome. Let us suppose that we are dealing with the rather crude informational structure of a cell of any organ. Contemporary fundamental science provides us with every opportunity to study it in great detail. From the informational point of view, in order to structure and process the information about these proteins, it is more important to understand to which informational level (or sublevel) the proteins belong: the DNA of the genome proteins, which conditions hereditary characteristics, or the protein progenitors (RNA) of the pathways of signal transduction (transcriptome) of the cell, which determine intracellular signaling. Or, these can be the proteins that determine the structure of the cell phenotype and form its proteome, or they may be complex proteins secreted by the cell (secretome). Alternatively, these could be the metabolome proteins, which are connected with the metabolism of a somatic cell. Today these terms are familiar to everyone and are clear even to the fourth year medical students. Hence, for better understanding and processing of the available data about cell proteins, the ranking of the molecular level of the cell into known information sublevels is optimal, and namely, into genome, transcriptome, proteome, metabolome, secretome (Figure 13). To my mind, the representation of these information sublevels as a Russian Matryoshka (nesting doll), whereby one level is placed inside another and is able to affect both upper and lower levels, is a good technical and design finding. When the levels are arranged according to the principle of a nesting doll, the available limitations of the interactions of the levels become clear.

From the information point of view, the genome is the project of a whole organism in every cell, reference programs to check the functioning of all informational levels in the cells, and system software for the processes of embryogenesis, ontogenesis, intratissular restoration and the sanogenesis of a somatic cell. Viewed from the angle of the information approach, the cell transcriptome can be presented as the resource for cell construction, repair and restoration. The cell proteome is an accomplished result of proliferative and differentiation processes in the body or a ready biological product (species), whose information speaks for itself. The cell proteome is expressed in a cell phenotype and permits cell recognition from 256 types of cells in a body. Cell metabolome is the power system and fuel and energy potential of a cellular system. The cell secretome is the functional information exchanged by the cells, or it fulfills the inherent regulatory or managing function directed at other cell and tissue systems. The names of the defined sublevels are clear and do not seem to require additional explanations. Moreover, when we compare these information levels with systemic biological data about the somatic cell and its basic intracellular elements (cell karyotype, signal transduction or intracellular signaling, cell phenotype, cell secreted biologically active substances, etc.), the correlating interaction of the information levels (sublevels) of cell functioning and main systemic evidence about the cell becomes obvious (Figure 14). If we study the interrelations of the information levels, we can see that the cell proteome depends on the state of the genome and the level of expression and deactivation of cell genes. The proteome is regulated by the genome by means of changing transcriptome functioning, as well as depending on the changes in cell metabolism or, from the information standpoint, from metabolome. The information function of a cell at the level of its secretome also depends on all downstream levels.

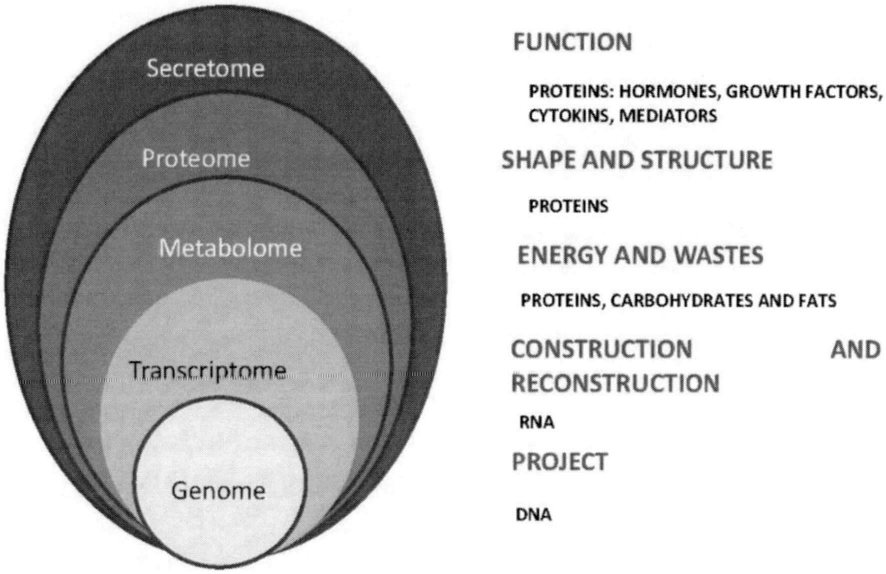

Figure 13. Structural hierarchy of protein components (proteins, protein progenitors and metabolites) of the information structure of molecular level of a somatic cell.

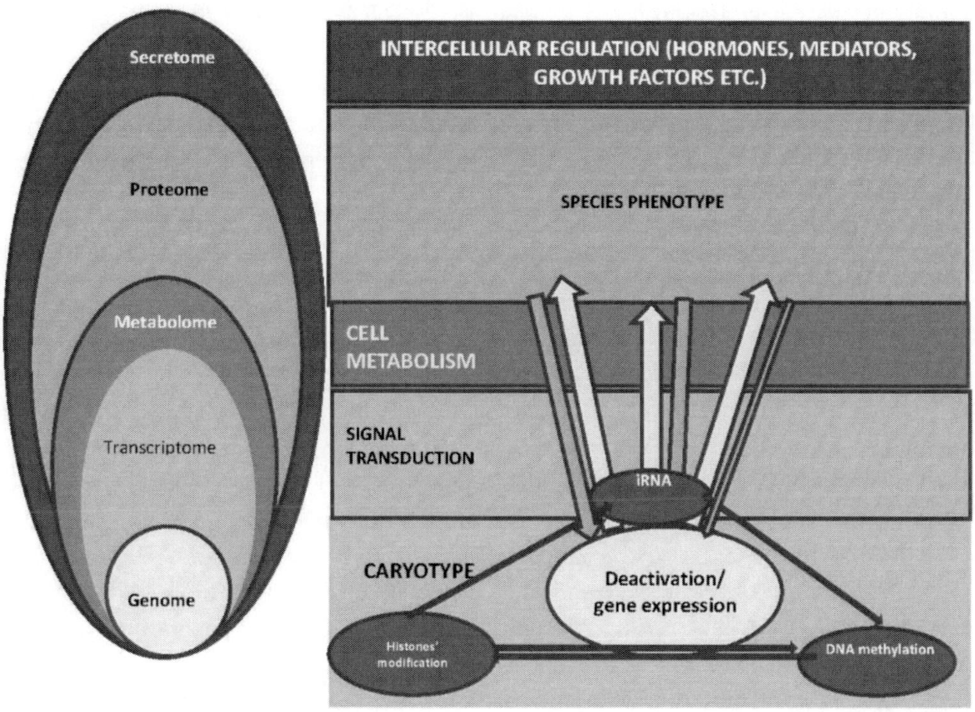

Figure 14. Information proteome structure of a somatic cell, its place in the information structure and functional significance for the cell system.

Hence, speaking about the information structure of a healthy somatic cell, we observe a rigid interdependent hierarchy of relationships of the information levels of a somatic cell whereby the slightest changes of activity at the genome level lead to programmed changes at all levels of the information structure, which is represented in changes to the profiled data of these cells (proteome profile of the proteins, complete transcriptome profile of gene expression, metabolome profile of carbohydrates, fats and protein metabolites, etc.). All previously described parameters of the information structure of the molecular level of a somatic cell (genome, transcriptome, metabolome, proteome and secretome) reflect only the biochemical machinery of a somatic cell. This ranking of the information sublevels of the molecular level of the nerve cell allows us to show how the information moves, only at the molecular level of all of its biochemical processes: at the genome level the information is transported by DNA; at the transcriptome level, by RNA; at the level of the proteome, by the proteins; at the level of the secretome, by the protein complexes (e.g., hormones, growth factors and neuromediators) too; and at the level of the metabolome, by the major metabolites, proteins and the products of carbohydrate cleavage. This would be right, if we perceived the somatic cell from the molecular positions of the system theory and only as a complex biochemical system. In this case, we could limit ourselves with these information levels or sublevels.

But the nerve cell is a living system in which biochemical processes form magnetic fields and transform into electric currents. The magnetic field level transfers the information to the genome level of the cell with the help of the magnetic field, which is formed by the movements of atoms, elementary particles, resonances and oscillations. Then the information is carried by biochemical carriers; it passes a whole biochemical cycle of transfer through intracellular structures, later to return to biophysical carriers of the information, i.e., to electromagnetic waves which can carry the information represented in electrostatic charges in the packages of electric impulses at extremely large distances. Electric currents in the neurons produce a magnetic field with 10^{-14}-10^{-11} Tesla induction, which can sometimes go beyond the borders of the body. As far as magnetic fields are the consequence of comparatively strong currents of the functioning organ or tissues, they weaken rapidly when the source of activity moves away. The magnetic fields of a living cell system can be a result of the following: 1) ion currents from the electrical activity of cell membranes; 2) the finest ferromagnetic particles introduced into the body voluntarily or involuntarily; 3) when an external magnetic field is superimposed, the heterogeneity of the magnetic susceptibility of different organs manifests and distorts the superimposed external field. The first two sources develop their own magnetic fields.

This phenomenon of the nerve cells can be illustrated by electroneuromyography, which registers the electric currents passing through the neurons, while the magnetic field of a living system can be visualized using contemporary computer magnetoencephalography. By analogy with other information levels of the cell, we named the genome preceding the biophysical information magnetic field level of tissue induction a cell *inductome*, and the level of the information exit from the biochemical level to the biophysical magnetic-wave level a cell *magnetome*. The names for these biophysical levels are given similarly to already known names (-omes) that characterize information levels of cell organization (genome, proteome, etc.).

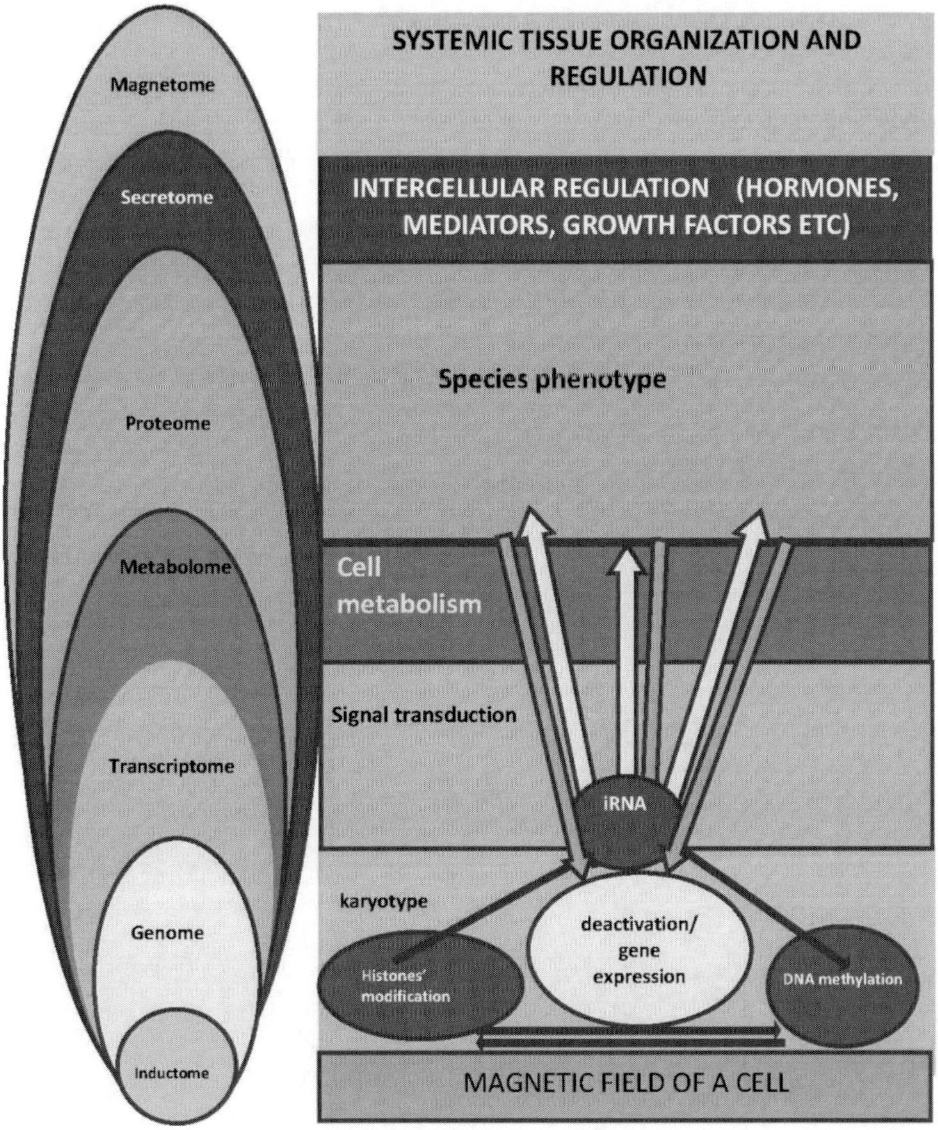

Figure 15. Information structure of a somatic cell, its place in the information structure and the functional significance for the cell system.

These words might have already been used but we utilize them to denote the newly described. These levels demanded some names and we simply proposed the terms that seemed to reflect their nature. These levels (inductome and magnetome) suppose that the cell system participates in the formation of system tissue organization and regulation (Figure 15). Obviously, the *inductome* of a somatic cell reflects the level and characteristics of the magnetization of the specific tissue and it is the controlling parameter of the action of the field information on the intracellular genome, and cell magnetomes provide the participation of the cell in the formation of tissue and organ levels and manifest in electromagnetic waves (EMWs) of super high frequencies (SHF). The works of the Russian biophysicists Oleg Betskiy, Mikhail Golant and Nikolay Devyatkov convincingly proved that the cell magnetome was represented by the EMWs of super high frequency of millimeter range at the biophysical level [132].

In a strong magnetic field, the magnetic field of a somatic cell intensifies, its intensity increases and biophotonic emission is registered; it launches a cascade of biophysical processes that manifest in several phenomena including illumination in the strong magnetic field. The illumination is described as Kirlian photography. In 1949 the Kirlians discovered and photographed the high-frequency illumination emitted by living tissues (Figure 16). The registered biophotonic emission of daphnias, which was calculated according to interference model (the curve) and experimental data, can serve as biophysical proof (Figure 17).

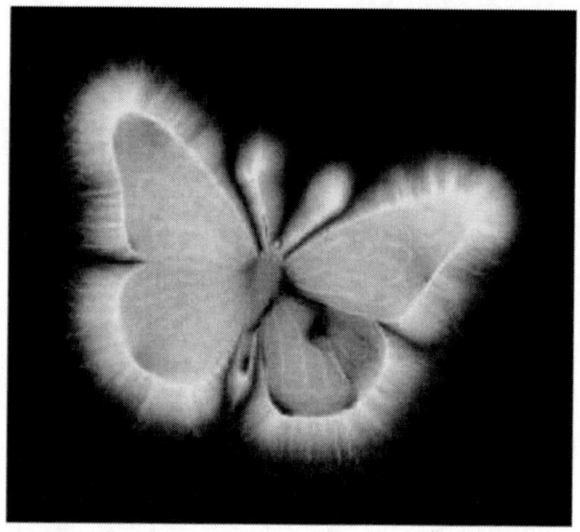

Figure 16. An example of Kirlian photography showing the magnetic field discharged by the biochemical machinery of living cells.

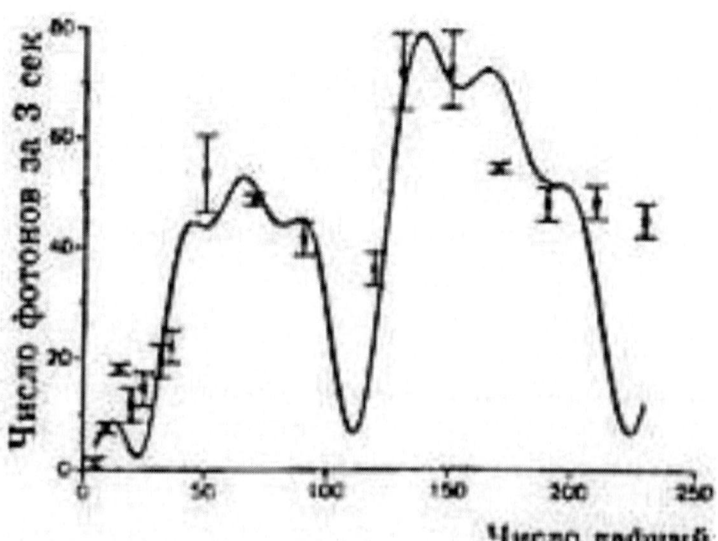

Figure 17. Biophotonic emission of daphnias calculated according to the interference model (curve) and experimental values.

Thus, the somatic neural cell systems, just as the majority of any other cell systems, have two more information levels that are formed by the magnetic field of the cell (inductome) and the biochemical machinery of the cell represented by the cell magnetome. This biophysical information issued by the cell must not be neglected in the informational tissue and cellular processes. So, we have denoted the magnetic-field and magnetic-wave informational levels of a somatic nerve cell, as of any other somatic cells, and called them inductome and magnetome, respectively, and consider that the information on them is transferred by means of material information carriers, just as at biochemical information levels. The magnetic field with such features as inductance, intensity and resonant-wave characteristics is the information carrier at the level of inductomes. The electromagnetic waves carry the information at the level of cellular magnetomes. The latter phenomenon has been vividly demonstrated by a biologist from Khabarovsk (Russia), Zhang Kanchjen [133]. In 1989 he developed a device that worked in the SHF range and recorded various electromagnetic oscillations of living systems on it. For example, he recorded the electromagnetic oscillations of duck spermatozoids that were later used to treat chicken eggs. The resulting effects were similar to those that would appear if a duck were hybridized with a hen (which cannot happen in nature as the two belong to different species). In another experiment he recorded the electromagnetic vibrations of peanuts and directed the EMWs with this information on sunflower sprouts. As a result, the sunflowers seeds tasted of peanuts. When the sprouted corn was treated with the signals recorded from the wheat, the spikes had seeds that were reminiscent of both wheat and corn. The seed yield increased twice, while the green biomass increased thrice. One should note that the results of these scientific biological experiments passed the expertise of 130 specialists from five independent institutes of the Siberian Department of the Russian Academy of Science. Due to the discrepancy of the data, these results stand apart from other biological research and were never coordinated with the biochemical parameters of a living somatic cell.

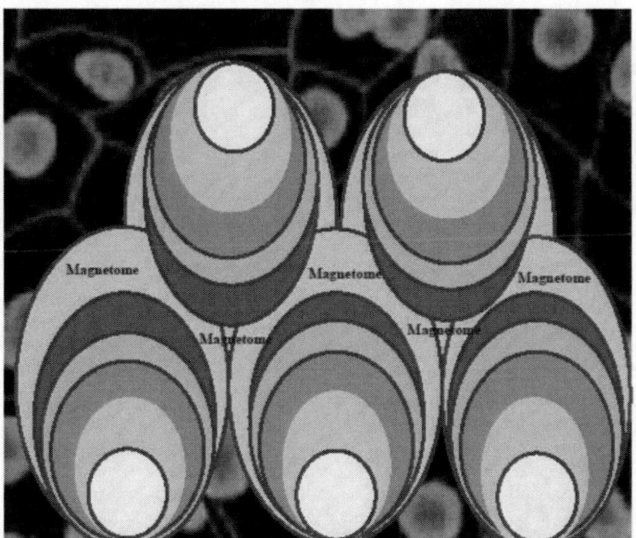

Figure 18. Information structure of the tissue against a background of visual microscopic tissue representation.

Hence, the information levels of the cell, which we called the inductome and the magnetome, are an inherent part of the information structure of any cell or tissue system and must be taken into account in our theory and practice. The role and meaning of the cell magnetome in sustaining the life of the cell must be appropriately evaluated. The main function of the cell inductome is its control of the genome, while the main function of the magnetome of a somatic cell is interaction with the magnetomes of other cell systems and the formation of general tissue magnetomes of tissue specific areas of informational activity of the cell systems in a certain organ (Figure 18). The interaction of the informational structures at the level of tissue magnetomes, and the existence and registration of the magnetome in the tissue let us speak about the signs of tissue viability and the formation of the organ information level.

The absence of the magnetome in the information structure of the cells renders the tissue dead and leads to its decay. The cellular magnetome conditions the main parameters for sustaining the life of the biological material. To my mind, the reason for the inefficiency of tissue engineering and artificial organs' growth lies in our disregard of the evidence about the inductome, cell and tissue magnetome in the cell's functioning and denial of the necessity for research and development of the specific tissue magnetome, which is a system forming framework and presents specific conditions in cultural work and matrices. We presume that in the living systems the cell systems integrate in a certain tissue and the ***tissue information level*** forms due to the interaction and interference of cell informational structures. Primarily, this interaction happens at the level of mutual influence of the magnetomes of the cell systems and development of the tissue magnetome, which is an integrated parameter of superimposition of the EMWs of the magnetomes of different cells (oligodendrocytes, astrocytes, microglia, etc.) of the nerve tissue (Figure 18).

The DARPA works in scaffold-free tissue engineering have convincingly proved this phenomenon [134]. The first samples of tissue engineered organs were developed from a magnetic field-effected mass of stem and progenitor cells without using any scaffolds or matrices.

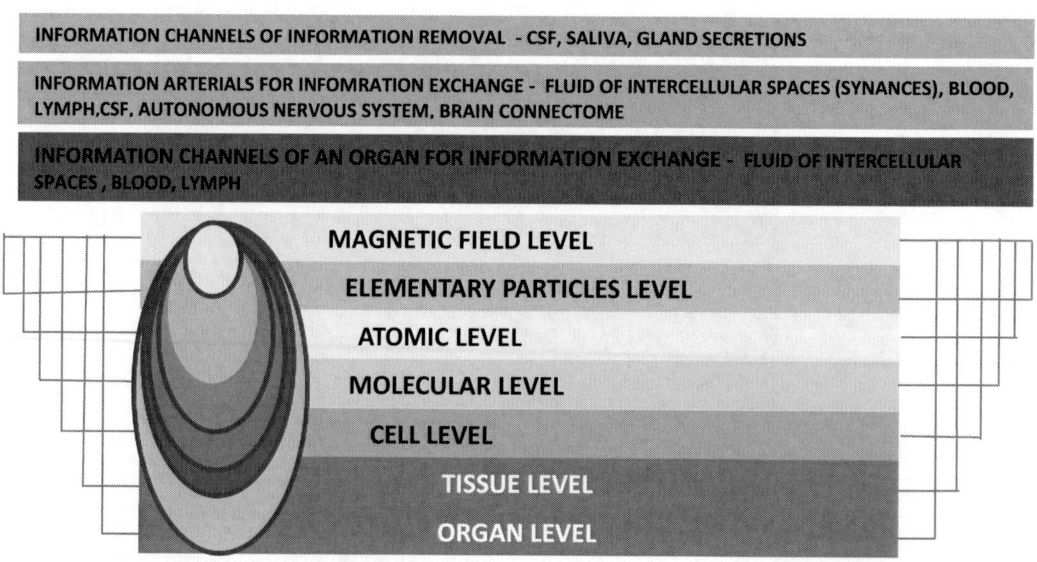

Figure 19. The model of the information structure of an organ.

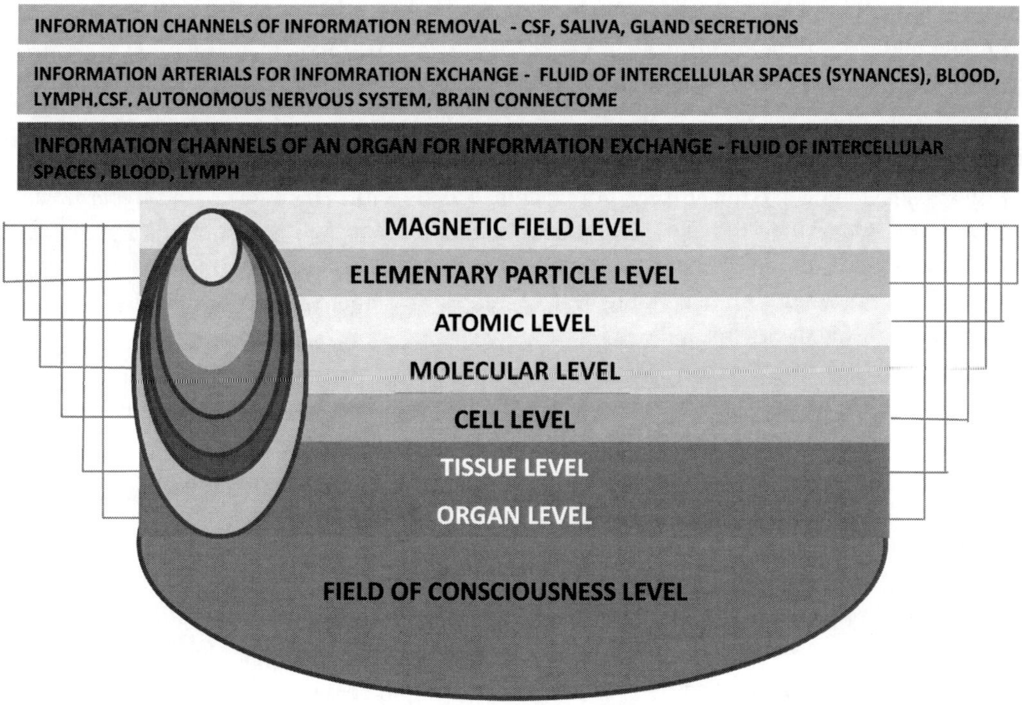

Figure 20. The model of the organ information structure of the human brain.

The informational structure of an organ forms as a complex multi-scale and multilevel bioinformation structure, which consists of various cell and tissue informational structures that are part of an organ. The organ informational structure includes supplemental informational structures of the blood supply system (arterial and venous), lymphatic system, connective tissue cells, nerve cells of the autonomous vegetative (sympathetic and parasympathetic) nervous system and tissue specific information structures of the cell systems of certain organs (e.g., neurons of the brain, hepatocytes of the liver and cardiomyocytes of the heart) (Figure 19). Obviously, at the level of organ informational structure the cumulative magnetome of different tissue parts conditions the presence of life and the viability of an organ. Due to the achievements in the transplantation of organs and tissues we have studied the terms and time-frame of the organ's survival outside the body; that is, limited life sustaining without organ information structure (IS).

What maintains different tissue and organ ISs? What integrates different magnetomes of phenotypically different 252 types of human tissues in one organ and one whole, an organism? They are controlled by the brain, and this fact found the scientific rationale in the information mathematical theory of system control [135]. According to this, the slowest process is controlling in any system. Every chemist knows it from their daily routine work, but to the doctors and neuroscientists it is usually explained with the example of a transport column (a tractor, a race car, a bus, a truck etc.), whereby the key system-forming factor is the speed of the involved vehicles. It is obvious that the controlling speed will be the speed of a tractor, the slowest vehicle; otherwise, the column will stop being a system. Although the general IS of the organism is formed due to the controlling biorhythm set by the heart of a healthy human, which is from 60 to 82 beats a minute, the slowest phase in a human/mammalian organism is the beat of the brain, which varies from 6 to 8 beats per minute. This is the slowest biorhythm of the contraction of the organs, and this rhythm is controlling all systems and subsystems of the body. On the one hand, the heart in the human/mammalian organism synchronizes the frequencies of different tissue magnetomes of the lungs, liver, kidneys, etc., of which the general electromagnetic field of any organ consists. On the other hand, the frequencies of different tissue magnetomes of the organs synchronize independently due to the law established by Norbert Wiener, the cybernetics inventor, who found that the close frequency oscillators of one system will inevitably synchronize. Today the frequencies and rhythms of these organs' contractions are well described and registered. But the brain beat regulates and controls the frequencies of the magnetomes of different organs and tissues of humans and animals. Thus, the brain is able to control all processes inside the organs and tissue at the systemic level. The principles of systemic control of the body organs and tissues by the brain lie at the informational level of all interrelations of the organs and systems.

Apparently, if viewed from the informational positions, the brain is an organ like all other solid organs of humans and mammals. But, as noted above, its basic difference from other organs of the human body is its slowest contraction; thus, it is able to control intratissular and organ processes. Its basic structural element is a neural cell that has long axons and is able to form neural networks in which the main means of information transfer is electric impulses and electromagnetic fields that form the bioelectric activity of the organ. The brain as the organ of a human and mammalian body has the most pronounced electromagnetic field of all organs, which is formed during the life activity and functioning of the neurons. Induction of this field is able to form a new information level and, namely, the level of the field of consciousness. These organ ISs of the brain are a controlled electromagnetic field. Its intensity depends on the specific influence of tissue magnetomes located in different parts of the brain that are formed from the set of modules of nerve cells consisting of neurons, vessels, fibers, and synapses of different brain structures. The main biological generators (neurons of different parts of the brain) that support the necessary intensity of the electromagnetic fields of the brain constantly change the values of the intensity of the magnetic field because of the information received online both from outside (from the environment) and from the depths of the subconsciousness (from the genome, transcriptome, proteome levels, etc.). Contemporary magnetoencephalography is able to register tissue magnetomes of the nerve tissue of the brain areas, and mathematical modeling of the integrated interaction of different tissue magnetomes permits its integration into a whole one and representation of data about the informational structure of a whole brain (Figure 20). We will describe the information organization, mechanisms and principles of the brain functioning as the information structure in the next chapter in detail. Interaction of the organ magnetomes of different organs of the body forms an inter-organ level of the information relations in the organism. Hence, we can suppose that generally the hierarchical system of the organism will take the shape of a mushroom in which the upstream level interacts with those downstream and *vice versa* (Figure 21). Such an informational structure provides an understanding of the role and place of the brain in the general information structure of the organism and the way in which the level of the field of consciousness (information level of a whole brain) correlates with other biochemical and biophysical information levels of the organism, controls them and influences their functions. The scheme lets us trace the relations of the upper information level (level of the field of consciousness) with other downstream information levels (levels of sub-consciousness). In the middle of the 19th century Sigmund Freud described the available relations of consciousness and sub-consciousness as looking like a mushroom, where consciousness is a mushroom cap, and the sub-consciousness is a mushroom stipe. So, understanding the structure of sub-consciousness as it was presented by Freud in his forecast can be the basis for understanding consciousness/sub-consciousness in humans and mammals.

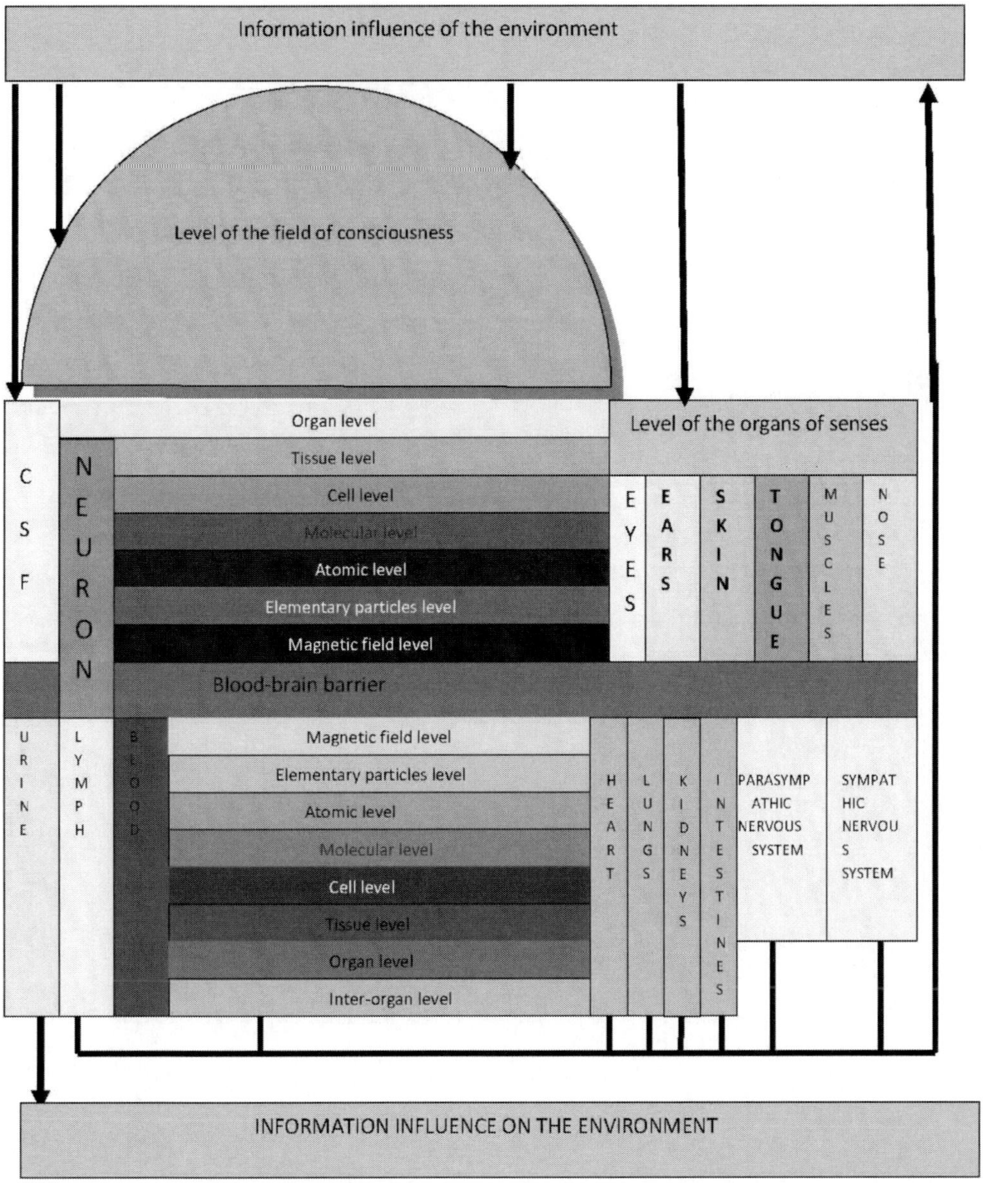

Figure 21. The scheme of the information structure and information levels of the brain levels and their relationship with information levels of the organs and system of a human body and the interrelationship between them.

Chapter 6

The Theory of the Information-Commutation Organization of the Human Brain and its Operational Principles

Abstract

The fundamentals of the information-communication theory of the human brain are stated in this chapter. No theory is perfect and needs no polishing. This material is not an exception and does not pretend to be an absolute truth; it needs elaboration and refinement. This chapter sets forth new conceptual principles of the information organization, architecture and operation of the human brain. It makes us look in a new light at existing dogmas and canons of clinical neurology. These are the personal scientific-theoretical and intuitive-practical views of the author on the structure and operation of the human brain. The author defines new concepts of the architecture of the human brain and information principles of its work. The theory is underpinned by an academic principle; to become classical and to influence the development of the science, the theory must not necessarily be true, but it must be radically different from conventional theory. The author presents his own opinion about the way in which the brain is organized, which radically differs from the theory that dominates in contemporary science, and the reader can look at the well-known structure of the mammalian head, its anatomy and functions of the subarachnoid and subdural spaces from the perspective of information-communication theory. The author presents the block scheme of the information organization of the human brain and the genius of the creator (Nature, God or Evolution) of a unique mechanism of holographic extraneural (located outside the brain) data processing in the human head. Rebellious ideas about the way in which the brain is organized are set forth, contradicting the universally acknowledged opinions of the great Russian physiologists (Pavlov, Sechenov, Vvedensky, Ukhtomsky and others) on the brain's operation. The author claims that the brain and the cortex are not the substrate of thinking and intellectual activity, but only an organic switchboard of the processes that develop extraneurally, outside the parenchyma of the brain. The author compares the human brain with a computer and shows that the memory disc in the brain is the pia mater, and not the hippocampus, and the system software disc is the arachnoid, while the gyri in the brain are necessary to implement the holographic principle of the record and reproduction of the data from the pia. The author offers almost no arguments, but it is so. Or, at least, so far they have almost no arguments; the author just supposes it to be so and in the book shares his ideas about the information processes in the brain.

Keywords: information approach, system approach, multilevel system, the methodology of the Human Brain Project, comparison of the methodology of system and information approaches

In this chapter I will dare to state the fundamentals of my uniform information-commutation theory of the brain, to describe the principal scheme of information setup of the brain, and, more specifically, my vision of it, which logically comes out of the proposed information concept of the brain's functioning and structure. Possibly, the proposed scheme of the information organization of the brain and the postulated information principles of the brain's operation can become the starting points for contemporary theoretical neurology and can facilitate the technical problem statement to develop a mathematical model of the virtual brain on the basis of the information approach, and work out the fundamental technological guidelines for new architectures of artificial intelligence systems.

Prior to the discussion of new or, to be exact, information principles of the brain's organization and operation, let us specify the main definitions, terms and available notions of the contemporary scientific paradigm of the organization and operation of the human and mammalian brain. Second, we will remind ourselves of all the existing dogmas, long-standing hypotheses and conventional theoretical concepts of the mechanisms of the brain's operation which had taken shape by the beginning of the second decade of the 21st century in the global clinical neurology and neurosciences. The main contemporary theories and hypotheses of the brain were described in the second chapter of this book, and in this chapter we concisely summarize available concepts within the framework of the systemic scientific morphofunctional paradigm that dominates in contemporary neurology and neurosciences. We would like to accentuate that we do not discuss the anatomical organization and physiological processes of the brain, but talk of the principles of the brain's operation and its physical and biochemical foundations.

Currently all conventional ideas of the human and mammalian brain's organization and functional principles can be generalized as several statements of contemporary scientific theory of the brain:

1. The brain is a multilevel, multifunctional structure of the central nervous system (CNS) of mammalian (including human) organisms intended to receive, transfer, process and store information received from the body's organs, systems and environment. The CNS regulates and maintains homeostasis in the organism, promoting its survival and adaptation under constantly changing conditions of extreme environmental factors [10, 12, 17, 30, 56, 90, 91, 136].
2. A number of systemic morphofunctional levels of the brain and CNS can be distinguished, i.e., the genome level, transcriptome level, proteome level and metabolome level, synaptic level, level of the cell, level of tissue circuits, level of brain regions, level of connectivity, level of the whole brain and cognitive level [1].
3. Nerve cells (neurons) of the brain are the basic information structural and functional units of the brain that, being connected through multiple synapses, form neural circuits [56], providing a morphological substrate for functional systems in the brain [22, 26]. Organized into neural circuits, neurons have strict topical localization and functional specialization (e.g., motor, visual and proprioceptive) in the CNS and cannot be restored if injured [7].

4. Inside the neuron, information is transmitted by electrical package-impulse transfer through the nodes of Ranvier on its axon; while between the neurons the information is transmitted chemically through neuromediators, growth factors and neurotransmitters [8, 137, 138]. Anatomic structures connecting neurons are called synapses and provide the morphological substrate for the formation of neural networks [1, 56].
5. Neural circuits are the basic information structures of the brain, and consist of neurons and synapses that support the basic functions of life support in a human/mammal, as well as memory record and storage, cognition and intellectual-mnestic activity [55, 72]. The cerebral cortex can be perceived as an information system consisting of hierarchical groups of neural circuits [33].
6. Overall, the brain is a multilevel neural network [53, 61] that receives, processes and stores information which is evenly distributed among all neurons of the brain due to the holographic principle [3, 26]. At the same time, the human brain can also be presented as a hologram capable of forming different functional systems to satisfy the needs of the organism and to achieve a useful adaptive result [22, 26].
7. Memory is one of the basic functions of the brain; it is evenly distributed among all cells of the brain cortex and subcortical nodes and is stored in the protein and genome networks of neurons [76] permitting the recording, storage and reproduction of the information in every region of this multilayered neural network [66, 139]. The main substrate of the brain responsible for memories is the hippocampus, the activation of which, by optogenetically manipulating memory engram-bearing cells, can result in false memories [77].
8. Morphofunctional systems in the brain are based on circuits providing the functional cortical neurodynamic integration [47, 48, 52] of different brain regions and brain formations, which is manifested in bioelectrical activity, oscillatory processes [34] and magnetoencephalographic manifestations of brain functioning.
9. Neurodynamic integration forms cognitive functions of neural circuits of the brain cortex [80] based on the principles of free energy [63, 140-142]. Perception and thinking are also circuit functions; it is the cooperation of different brain areas that keeps constantly adapting on the basis of the solved task, internal resources of the brain and biological limitations [69].
10. Information is processed in the brain cortex at the level of neural codes [43, 45, 46] by activation of the cortex, as well as the simultaneous interaction of different cell levels of the cortex [71], which is manifested in cognitive functions. Quantum mechanisms of consciousness formation [2, 37, 40] and neuroconnectivity of the cerebral cortex [74, 83] underlie the information processing.

That is how a contemporary paradigm of the global fundamental neurosciences, neurology and neurocomputing can be presented. The mathematicians and engineers involved in the studies of the principles of brain operation share this opinion, as well as the members of a socially active neurocommunity and popularizers of neurosciences. These very principles have been laid in the basis of all computational and neurobiological models of the brain, but, as we show further, have not brought the results that were anticipated. The inefficacy of the mathematical models seems surprising, as today all mathematical models of the virtual brain have a number of neurons and synapses which are technologically comparable to those of the natural brain. Apparently, the reason for the inefficacy of the available brain models lies in a misunderstanding of the information interrelationships of neurons and the synapses between them, and not in the expansion of the number of these morphofunctional formations in the brain.

What is the strategic reason for the failures in our studies of the brain? Maybe we make it too complicated and explain to ourselves that "the human brain is not able to understand itself"? Probably, we miss something very simple, banal and obvious. We repeat a commonplace dogma "the brain thinks" so frequently that we have no doubts about it, although we clearly understand that the speed of the information transfer in the nerve tissue cannot be compared to the speed of our thought flow. Our eyes are "glazed over" and we do not notice the things on the surface; they seem obvious and we dig into new scientific depths of theory and experiments.

We propose revising the established concept and studying the information functions of well-known neuroanatomical formations (brain meninges, CSF spaces) of the human and mammalian brain from a new angle. Namely, we plan to evaluate their functions not from the viewpoint of the neuroanatomist, morphologist or clinical neurologist, but from the position of the theoretical neurologist (similarly to that of the theoretical physicist) and the existing theory of information, as well as describing the role that these formations play in the information-commutation organization of the brain. It seems that, having no terms or definitions of the information theory, our outstanding predecessors – famous morphologists, neurophysiologists and neurologists – evaluated the main functions of "accessory" structures in human and mammalian heads (brain meninges, CSF, skull) only as mechanical (supportive and protective) or physiological (secretory, excretory, regulatory, nutritive, etc.) They could not imagine the brilliant simplicity and harmony of the information theses that are implemented in the brain by the Creator (God, Nature or Evolution – as you like it).

I propose reflecting on the long-standing classical statements about the brain that prevailed for a hundred years ever since they were claimed by the Nobel laureate Ramon y Cajal. It seems appropriate to evaluate the achievements and failures of our recent neuro-research, and to discuss certain inaccuracies in the available terms and notions in global theoretical neurology, as well as considering the methodological and technological discrepancies and errors observed in the contemporary neuroscience paradigm. This will help us to critically evaluate the results of the previous stages of research and to propose an alternative viewpoint on the information processes in the brain and develop it as a novel information-commutation theory of the brain's organization and functioning.

Therefore, we will proceed with a revision of the basic neurological dogmas about the brain.

First, the neurological dogma that the neuron is everything in the brain and, namely, the neuron is the main information-commutation unit of the brain, is, obviously, an exaggeration, and, possibly, a mistake. A neuron cannot be the main information unit as it is only a somatic cell of nerve tissue with several short branches (dendrites) and a long branch (axon). The conventional perception of the neuron as the main information workhorse of the brain seems to reflect incorrectly the essence of information relations in the brain. Apparently, a neural cell is an important morphological unit of the brain tissue, but it cannot play a key role in the information continuum of the brain processes as, until now, no convincing evidence has been received to confirm its isolated individual meaning in the global information processes of the brain. Mathematical modeling and the technical realization of the neural network that consists of neurons convincingly prove the low functional performance of a neuron in the commutation processes of the brain. A neuron and neural networks cannot stay isolated without the tissular micro-environment that conditions the communication capacities and information opportunities of the nerve tissue. We endow the tissular micro-environment of a neuron with mechanical, support and nutritive functions and do not recognize their meaning and information significance in the global commutative processes in the nerve tissue. In fact, today it is obvious that only the combinatory capacities of different cellular systems of nerve tissue (astrocytes, oligodendrocytes, microglia, synapses, vascular cells, etc.) with neurons permit adequate information transfer to the neurons. The idea can be explained as the following: the neurons without a micro-environment are an army without a rear. And the absence of support area leads to defeat.

Another aspect of neuro-research that requires revision is the available technical and technological limitations of the studies of neurons and neural networks. So, today it is technically impossible to isolate only one separate neural cell to structure all of its information levels and correlate them with its functions. This is the reason why most researchers start talking of neural networks, protein networks, genome networks of neurons, etc. In reality, it looks even more complex. We are confused by genome, proteome and neural networks and cannot see their practical realization. Neural networks in their pure form do not exist in nature; there exist specific information-commutation complexes or, to be exact, *information-commutation modules of the nerve tissue* consisting of different cell systems that form nerve tissue (various types of neurons, neuroglial cells, fibroblasts, endotheliocytes, synapses, fibers, etc.) and targetedly transferring information between different regions of the brain. Therefore, the isolation of neurons or neural networks and the evaluation of their information levels is almost impossible (and not necessary) and we must frankly admit that this method is unsubstantiated. These technical limitations of neural research are primarily associated with the technological difficulties of the analysis of a single neuron by contemporary methods of genome and post-genome tests of somatic cells, and the range of formal and quantitative limitations of existing biotechnologies in brain cell research. I would like to dwell on it in more detail to make myself clear. All available data about the information structure of a neuron were received from isolated cultures of nerve cells. To obtain such a culture of the nerve cells it is necessary to isolate neurons selectively, and then to culture them in vitro for 5-7 days. Finally, the biological structure of the resulting culture of nerve cells does not have anything in common with the structure of the nerve tissue of the brain. Another limitation of our opportunities in neuron research is embedded in the technology of genome and post-genome mapping and profiling. For the complete gene mapping and profiling of all DNAs of a nerve cell at the contemporary level of the development of sequencing and PCR diagnostics, one requires no fewer than one million neural cells of which the requisite material for analysis will be obtained. Complete transcriptome assay to study the gene expression of a nerve cell can be received only with a minimal number of nerve cells from 2 to 2.5 million in a sample. The mapping and profiling of a cell proteome can only be done using no fewer than 2 million neural cells. A standard metabolome test as the analysis of the activity of radioactive glucose of nerve cells requires tens of millions of cells of nerve tissue. To analyze their metabolism the distribution of radioactive glucose in PET is studied and technically it registers a metabolic activity of a rather large area (no less than $3mm^2$), which involves not only several million neurons but also no fewer than 10 million different cells of nerve tissue (neuroglia, vascular cells, fibroblasts, synapses, etc.). Similarly, in the study of the magnetic field of neurons in the brain MRI where the minimal size of magnetized nerve tissue makes one pixel, equaling one voxel or 3mm^2 of nerve tissue, thus consisting of several million different cells of nerve tissue. Magnetoencephalography is also unable to estimate the electromagnetic characteristics of one nerve cell; it can only localize and describe the magnetome of a tissue section of no less than 10mm^3. These rough calculations permit us to say that the information levels of contemporary research are only specific sections of nerve tissue consisting of standard cell elements. This fact should be taken into account in our information analysis of the neuro-research data.

Therefore, the research of the information relationships in the brain should deal with the information modules of nerve tissue capable of commutation networks in the brain and not with a neuron as its basic information unit or its neuron networks. The module of nerve tissue which is able to commute information is the complex of basic tissue elements: different types of neurons (motor, sensory, proprioceptive, etc.), oligodendrocytes, astrocytes, the cells of microglia, of vascular epithelium, of muscular and fibrous walls of vessels (arteries, arterioles, veins, venules, venous sinuses, etc.), axonal nervous fibers, dendrites, autonomous nervous system fibers, and synapses. It is this very module of the nerve tissue, and not one neuron, that performs the main commutative function of routing information in the nerve tissue providing the preferable direction and intensity of the transferred information. Specific modules of nerve tissue fulfill the functions of information reception, transfer and guidance. The synapses between the neurons help to develop the neural networks but in these networks not only synapses but also other auxiliary structures (cells of neuroglia, vascular endothelium and epithelium, fibroblasts of connective tissue, nervous fibers, etc.) play an extremely important role. Meanwhile, every cell of the nerve tissue module changes all of the information structure of the nerve tissue at transcriptome, proteome and metabolome levels because all have their transcriptome, proteome, metabolome, etc., which influence the communication and information components of a whole module.

Second, although the brain on the whole is a multilayer system with complex neural-glial-vascular networks, it is not technically capable of providing for the reception, processing and storage of incoming data by means of even distribution throughout the brain. Recent research did not detect centers for thinking and memory in the brain cortex, or the specific structures to realize these functions. Thinking and long-term memory cannot be implemented by the pathways of nervous impulses conduction through neuron networks of the brain, as the speed of action potential transfer along nervous fibers and the time of synaptic transmission are not able to provide for the existing operation speed of memory and thinking. Hence, the dogma that neural networks process information in the brain is erratic – just as the ubiquitous dogma of neurology that nerve cells do not restore is also erratic. To date, it has been proved that under specific conditions the nerve cells can restore and this fact is not doubted by the experts in regenerative medicine.

Third, the majority of researchers admit the holographic principle of information processing in the brain, as well as sharing the idea of Karl Pribram that the brain may be a hologram. However, so far the physical basics of the holographic identity of the interference within the framework of bioelectrical activity of the brain are not clear, just as the main substrates of hologram formation are not shown. How are the reference and object waves formed? Where does the interference of bioelectrical signals happen, and what are the splitter and reflector of these bioelectrical waves in the brain? The ideas of Karl Pribram that the brain is a lens and a hologram at the same time, and that the hypothalamus houses the memory, seem out-of-date and erratic, and they can be explained only by a lack of knowledge of informatics and 3D holography.

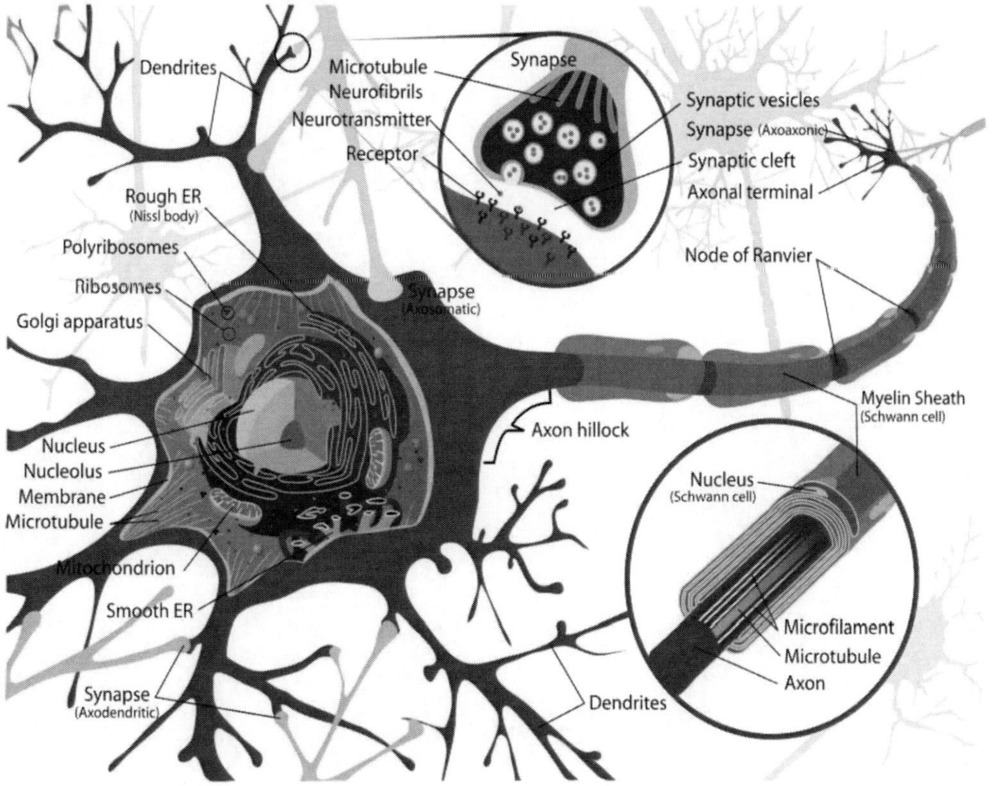

Figure 22. A biological model of a neuron as the main structural element of the brain.

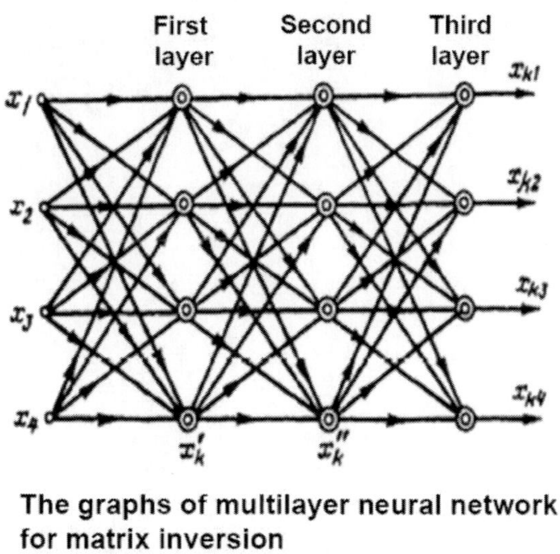

Figure 23. The first experience of solving mathematical tasks from a neural network logical basis, 1972-1974 (The model of a neuron as a biological system).

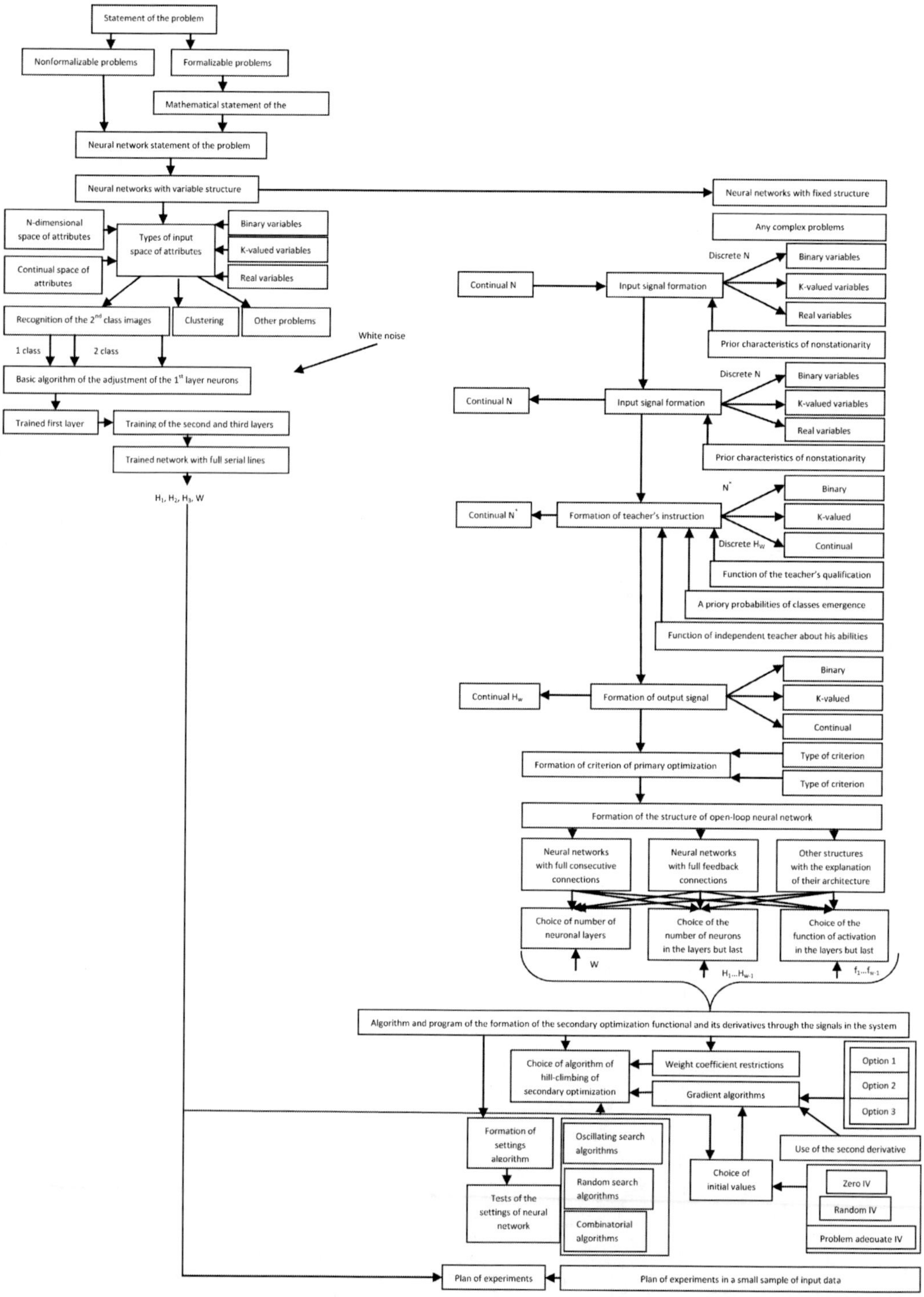

Figure 24. The structure of a general method of system problem solving in the neural network logical basis (2010-2013). The model of a neural network as the complex of cell biological systems.

Fourth, memory cannot be evenly recorded in all neural and protein networks of the brain; in this case, its rapid retrieval is problematic. The storage of information as distributed engrams inside the brain cortex requires larger biological structures than the square of 2.2m^2 (the square of the brain cortex) and three to six millimeters' thickness. In that case, the volume needed to store all of the information should be significantly different.

Fifth, the morphofunctional systems of the brain can provide the integration of different regions and brain formations (hemispheres, lobes, gyri, etc.) at the level of a whole brain. But the bioelectrical activity of the brain manifested in EEG oscillations and magnetic encephalographic activity does not reflect information processes between various brain formations and almost does not correlate with cognitive functions of the brain. They are unable to explain the mechanism of different structures of the brain by electricity. Impulse electrical current in a neuron can carry information but so far the patterns of formation of electrical commutative interrelations and self-management of the amplitudes, frequencies and voltage have not been described. This function should be fulfilled by other carriers of information.

Hence, the main revisionist scientific fact established in our theoretical investigations with the information approach methodology is the proof of the existence of the information structure of a nerve cell (neuron), and, most important, the detection of the information structure of the nerve tissue information-communicative module (NT ICM). What differentiates the information structure of the NT ICM from the biological model of a neuron used in science until now? First, the neuron as the main information foundation of the brain was perceived only as a biological cell system with a nucleus, membrane, cytoplasm, organelles and the rest in all theoretical scientific constructs in classical neurology and theoretical cybernetic research involving neuromathematics and the theory of neural networks. Therefore, the neuron as a living system is connected with other neurons by means of synapses that transfer the information in neural networks of the brain (Figure 22). At the end of the 20th century these theoretical views were taken as the basis for neuromathematics, mimicking the morphofunctional structure of the brain (Figure 23), which actually remained unchanged until now (Figure 24). Everything new that can be extracted from a biological model of a neuron lies in the expansion of the capacities, levels and layers of the neural network, which considerably limits the opportunities for calculations. On the one hand, mimicking the neural networks of the brain led to the development of extremely powerful superneurocomputers able to process huge data amounts in minimal time. On the other hand, the ideology of biological neural networks led to the methodological problems of further limitations in big data processing. In all existing mathematical models of a neuron, synapses and neural networks, the neuron and its ensembles were perceived as a biological cell system that consists of the morphological substrate that copies the shape and work of a cell and its connections. Systemic representations of a neuron as an analogue and image of a living cell, and of neural networks as the systemic structure, significantly limited understanding of the brain's operation and prevented us from understanding its information structure and identity in all scientific projects. This is the reason why, in the second decade of the 21st century, we are not able to overcome the main scientific contradictions hidden in the available paradigm of computation. This caused a global technological dead-end in the development of computer technologies and artificial intelligence systems and a global Power Wall, as mentioned previously. Obviously, the NT ICM model must rely on different methodological and biotechnological principles as an alternative to the biological principle. Only the information principle of the brain model construction will allow for overcoming the main problems of mathematical modeling of the virtual model of the brain. The experts think it necessary to change the entire paradigm of computation to find the solution to the Power Wall problem. A new paradigm can rely either on the principles of quantum mechanics, or on the neuromorphic technologies based on the algorithms of the human brain's operation, which is able to perform asynchronic and stochastic calculations and process petabites of data in milliseconds, while it is impossible for all of the computers of the world taken together.

What is specifically different between the information structure of somatic tissue and, namely, that of the nerve tissue represented as the NT ICM and the biological model of a neuron constructed by contemporary science and technology? What can be helpful in the seemingly primitive arrangements (inductome, genome, transcriptome, proteome, metabolome, secretome and magnetome) of the information levels of nerve tissue structure for the theoretical neurology, computation and development of a new generation of supercomputers? It turns out they can really help and have great potential to significantly alter our ideas about brain functioning!

To date, the concrete objective and individual digital data lie behind every information level of a somatic cell or a neuron information structure, and they characterize specific manifestations of this level that are received with the help of contemporary and super-accurate laboratory equipment for genetic research or innovative equipment based on post-genome technologies (Figure 26). And when we are able to digitalize something, it can be easily modeled. The information level of the genome can be fully digitalized by a complete genome sequencing of DNA and genome mapping of a somatic cell, and, particularly, a neuron, and detection of the sequence of nucleotides located in it and its mutations. The Global Human Genome Project made it technically possible, and to date the high research technologies and description of nucleotide sequences of the genome of mice, rats, monkeys and humans are put into practice. Currently, a complete genetic analysis of the sequencing of chromosomes of human somatic cells, including neural cells, does not take longer than a week and its price has considerably reduced.

The information level of the complete transcriptome of a nerve cell is presented as the expression profile of 25000 genes, which was received in a microarray complete transcriptome analysis of RNAs of the cell. The time needed to obtain the RNA microarray is about two days. Approximately the same time is required for the proteomic microarray. The proteome mapping and profiling of the proteins of somatic cells with mass-spectrometry take about a week or two. The data received in the proteome analysis of the protein lysates permit the complete mapping and profiling of the proteome of the studied cells and further bioinformation analysis of proteome maps permits research into the expressed proteins of the proteome and proteins of metabolism. Today the protein microassays permit the characterization of up to 9000 proteins of any somatic cell in two days. The same can be said of the proteome of a neuron. These digitalized data of normalized signal intensity of the proteins are very specific, and allow for the complete mapping of the information protein structure of all cell structures. The MRI spectroscopy characterizes the metabolome of any cell systems of nerve tissue, which can also be characterized by the positron-emission tomography of the brain. Contemporary methods of analysis of the concentrations of cytokines, neurotrophines and mediators in the tissue can characterize signal and regulatory proteins expressed by the cell or the cells of specific parts of the nerve tissue, so that we can profile their secretome. The use of a biophysical method of magnetic field registration (induction, magnetization intensity, frequency, etc.) of the cell systems, including neurons, provides the digitalized information structure of the cell magnetome. Description of electromagnetic parameters of every cell and tissue is routine for biophysicists today.

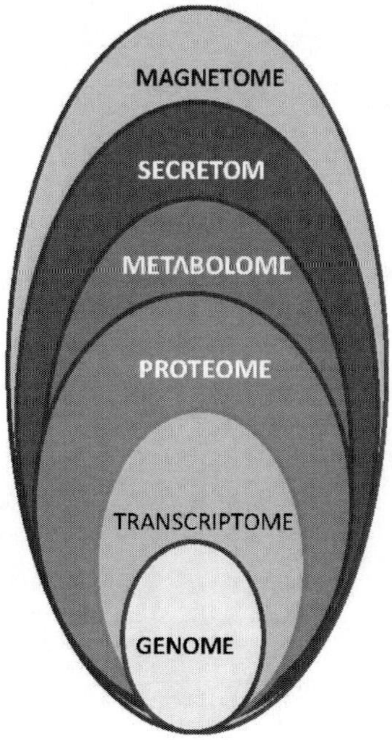

Figure 25. The method of objectification of the information levels of any somatic cell, including the neuron.

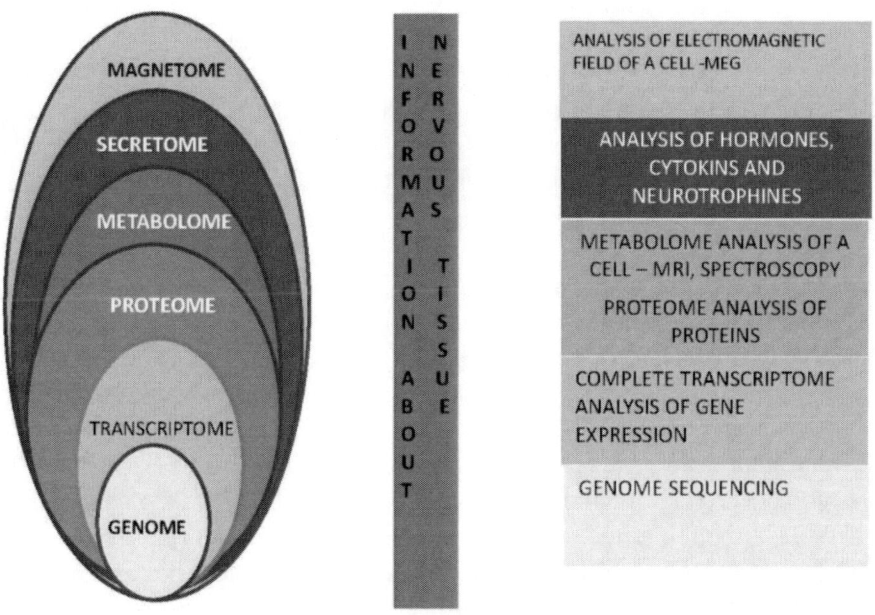

Figure 26. The method of objectification of the information levels of a somatic cell, including the neuron.

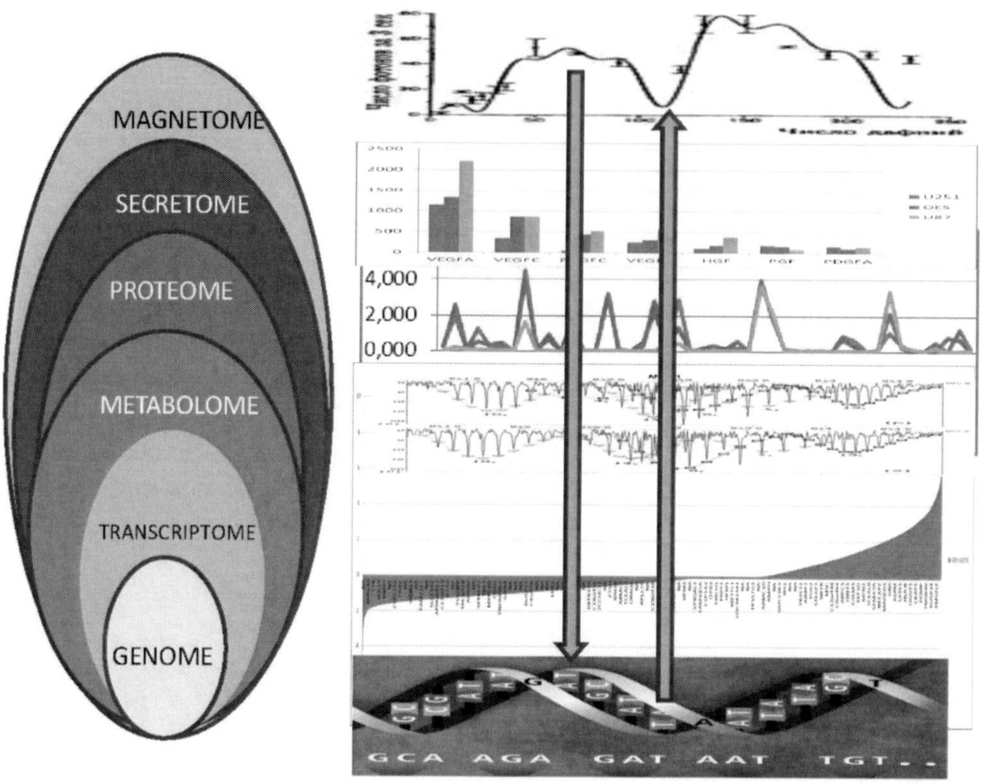

Figure 27. Multilevel mapping and profiling of information structure of a somatic cell are a reality in contemporary biotechnologies.

Therefore, the proposed information levels of the information-communication module of nerve tissue can turn from abstract and meaningless color circles nested inside each other as in Matryoshka, a Russian nesting doll (Figure 13), into a rigidly interdependent multilevel and multi-scale structured information construct in no time. Each level has a digitalized profile and a map chart of very specific information (Figure 27); it can be integrated into a mathematical database as an "information image" which is very specific, depending on the localization of the information construction of this tissue area. The interactions and interrelationship of different information levels of a cell and different information tissue structures from the abstract theoretical sphere acquire concrete digital representation in the individual 3D-maps of the objective data or digital profiles of the proteins, their precursors or metabolites, which reflect the changes of any of the information cell levels of the exact information structures of tissue samples under a targeted endogenous influence or, on the contrary, under external influence on a whole structure. Examination of the interconnected changes in the information levels within the information cell structure of nerve tissue and mathematical modeling of the information structure of a cell permit an understanding of the dynamical changes of all information structures of a living cell system at each level. Thus, we are able to understand the main laws of their existence, and tendencies and patterns of the changes, and to follow up how the influence on the magnetic field of the cell and tissue affects the genome and changes the profiles of gene expression, as well as the changes of phenotype that result from these proteome modifications. And, on the contrary, we can follow how transitory changes in the activation or inhibition of gene function alter the secretome and the magnetome of a cell. Therefore, we can understand how they modify its function and change the tissue-forming potential of a cell. Modeling the interaction and relationship inside the information structure of the studied module of the nerve tissue permits the answers to the researchers' questions without experiments with a living cell or nerve tissue in vitro, when these experiments are impossible or dangerous.

The information structure (IS) of the nerve tissue represented as the ICM differs from the IS of a nerve cell (neuron) also in the fact that it represents the integrated data of the information (inductome, genome, transcriptome, proteome, metabolome, secretome and magnetome) levels of all cells contained in the tissue and obtained from the tissue sample. The NT ICM contains the cells which are at different stages of the cell cycle, at different differentiation stages, of different phenotypes (tissue-specific, supporting, stromal connective, vascular and neurogenic) and of different functional mission. Moreover, the secretome of the information structure of the studied tissue will contain the heterogeneous range of regulatory and signal agents of various cells, and the magnetome of the studied information structure of the tissue is the integrated magnetic field that developed from the interference, overlapping and interaction of all magnetomes of the cell systems that constitute its morphological structure. For example, the information structure of a nerve tissue sample sized 1cm x 1cm from the frontal cortex of the brain will consist of the information structures of the nerve cells of all six layers of the brain cortex, neuroglial cells (oligodendrocytes, glial cells, astrocytes), vascular cells of the pia (endotheliocytes, myocytes, fibroblasts, epitheliocytes, adipocytes, etc.), synapses and formations of cell gap junctions, as well as the axons from the periphery. Undoubtedly, the research of the information structure of every living cell system is very important for bioinformation analysis, but the information structure of the tissue as a whole has decisive practical significance (Figure 28). We can refine and itemize this information deeper and more profoundly, and elaborate the information structure at the level of inductome further. For this, the level should be worked out in more detail and disaggregated to the atomic level, which we named "corpusculome", to the level of the elementary particles, which we named "quantome" and the level of the magnetic-resonance field of the cell. The last information level can be called femtomagnetome (micro is 10^{-6}, nano is 10^{-9} and femto is 10^{-14}) of a cell or tissue. Thus, the femtomagnetome is a cell magnetome with the level of induction that equals 10^{-14} Tesla. Consequently, the scale of cell and tissue magnetization, or, in other words, the scale of the induction and existing energetic transitions of cell systems lies in a rather broad range from 10^{14} Tesla to 10^{-14} Tesla.

Apparently, we would be able to describe the extended information structure of a separate cell, as well as of separate tissue or part of it (Figure 29). As seen from Figure 29, we propose the integration of three basic biophysical levels (corpusculome, quantome and femtomagnetome) of the information structure of a cell and tissue within the framework of the magnetic field level of a cell and tissue (the level of inductome) and verify it with magnetic-resonant tomography as the main biotechnology of choice. Why do we presume that magnetic-resonance imaging is able to objectively describe the atomic level, the elementary particle level and the level of the magnetic-resonance field of a cell and tissue? Remember that MRI is the method of layer-by-layer nuclear magnetic resonance imaging of a human body. Every section has its thickness. To a certain extent this method of imaging consists in the removal of everything under and above the section. The section is composed of the volume elements or voxels. The size of every voxel is $3mm^3$. A magnetic-resonant image consists of separate elements of the surface known as pixels (picture elements). The intensity of a pixel is proportional to the MR signal intensity, which consists of appropriate volume elements or voxels of the imaged object. It used to be thought that it was impossible to see an object smaller than the length of the wave used for imaging. MRI overcomes this limitation due to the imaging based on spatial variations of the phase and frequency of radio energy absorbed and issued by the imaged object. One should note the microscopic properties of the cells and tissue involved in the formation of the image. Predominantly, a human body consists of fat and water. Fat and water consist of a multitude of hydrogen atoms, so that 63% of a human body is composed of hydrogen atoms. The nucleus of the hydrogen atom emits a nuclear magnetic resonant signal. So, the MRI mostly represents a nuclear magnetic resonant signal from the nuclei of hydrogen. Every voxel of a human body image contains one or more tissues. For example, we have a voxel with one tissue. Using zoom, we can see the cells. There are molecules of water inside every cell. Every water molecule consists of one atom of oxygen and two atoms of hydrogen. If we magnify one of the hydrogen atoms, we will see a nucleus with one proton behind an electron cloud. The proton has a characteristic called spin, which can be qualified as a weak magnetic field, and it makes a nucleus emit a nuclear magnetic resonant signal. The MRI is based on the absorption and emission of energy in the range of radio frequencies of the electromagnetic spectrum, so that we can measure tissue magnetization caused by the change of spin location and the transfer of elementary particles to different levels of energy. The level of the total magnetization of tissues lets us judge the integral state of all three subjacent biophysical energetic levels of a cell and tissue (Figure 30).

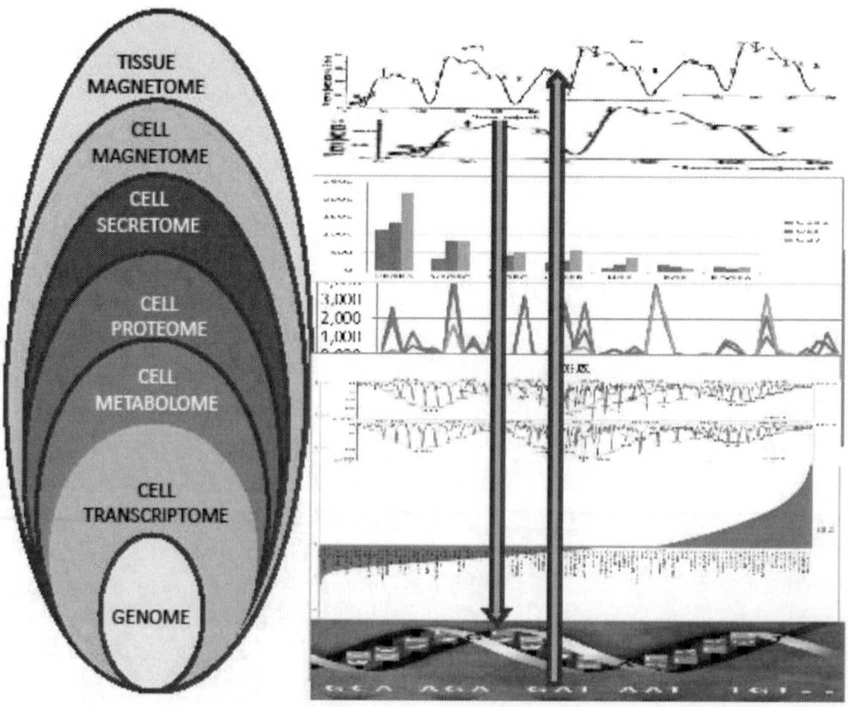

Figure 28. Multilevel mapping and profiling of the information structure of a somatic cell is the reality of contemporary biotechnologies.

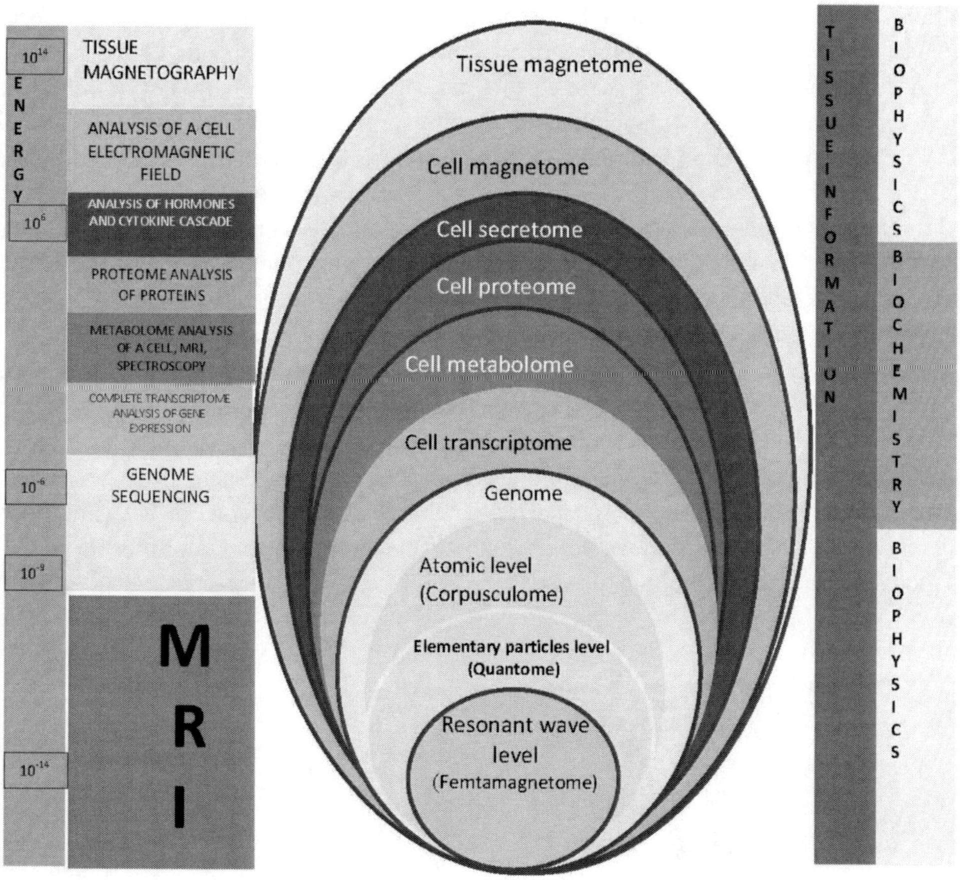

Figure 29. Complete information structure of somatic tissue and the methods of its registration.

Therefore, using MRI we can evaluate the direction and parameters of the vectors of magnetization of the hydrogen atom spins of water molecules in the imaged cells and tissues. So, the obtained maps of cells and tissue magnetization can be used as an integral parameter of cell energetic levels and substantially enrich us with new objective biophysical data, which are important for the systemic and information relationship of the studied cell or tissue structure of the human/mammalian brain. Hence, the division of the magnetic field level of a cell and tissue into atomome, quantome and femtamagnetome is important only from the standpoint of accuracy. The term that we proposed earlier, "cell inductome", satisfies our needs completely, and the possibility of its registration can be realized. In the final version the information structure of somatic tissue (including nervous) will be represented by the data of all information levels and will look as shown in Figure 31.

Hence, the model of the NT ICM proposed here is an alternative working model of the information structure of human nerve tissue, which has many advantages over a biological model of a neuron for mathematical modeling and the modeling of the neural network structure. The model permits studies of the physical laws and mathematical patterns of synchronic and interdependent change of parameters of the information levels of a human/mammalian cell and tissue in health. Using this, we can also model the detected interdependencies of dynamic changes of the parameters of the information levels depending both on the influence of the micro-environment and the environment on the cell information structure as well as on the influence of the endogenous effect on one of the levels of the information structure; for example, in the genetic engineering of cell systems or intoxication.

The opportunities for mapping and digitally registering the information structure of different areas of the brain in normal state and in various functional states (sleep, thinking, stress, etc.) permit us to develop information maps or matrices of these brain areas in health and in disease (depression, atrophic degenerative organic disorder of neurons, demyelinating diseases, etc.). To facilitate the bioinformation processing the maps/matrices of different tissue areas can be integrated within the framework of 3D models of conventional anatomical brain formations (frontal cortex, occipital lobe, cerebellum, brainstem, pons cerebelli, etc.).

The next stage of the data processing is the study of the information structures of different regions of the brain. It can be achieved if all available results of the research of the information structures of the examined brain region are united. The tool for this integration can be the mathematical modeling and development of virtual mathematical 3D models of a whole brain and their storage in specialized databases as the versions of working models of different functional states of the brain in health, as well as development of the working virtual 3D models of the human brain in disease.

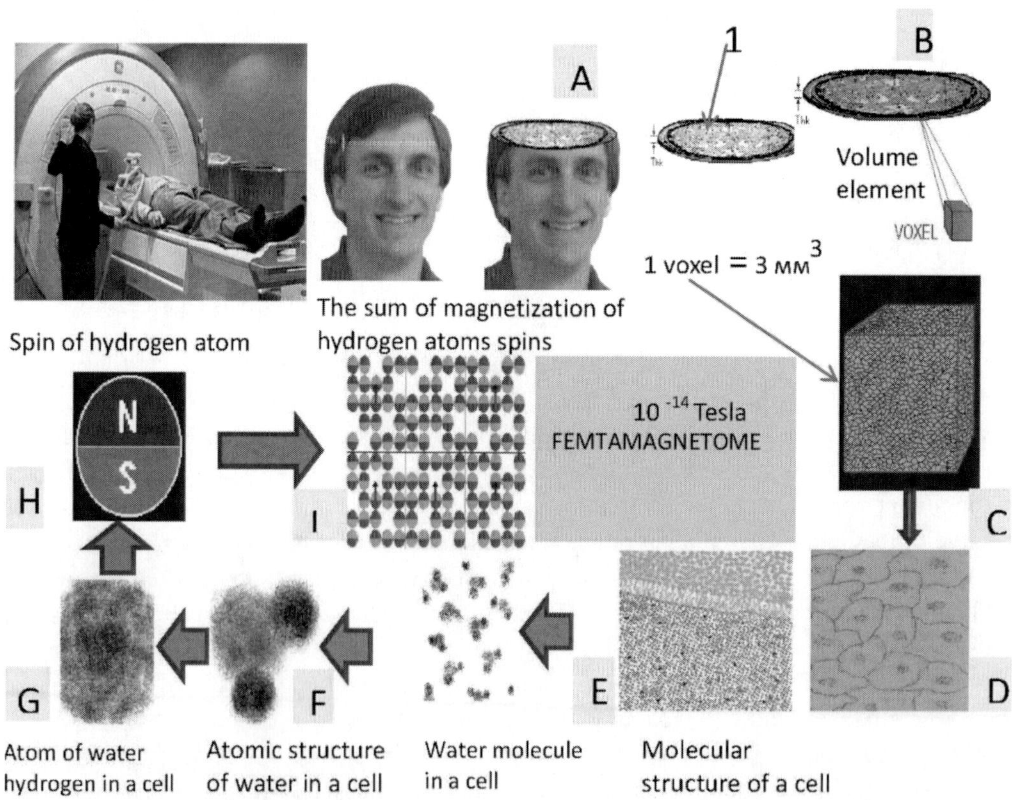

Figure 30. Brain MRI is the method used to objectify atomic structures, elementary particles and resonance wave processes in a cell and tissue and mapping femtamagnetome; that is, the magnetization of a cell or tissue (inductance at the level of 10^{-14} Tesla).

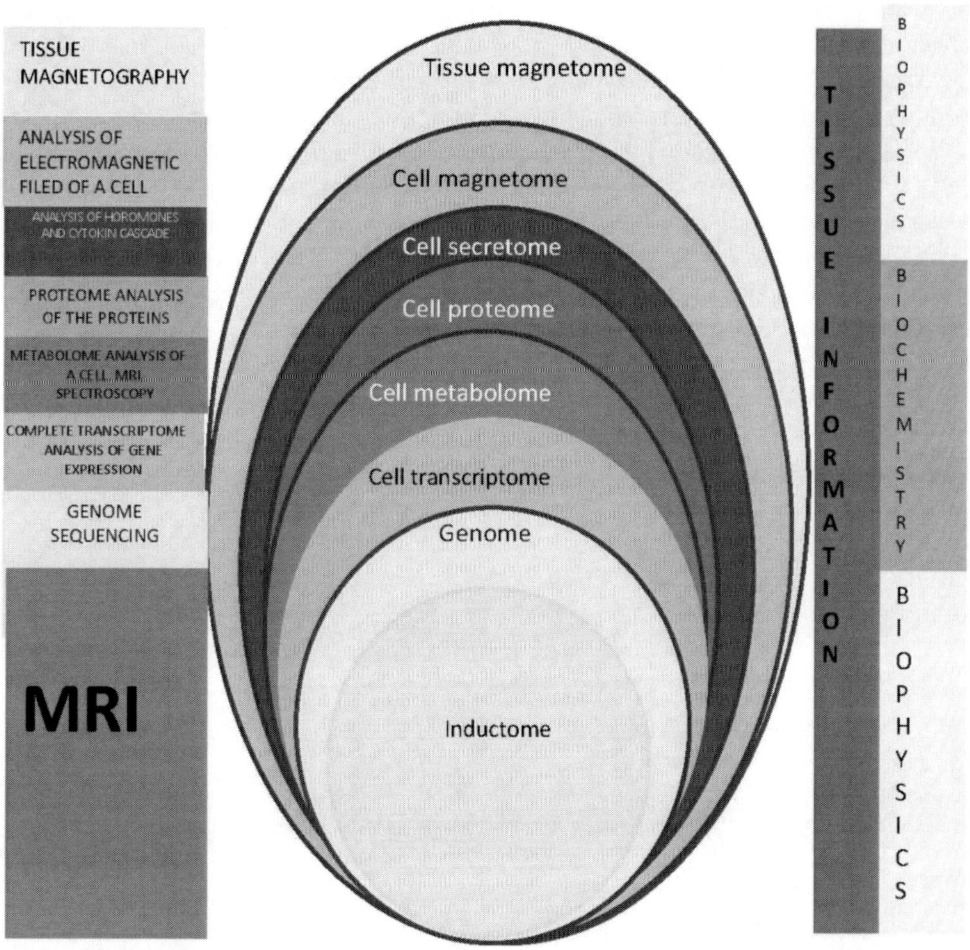

Figure 31. The scheme of the information structure of a somatic tissue and the methods of its registration

The information approach to the processing of information received from a whole brain cannot be realized only by means of neural networks connected through many meters of conducting axons and dendrites of the nerve cells; it demands rather large volumes of memory and calculating resources to process this information.

The neural networks, even if super-multilayered, are able to receive and to store a huge quantity of data biotechnologically, but other quantitative resources are required for their processing, those that exceed the biological capacities of these anatomical formations of nerve cells manifold. John von Neumann, a genius physicist and mathematician born in Hungary, calculated that in a lifetime the human brain can store up to 280 quintillion memory bits (280000000000000000000) [143]. This incredible amount does not agree with the traditional image of memory storage. Apparently, for the practical – or, to be exact, the technical – implementation of the processing, analysis and synthesis of the endogenous information which comes to the neural networks of the brain cortex (from 1.5 to 5 cm thick and consisting of 5 billion nerve cells) from the inner organs and systems, and exogenous information from the environment, the information capacity of neural networks should be expanded by one hundred thousand times. Simple arithmetic tells us that the existing number of neurons in the brain cortex cannot store these amounts of data. And, one-third of this amount is already being used in contemporary mathematical models of the brain and they are obviously insufficient for neurocomputing and processing all input information

I presume that the solution that the Creator (God, Nature, or Evolution – as you please) offered for this problem was brilliantly simple: the information processing was placed outside the neural networks of the brain. And the technical and technological implementation proposed by our Creator is simple, original and energy-saving. This solution is in the principle of holography realized in the subarachnoid and subdural spaces of the brain and not in the brain. These two spaces located above the brain in the skull of humans and mammals became that very information-cellular space that provides extraneural processing of the information based on holography.

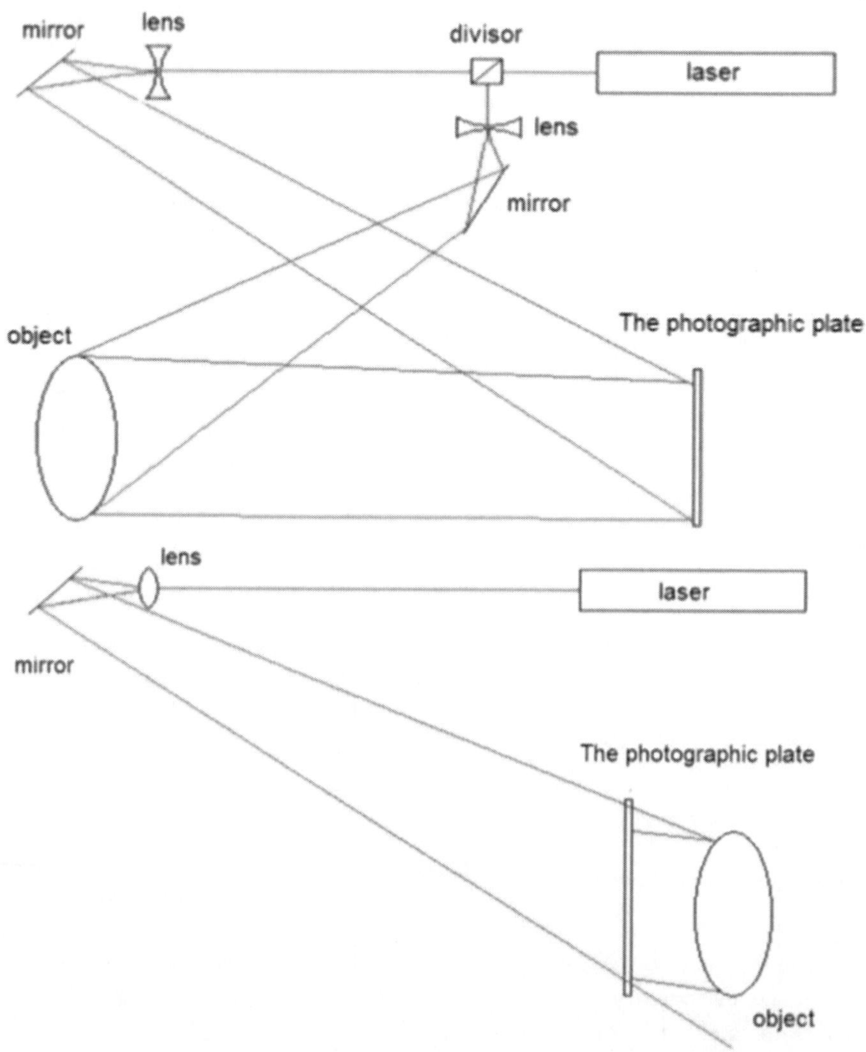

Figure 32. Holographic schemes: A. The scheme of Leith-Upatnieks; B. The scheme of Yuri Denisyuk.

Let us remind those who know, and explain to those who never knew, what holography is. Wikipedia explains the details so simply that they are clear even to non-specialists. The principle of holography relies on the fact that the electromagnetic or optic waves scattered by the object are characterized by the amplitude and the phase. To register these parameters is not hard: regular photo film registers amplitude and transforms its value into appropriate blackness of photo emulsion. The phase relationship can be registered by means of the interference, which transforms the phase relations into the corresponding amplitude. The interference develops when several electromagnetic waves with coinciding frequencies overlap in some area. When a hologram is registered two waves overlap in a certain part of the space: one is emitted directly by the source (reference wave); the other reflects from the object of the record (object or signal wave). In the same area the photo plate (or other registration medium) is placed, and, as a result, the complicated image of dark stripes appears on the plate where the dark spots correspond to the distribution of electromagnetic energy (interference picture) in the space. If this picture is lightened with the beam close to the reference wave, it transforms this beam in a beam close to the object wave. So we will see the same light as it would be reflected from the object of the record.

To model the physical principle of holography in an experiment (Figure 32), a laser beam should pass through the lens and scatter. In the way of this scattered beam the mirror is placed; the beam is reflected from it and is forwarded to the photo plate (recording medium), passing through it and lightening the object. Both beams (reference and object) get on the photo plate on one side and a transmitting hologram forms. For its restoration it requires a light source with the same wave length (Leith-Upatnieks scheme) [144]. In 1962 Yuri Denisyuk, a Russian physicist, proposed a method to record holograms in a three-dimensional medium [145]. According to this, the laser beam is expanded with the lens and directed to a photo plate by means of a mirror. Passing through it, a part of the beam lights the object. The light reflected from the object forms an object wave. The object and reference waves get on the plate from both sides (a so-called colliding beams scheme). In this scheme a reflecting hologram is registered; it cuts out a narrow part (or parts) of the constant spectrum and reflects only it (or them), functioning as a filter of the light. So the image is seen in white light (of the sun or lamp). Primarily, the hologram cuts out that wave length on which it was recorded, but while the hologram is processed and stored, the emulsion can change its thickness and the wave length changes too. It permits the record of three holograms of one object with red, blue and green laser on one plate, receiving a color hologram that is hard to distinguish from the original object.

Therefore, a general understanding of holography makes it clear that the multilevel information structures of different parts of the nerve tissue of the brain cannot be involved in the realization of holography in the brain. Anatomically, the brain regions and various intracerebral structures are separated from each other by the branchings that protrude out of the dura mater (falx cerebri, falx cerebelli, tentorium cerebelli, etc.) or separated by a CSF space (brain hemispheres). So, direct communication of the information between them is considerably limited. The only material substrate that integrates these large morphofunctional brain regions though they are different in morphology and functional meaning is pia mater. The pia ensheathes the gyri and the sulci of the brain at all sides adhering to bordering the glial membrane of the brain. The glial membrane, which consists of different types of nerve cells, separates the brain cortex from the pia and its square within the brain equals the square of the brain cortex, making 1600cm^2. It is firmly against the exterior surface of the brain and consists of loose connective tissue, pia cells, its own capillary network, sympathetic fibers, and nerve plexuses of brain arteries and terminals of III-XII pair of cerebral nerves. The pia is the main "material border" and main information substrate in the brain, where the main biochemical processes transfer into the main biophysical processes of the brain, and *vice versa*. Moreover, it is a natural intensifier and resonator of electromagnetic oscillations (magnetomes) of all information structures that come with their magnetomes to the surface of the brain. So its role in the realization of the principle of holography in the brain is obvious and well justified.

Another important feature of the constitution of a human/mammalian head, which is important for holography realization, is the arachnoid mater, which stretches over the brain gyri but does not go inside the gyri or the sulci. This membrane does not have blood vessels; it is formed by arachno-epithelial cells and clusters of collagenous fibrils, the number and thickness of which varies. Mostly, it is thin, half-transparent, smooth and glossy. It has so-called reactive structures on its surface, which are cell spots, cell hills and arachnoidal (pacchionian) granulations. The functional meaning of these formations is considered to be in securing (suspending) the brain in the skull cavity, as well as in slowing CSF outflow from the subarachnoid space in the cavities formed by these structures. Meanwhile, the arachnoid is able to function as a mirror (reflector) of electromagnetic waves (magnetome) of the information structures, and the confined spaces with slowed CSF flow in subarachnoid fissures are an ideal lens able to split electromagnetic waves emitted by the cortical NT ICM magnetomes.

If one looks attentively at the structure of cerebral meninges in Figure 33, it becomes clear that they are ideal for the realization of the principle of holography. Considering that the electromagnetic waves of somatic cells (including nervous) have a millimeter range of frequency drifts, the space between brain membranes serves as an arena for information processes in subarachnoid and subdural spaces of a human/mammalian skull.

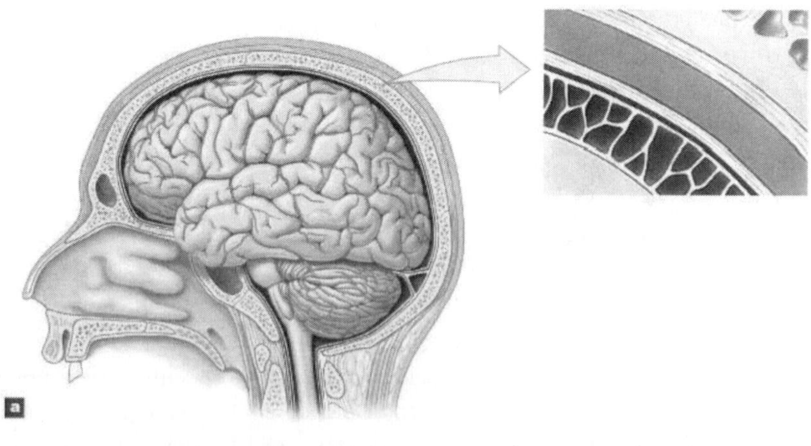

Figure 33. Meninges and cisterns of the brain (sagittal section): 1 – brain hemisphere (hemispheria cerebri); 2 - corpus callosum; 3 - corpus pineale; 4 - lam.quadrigemina; 5 – cerebellum; 6 – spinal cord medulla spinalis; 7- medulla oblongata; 8 - pons; 9 - hypophysis; 10 –chiasma opticum; A - sinus sagitalis sup.; B - cisterna corporis callosi; C - cisterna circumcruralis; D- sinus transversus; E - cisterna cerebellomedullaris; F - cisterna pontis; G - cisterna interpenduncularis; H - cisterna chiasmatis; L- cisterna terminalis (quoted by the atlas).

So, we have already noted that all neural networks of the internal and external surfaces of the brain are covered by the transparent membrane, or the pia mater, and this provides the conditions for the realization of the principle of holography for the interaction of multilevel information structures of the brain cortex. The pia mater is a unique holographic screen of the brain. On the one side it is closely adjacent to neural networks on a large surface of the brain and the information from nerve cells' networks transfers to this membrane directly in the shortest possible way. On the other side, the processed information can be easily transferred to the pia for storage, and not to the neural networks of the brain. The pia mater surprisingly fits all demands to holographic films and it is universally adjusted to receive and to yield biological information, as well as to carry it to the information field for processing and synthesis (Figure 34). It is a smooth biological membrane able to project any holographic images on itself and to function like the hard drive of a computer. As we have already mentioned, it receives and emits a huge amount of information from the neural networks of the brain. It is penetrated by large and small vessels: major arteries of the brain, arteries of average and small size and arteriolas, as well as a branched network of major veins, venous collectors in the form of sinuses and various veins and venules. Thus, it able to receive and to process the information not only from the neural network but also directly from the blood and CSF. And its proximity to the venous sinuses and CSF which flows about the pia provides unique conditions for the rapid removal of unnecessary data from the information field of the information processing and circulatory transfer of the formed holograms around the brain without energy consumption only due to the natural CSF flow. The direct contact of the pia with neural structures of the vessels opens up unlimited opportunities for the regulation of cerebral vessels and the pairs of cerebral nerves from III to XII entering the pia permit the control and regulation of all brain functions performed by these pairs of nerves.

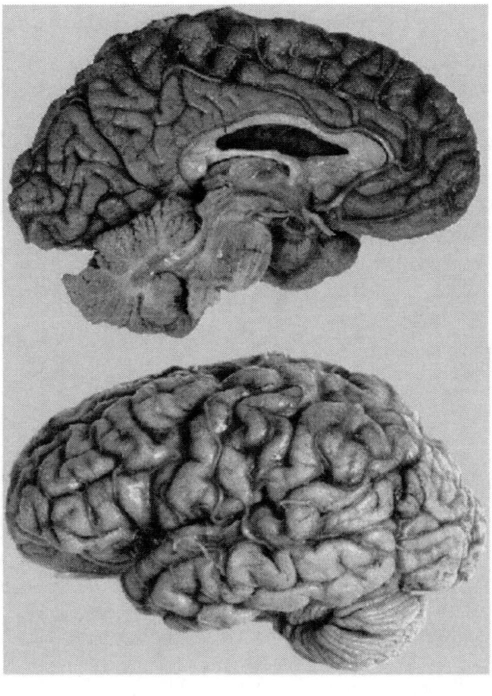

Figure 34. Appearance of the pia mater covering the brain – a universal holographic membrane.

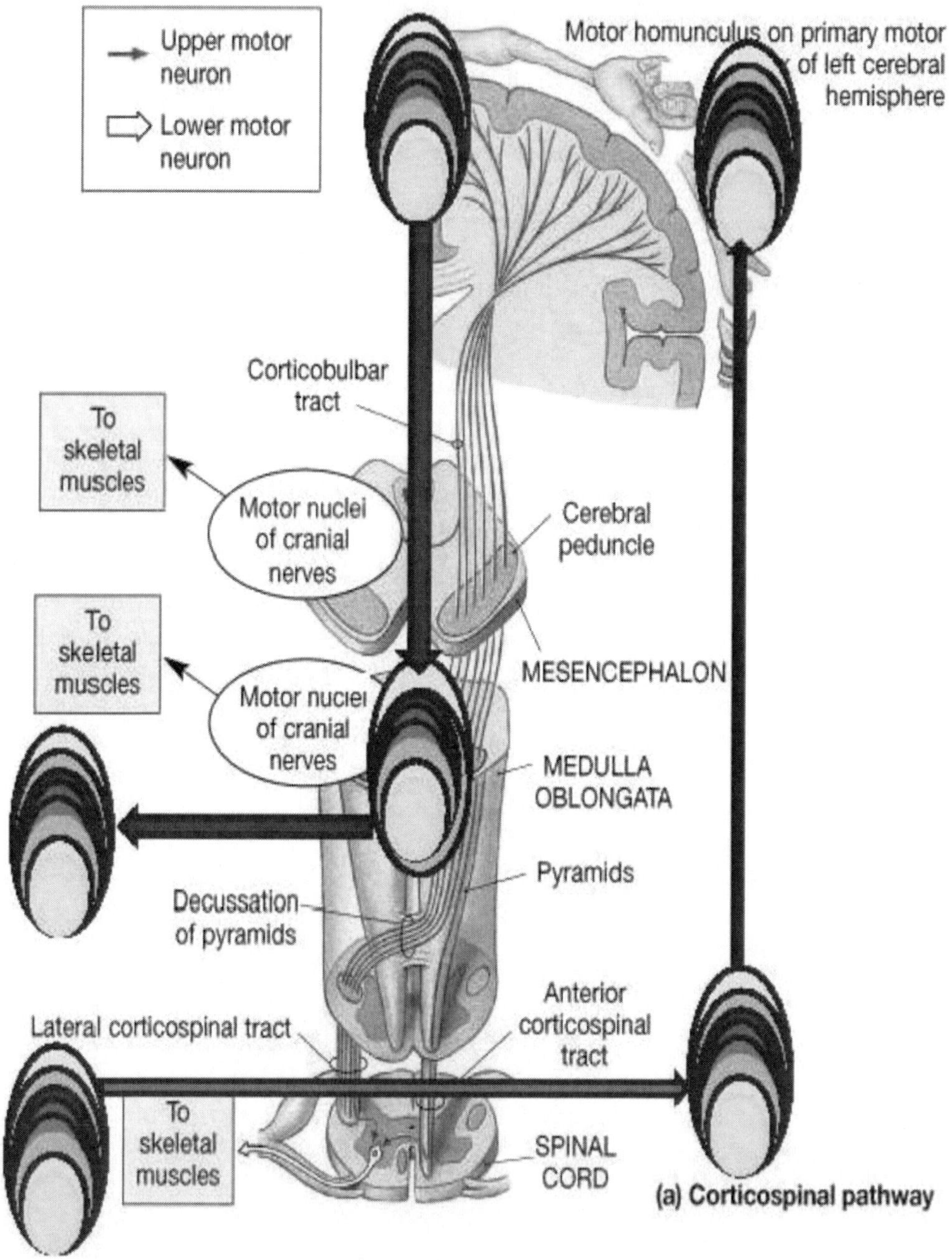

Figure 35. The scheme of information-communication modules located on an input information line (green) and output information line (red) with regard to the system of motor analyzer; 1 - Darkshevich ganglion, 2 – brain stem reticular formation, 3 - dentate nucleus, 4 - prenucleus, 5 - nucleus of dorsal columns, 6 – muscle spindles, 7 - muscle, 8 - major motor nucleus Renshaw cells, 10 - motor neuron, 11 - interneuron, 12 – gamma-motor neuron.

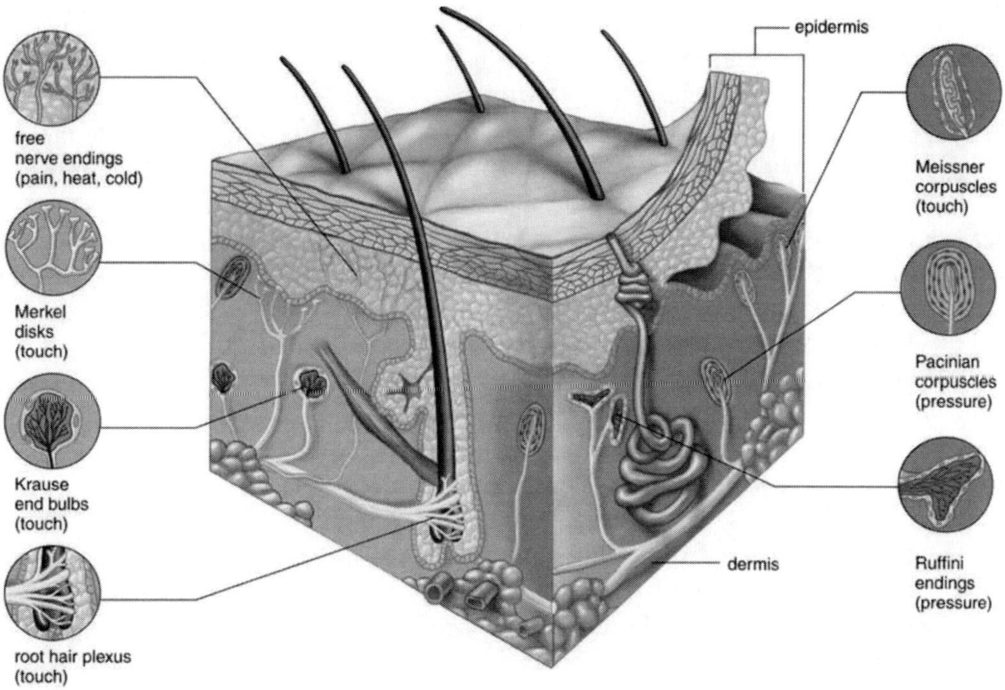

Figure 36. The receptors of different types of sensitivity of the human body.

Therefore, the pia mater of the brain is a unique anatomical substrate and the main material carrier for information recording, storage and reproduction in the human body. The fact that the data are recorded, stored and reproduced from the pia, and not from the neural networks, explains the amazing (but still unexplained by conventional theories) fact of the intact memories in patients after clinical death, when the energetic potential of the brain cortex is reset to zero, and a person, upon regaining consciousness, remembers all events that preceded the clinical death and recognizes their friends and relatives. If the memories were stored in the neural networks or "field forms", they would be completely erased in clinical death, which is characterized by the complete absence of bioelectrical activity and disintegration of the magnetic-encephalographic manifestations of the brain.

After this deviation from the main theme, we would like to discuss how the information from the regional tissue level goes to the level of the information structure of a whole brain. We have already determined that the information structures of the nerve tissue of the brain regions are separated by the branching of the dura mater and are united only by the pia and CSF washing them. Further, we discussed the organization of the brain at the level of nerve tissue, but in this section I would like to explain the formation of the field of consciousness.

The information received from the sensory receptors (Figure 35) - visual, auditory, olfactory, gustatory receptors, receptors of balance and other body systems - is sent to the communication nodes, the NT ICM receivers, consisting of the tissue of the receptors and tissue of the peripheral nervous system. Then, the information is forwarded to the NT ICM transmitters located in the vegetative ganglia, spinal cord or subcortical nodes of the brain, and then to the NT ICM subscribers, which send the information to the muscles for execution or to the information-cellular space of the brain for processing. Different NT ICM form input and output information lines of the organism (Figure 36) and provide vertical commutation of the NT ICM in the brain. The information line consists of several information channels formed by the axons and connects NT ICM in the following strict order: NT ICM receiver, NT ICM transmitter and NT ICM subscriber. Figure 36 shows the localization of the main NT ICMs on the input and output information lines of the motor analyzer. As we can see, the NT ICM subscriber of the input information line of the motor analyzer is located in the precentral gyrus of the cerebral cortex, and the NT ICM receiver of the output line of the same system is located in the post-central cortex of the brain (Figure 37). Hence, the brain cortex has a uniform monotonous structure that involves the NT ICM subscribers of the input and the NT ICM receivers of the output lines of different analyzers (visual, auditory, motor, etc.) and the brain cortex functions as a high-speed biological switch-board. Horizontal commutation of the NT ICM forms the information-commutation platforms (ICPs) of the brain: the central ICP in the brain cortex, the intermediate ICP in subcortical nodes of the brain, spinal cord, autonomous nervous system and peripheral ICPs in the organs of senses (receptor ICP) and the ICPs of neuromuscular apparatus (executive ICPs).

But the main characteristic of the human/mammalian brain is not the commutation capacities of the brain cortex but the fact that the information is processed extraneurally; that is, outside the morphological architecture of the nerve tissue of the brain. The information is processed in the subarachnoid and subdural space of the brain millimeter electromagnetic waves (EMWs) of NT ICM subscribers of different input information channels and lines interact with the brain membranes, which reflect the EMWs, so that they get to the NT ICM receivers of the same analyzer (Figure 38). This mechanism provides the commutation of the reflex activity of the specific analyzer without extra energetic expenses. The EMSs of millimeter range pass through CSF, scatter, reflect from the mirror-like surface of the arachnoid and form reference waves. The information from other information structures, when getting into the CSF, form the object waves and the waves interfere, thus forming a standard EMW hologram, which is transferred over the pia by CSF. It is then projected onto various parts of the pia and interacts with the NT ICM receivers of the output lines of different analyzers. So, the flow of CSF permits the commutation of the information in the hologram by the input and output lines of distant analyzers of other cytoarchitectonic fields. The holograms circulate around the brain in subarachnoid and subdural spaces in several cycles, so they can leave traces on a significant square of the pia, as the holographic image of an object reflects on the pia during all its route and registers on it just as it is registered on a holographic film.

That is why the pia is the main hard disk that registers all holograms with the input information. The hologram is produced immediately when the information structure of the NT ICM under the pia is activated due to the stimulation of the memory engram by the EMW of the magnetome of the NT ICM subscriber of an appropriate analyzer in the cerebral cortex or at the activation of the hologram record by the EMWs of the same phase and amplitude reflected from the brain meninges of the NT ICM subscriber of other analyzers. The principle of recording and reproducing the holographic information images in three-dimensional space is based on the previously described scheme of Yuri Denisyuk [145].

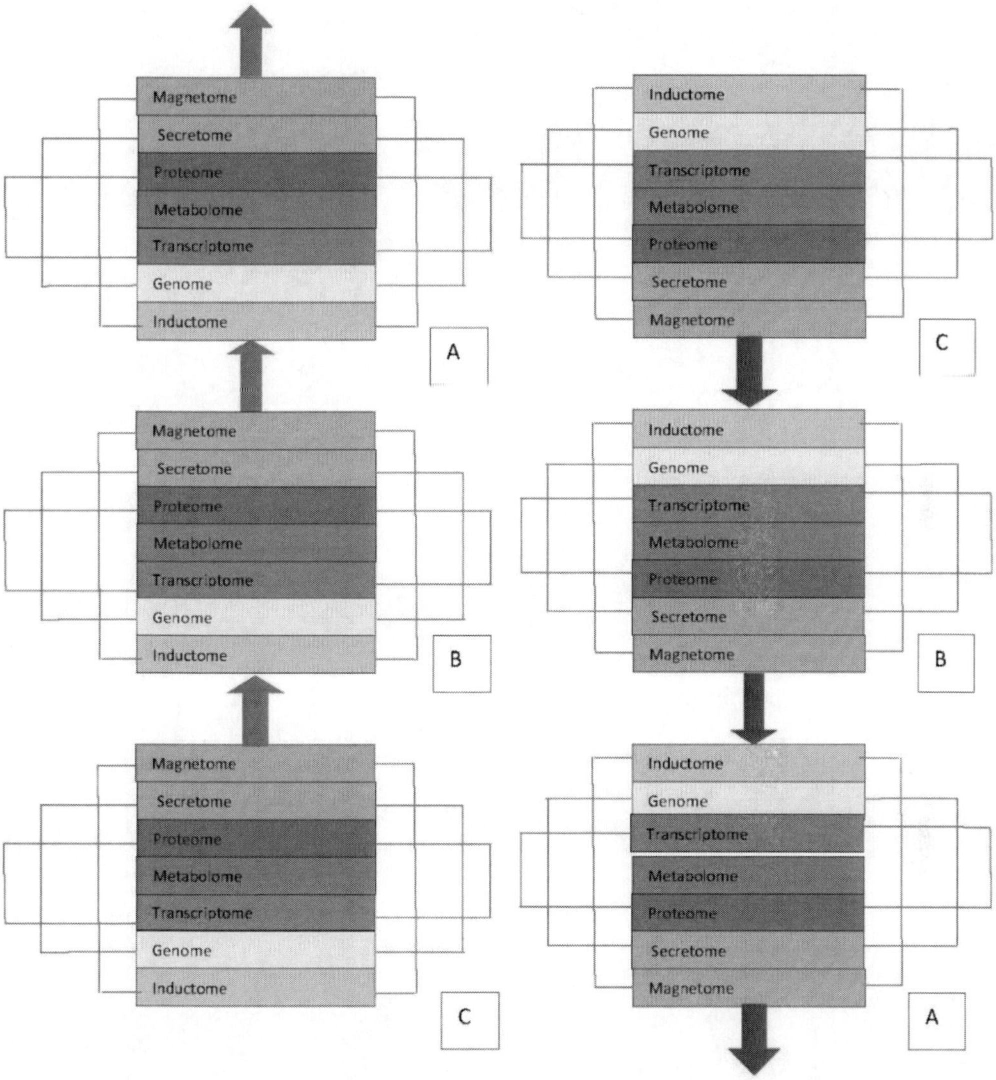

Figure 37. Input (green) and output (red) information channels (information lines) of the human and mammalian brain with information-commutation modules of neural tissue (ICMs of NT): A – ICM-subscriber, B – ICM-transmitter and C – ICM-receiver.

So, we claim that the processing of the brain's information happens outside the brain at the holographic level of the information field of consciousness and not in the neural networks of the brain. The size of the information field demands further specification. Possibly, it is limited by the subarachnoid or subdural space, or the boundaries of the information-cellular space of the consciousness extend slightly beyond the human/mammalian skull and some holograms form outside the skull in some people. The fact can be indirectly supported by the images of the "holy" people at the icons with the nimbi over the head, and the possibility of registering the EMWs of the brain with paramagnetic resonance methods of imaging when the illumination over a human head is registered, which is caused by the EMWs of super high frequencies (SHF) characterized by the wave length of millimeter range.

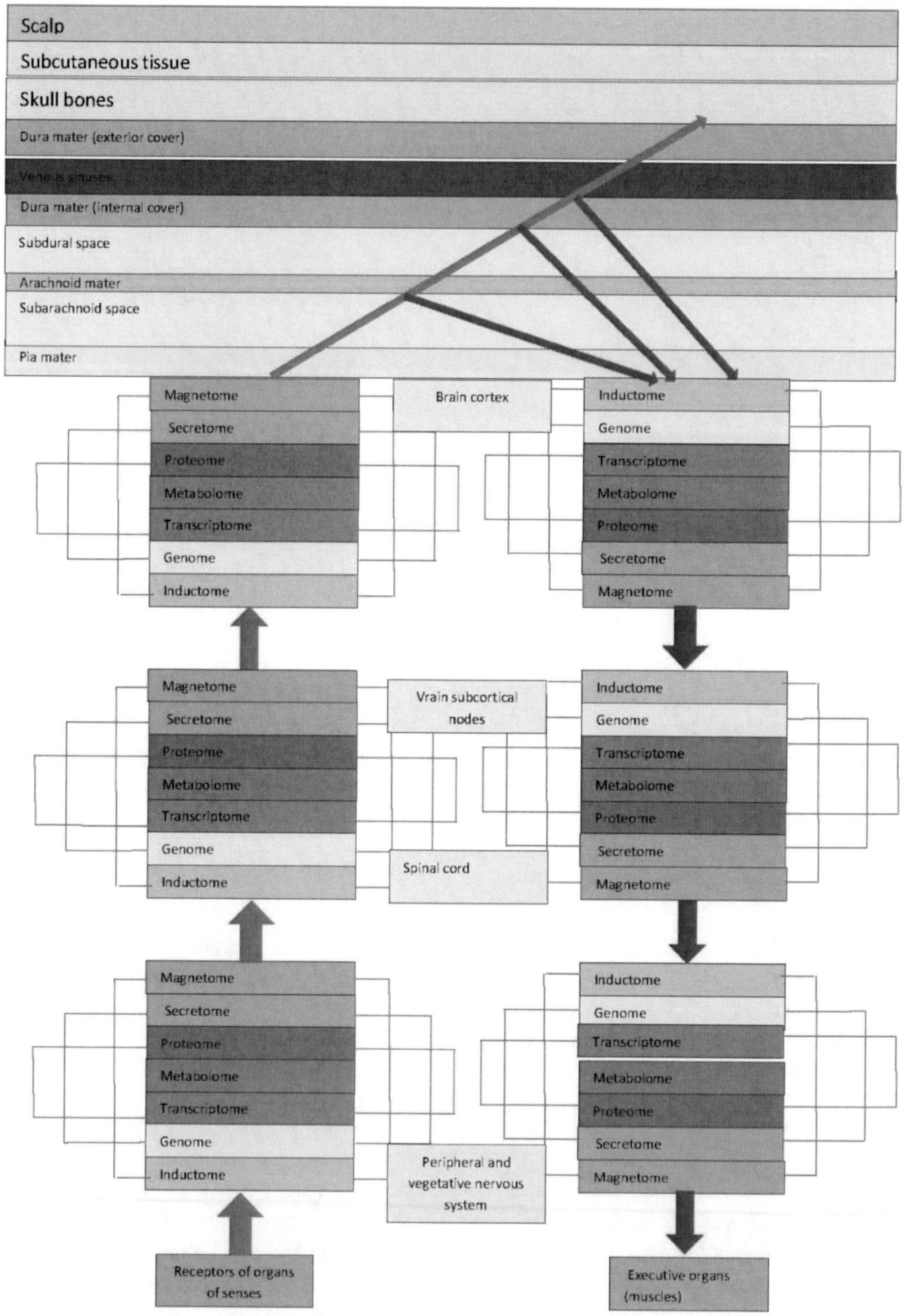

Figure 38. Extraneural mechanism of the reflex activity of the brain (for details see the text).

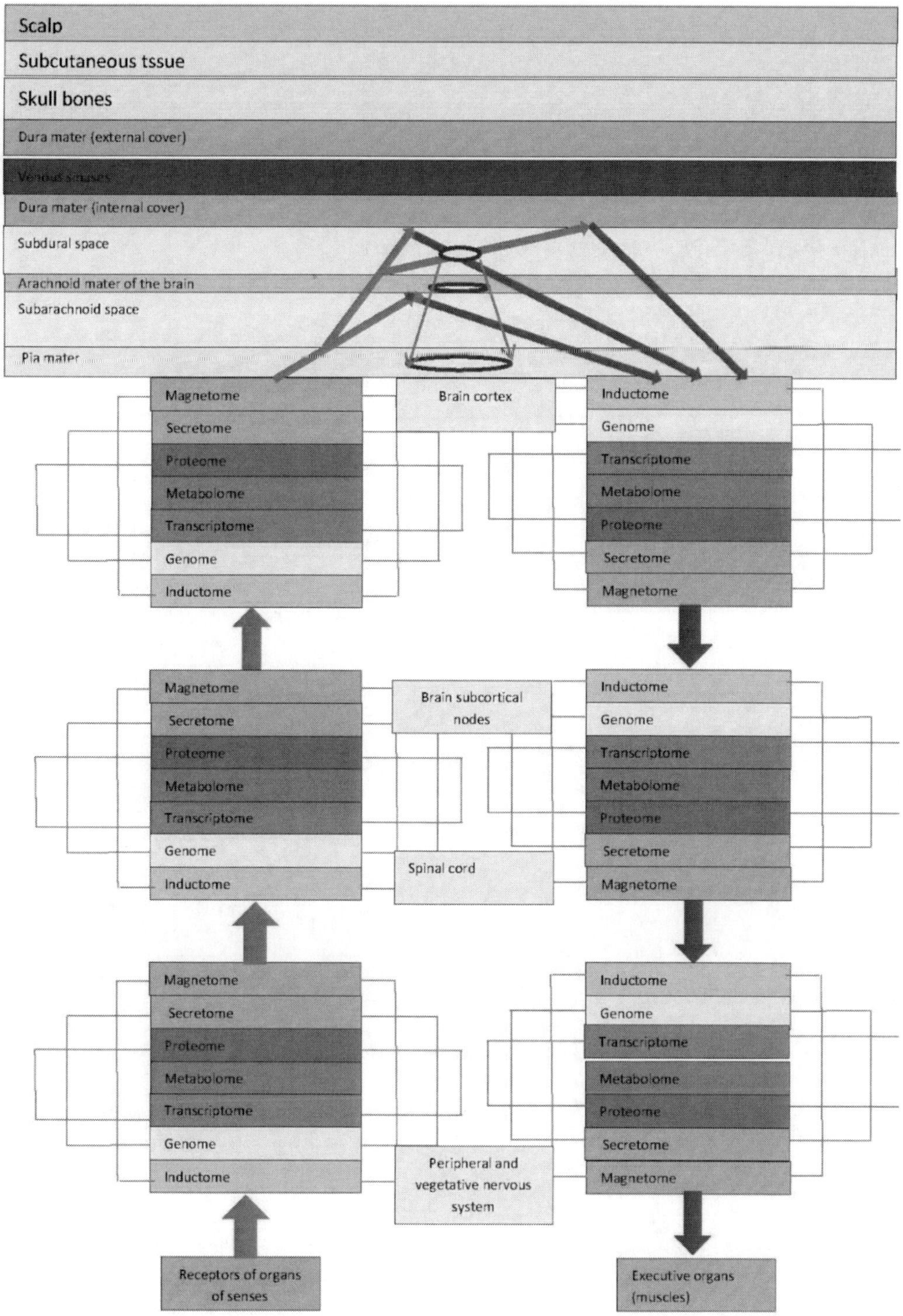

Figure 39. Extraneural mechanism of intellectual control of the reflex activity of the brain: 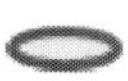 - hologram.

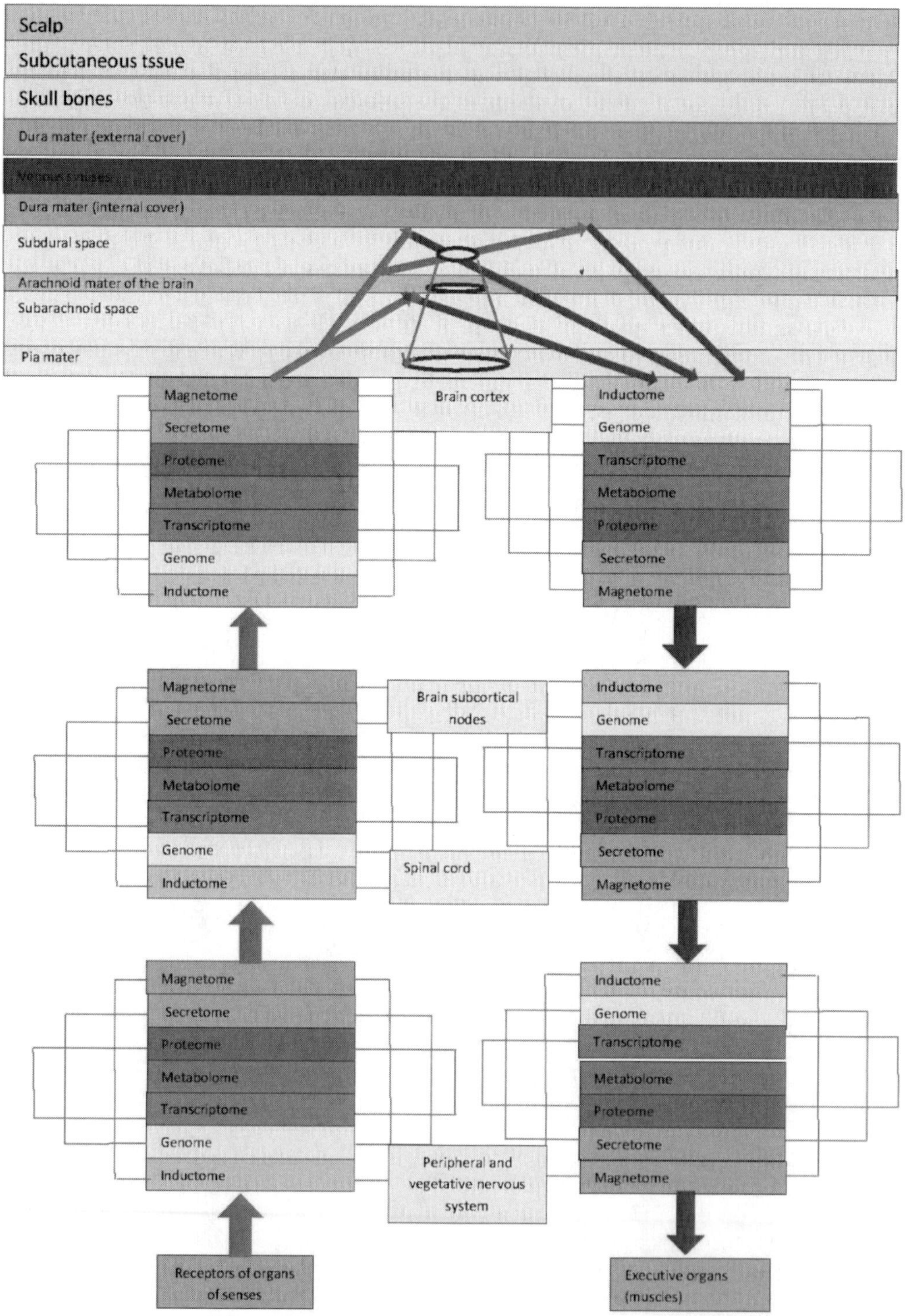

Figure 40. Formation of vertical systemic commutation connections of intraneural information-cellular space by the hologram formed in the extraneural information-cellular space.

The genius of our Creator manifested in the expansion of the information-cellular space of consciousness due to the gyri of the brain covered by the pia, which significantly increases the technological surface for the data recording (by 30%) without an increase in the number of cortical neurons and general brain substance. The holograms on the pia are recorded at different angles due to the architecture of the gyri, thus enhancing the recording capacity one hundred times. So, we come to the conclusion that the information level of complex evaluation of the information from the brain is not a cognitive level (from the viewpoint of the system approach of HBP scientists), but a holographic information level of the field of consciousness.

The holographic representations are realized through the formation of the information image matrix (IIM), which develops due to the interference of the EMWs of the magnetomes of NT ICM subscribers of the input line of various analyzers (visual, auditory, motor, etc.). The interference, diffraction and imposition of EMWs of different magnetomes of the NT ICM in the intermeningeal space of the brain represents the holographic level of consciousness, where the holographic images of reflected objective reality and projections of transcriptomes, proteomes, secretomes, metabolomes and magnetomes of the NT ICM of internal organs interfere and interact, forming the reference IIMs of the objective and subjective reality (Figure 39). Every MIO is assigned to the hologram of a real object or action in a person's lifetime. The hologram of electromagnetic radiation of the nerve tissue modules is an integral function interacting with numerous input and output information channels and lines. To illustrate it, I would represent the process as a spider crawling on the pia, the shadow of which leaves traces on its way on the pia. The body of the spider is a hologram of an integrated information image, the IIM, and its legs form the multilayered horizontal commuting bioinformation structure of the IIM and have the exact coordinates of input and output information lines of different analyzers. However, unlike the spider's eight legs, a hologram can have more support on various information lines and channels of the cortical switchboard of the brain. In other words, the interaction of information systems at the level of the magnetomes of these systems leads to their interaction at the level of all multilevel relations and provides horizontal commutation of information from different brain areas. A formed hologram of the IIM has its own coordinates at all information levels (at the level of inductome, genome, transcriptome, proteome, etc.) involved in the construction of its information structures of the various parts of nerve tissue from different brain regions. Possibly, the IIMs are those very engrams of the brain mentioned by Anokhin, Sudakov and some of the European scientists in the '80s. The holograms synchronize and coordinate the necessary level of changes of the DNA profile, transcriptome profile or proteome profile (Figure 40). The formation of the IIM holograms and their fixation and reproduction on the pia is the main system-forming start of the work of a whole brain (Figure 41).

Human speech helps linguistically (with words and phrases) to denote the main dominating IIMs of the environment and the sense of self and to compare new IIMs that were developed due to life activity and under the effect of the environmental factors with the existing set of holographic IIMs registered in the memory of the pia as the activated engrams of excited neurons in certain zones of neural networks. The set of standard IIMs of physiological standard and social well-being forms in humans from the age of seven to ten years and is registered at all levels of the distributed information of the parts of the nerve tissue of the brains of humans/mammals. That is, the memories of the IIMs received in childhood are registered at the genome, transcriptome, proteome, metabolome and magnetome levels of a cell and nerve tissue and distributed through different parts of the brain tissue. The topical distribution of the information in the tissue of different brain regions and its localization at different levels of the information structure of nerve tissue permit the storage and reproduction of numerous IIMS at different levels of neural networks of the brain. During a lifetime, when the holographic IIMs obtain their linguistic and semantic meaning, the inborn mechanisms of the IIMs recognition are engaged, as well as their arrangement and ranking in our hard drive with the acquired information. The ability of the arachnoid to establish the algorithms for the activation of specific sets of holograms on its surface led to the formation of the notions and relationship between them, providing the basis for consciousness. Consciousness can be viewed as a self-developing *sense model* of the surrounding world, having a material substrate on the arachnoid. The sense is not the information. *The information exists only on the material carrier and this carrier is the arachnoid.* The human consciousness is considered immaterial but, as we can see, it has material carriers: holograms, the pia and the arachnoid. Algorithms of the IIM holograms' management determine our consciousness. Sense exists in the human consciousness in the form of words, images, feelings or in other information terms, in the algorithms of holograms. A person pronounces words not only aloud, but also silently. Also, silently, we can remember or create images and feelings. However, we can restore the information corresponding to the sense by pronouncing the words or writing them. Speech permits humans' development of the amazing system of holographic matrices for recognition of the information images and their operation in the information field of consciousness located in the intermeningeal space of the brain. One of the most important characteristics of the speech is its denotation of objects. No less important is the denotation of the relations between the objects; in other words, the objective personification of these relations, abstractions that cannot be pointed at or mimicked. To denote this characteristic, it seems appropriate to use the psychological term *objectification*. Objectifying abstract notions, speech creates the artificial objects presented as words to enrich and develop personal communication [146, 147]. In our brains we form a set of very specific holographic engrams, recorded on the pia of the brain, and are able to activate these engrams by activation of the cortex. And the arachnoid permits manipulations by these holographic images at the level of ready algorithms. In its turn, this is a potent incentive to develop the framework of concepts of the psyche and, primarily, the long-term memory, intellect and speech. Consequently, positive feedback forms and leads to the intensive development of all cognitive processes with certain program sets of holographic carriers, which can be activated both from the brain and indirectly as a reflection of the information processes in the organism or environment.

So, the level of the field of consciousness is the holographic information level; that is, the higher information level of the information processing in the brain by means of manipulation of the already commuted holographic IIMs. The holographic IIMs can be further manipulated on the basis of the mathematical theories of commutations, machines, image recognition and many other contemporary theoretical approaches of mathematics and cybernetics.

The main scientific fact and fundamental basis of our theoretical study lies in the interaction of all information structures of the brain tissues and the information structures of other solid organs at the level of their magnetomes of information structures according to the holographic principle. The formed hologram integrates the specific subpopulation of the information structure of the brain and other organs of the human body and is the main regulator of their information exchange, interinfluence and interaction. The formation of a specific hologram of the IIM provides cognitive functions (thinking, learning, etc.) in the brain. Moreover, the thought becomes material as it has its own IIM, which is formed by the specific set of information structures and organs of the human/mammal body. Thus, the mechanisms of the therapy with words and psychotherapy become clear. In other mammals, the IIMs also form as exact holograms integrating the activity of multilevel information structures and are associated with certain emotions, shouting, type of barking, wailing, etc.

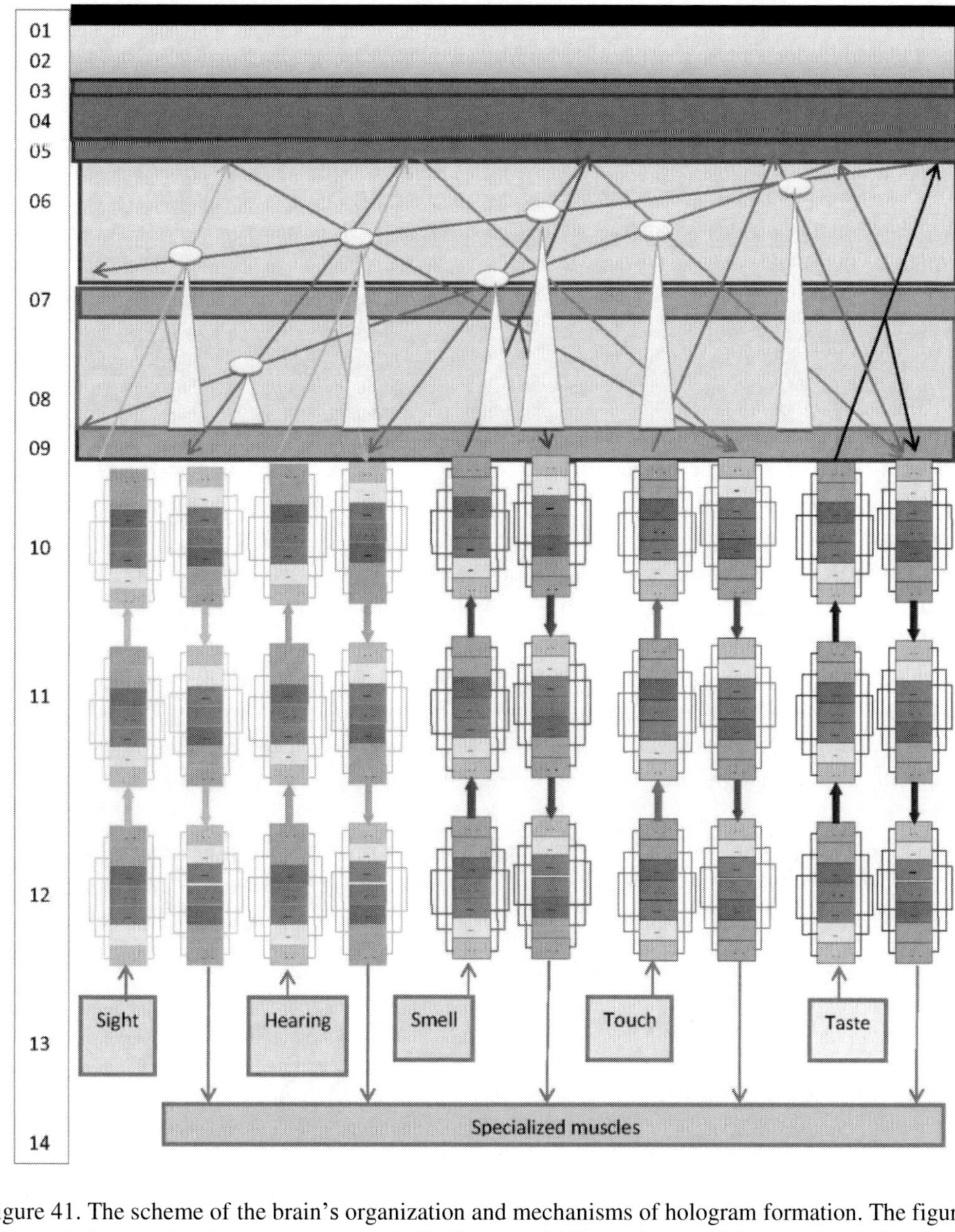

Figure 41. The scheme of the brain's organization and mechanisms of hologram formation. The figures denote: 1. Scalp and subcutaneous tissue; 2. Skull bones, 3. External layer of dura mater, 4. Venous sinus, 5. Internal layer of dura mater, 6. Subdural space, 7. Arachnoid mater, 8. Subarachnoid space, 9. Pia mater, 10. Cerebral cortex, 11. Subcortical nodes of brain and spinal cord, 12. Peripheral and vegetative nervous system, 13. Sense organs, 14. Executive organs.

Our supposition that the pia of the brain functions as the display of a human/mammal biocomputer and simultaneously as the hard drive for the storage of huge volumes of data explains the available evidence of the brain's functioning. Let us remember the works of the pioneer of the holographic theory of the brain, Karl Pribram, who, due to his studies of the memory mechanisms in rats, came to the conclusion that the memory was concentrated in the hippocampus and that its teta rhythm controlled memory processes. As we have already discussed, Pribram removed different parts of the rats' brains and showed that their memory was not damaged. But for the dropout of some motor functions, the operated rats demonstrated intact memories in the labyrinth tests. Obviously, the hippocampus is not able to regulate or control the memory processes as it does not have the biological resources to store it. Meanwhile, a minimal part of the preserved pia on the retained regions of the brain is able to reproduce it completely according to the principle of holography.

From this standpoint, it becomes clear why, after surgical removal or severe traumatic injury of the major part of hemispheres, a human still demonstrates correct behavior, remembers their friends and relatives and the circumstances of injury. The holographic principle of the reproduction of the information that was previously recorded on the pia permits the usage of the major part of the memory for life and self-service, even if the minimal part of the pia is left, and almost 90% of the cortex and white matter are injured or removed.

The proposed organization and information-commutation principle of the brain's functioning gives a sensible explanation for the significant mnestic defects in a slight injury of the brain with the manifestations of cerebral arachnoidites or even minor cicatrical degeneration of the pia in X-ray. Also, the development of global amnesia in transitory ischemic attack or vascular cerebral crisis can be explained by the angiospasm, angiospastic and angioparalytic condition of the arterioles of the pia, which lead to disorders in the recording and reproduction of the IIMs because of the pia's disrupted tension and its slackness, caused by angioparalysis. Memory disorders in the initial manifestations of the cerebral sclerosis of the brain cortex, in clonidine intoxication and senile atrophy of the brain are associated with changes in the shape, structure and surface of the pia, interfering with the process of image recognition and their reproduction. We will dwell on it in detail in Chapter 8.

As a result of our studies in theoretical neurology, we formulated an *alternative information-communication paradigm of the setup of the brain and its principles of functioning.*

INFORMATION-COMMUNICATION ARCHITECTURE OF THE SETUP OF THE BRAIN

1. The human/mammal brain is a life-time, multilevel module information-commutation structure programmed in the upbringing and education, with an open type of communication architecture that fulfills the functions of receiving, transmitting and routing information through the nerve tissue. The brain is a universal switchboard of the information received from the external world and internal organisms and systems of the body. All information processes of

management, processing (calculations, synthesis, analysis) and storage happen extraneurally (outside the brain's nerve tissue) in the intermeningeal CSF space around the brain located between the pia, the arachnoid and the dura mater.

The system-forming, transporting and communicative fundamentals of the communication architecture of the brain's informational organization are the information-communication modules (ICMs) of the nerve tissue (NT), which are the interim basic bioinformation stations of the brain that receive, transmit, modulate and route the information in the brain, and morphologically represent the complex of the main NT elements: neurons (motor, sensory, proprioceptive, etc.), oligodendrocytes, astrocytes, microglia cells, vascular epithelium cells, cells of muscle tissue and brain vessels, synapses, nervous fibers, ganglias, etc. The NT ICMs (rather than separate neurons or neural networks, as was previously thought) fulfill the main commutative function of routing information in the NT, providing the necessary direction and regulating the characteristics of the transmitted information. The main function of the brain's neurons is their network commutation to form nervous fibers of conducting pathways, to connect different ICMs and for them to interact, as well as providing targeted inter-modular transfer of the information.

2. Every NT ICM of the brain has a tissue-specific information-cellular structure that consists of interdependent and interregulated information levels: the level of inductome (magnetic field level), genome level, transcriptome, proteome, metabolome, secretome levels and the level of cell magnetome (magnetic-wave level). Every cell system involved in the NT ICM occupies its information sector and has information levels which are analogous to the modules which, on the one hand influence general communicativity and condition information characteristics and the information constituent of the module. On the other hand, it is affected by the NT ICM in a regulatory and controlling fashion. The tissue-organizing factor of the NT ICM is the level of tissue magnetome that unites magnetic-wave levels of all information sectors of cell systems that are the constituent parts of the NT ICM. The tissue magnetome of the NT ICM forms due to the composition, imposition, diffraction, interference and integration of cell electromagnetic waves of super-high frequency range. The EMWs of tissue magnetome are manifested in the millimeter range of extremely high frequencies (EHF) and form the main controlling unit to route the information.
3. All NT ICMs are subdivided into NT ICM receivers, NT ICM transmitters and NT ICM subscribers, depending on their localization in the 3D space of the human/mammalian brain and depending on their functional destination and their role in the information transfer. In different combinations they form input and output information channels of data, which form the fibers of NT and appropriate input and output information lines.
4. The central NT ICM subscribers of the input information lines and the NT ICM receivers of the output information lines form the brain cortex, where they are located in maximal proximity to each other to facilitate the functional interaction of the signals of one functional analyzer. In some cases, the commutation between the input-output information lines can be established by synaptic contacts between their sectors of neural cell components, but mostly the commutation of horizontal information of cortical NT ICM happens outside the parenchyma of the brain NT,

extraneurally, in subarachnoid and subdural spaces. The biological substrate of the brain, which permits extraneural integration of reflectory and cognitive information via the central NT ICMs, is the part of the brain cortex united by one function as cytoarchitectonic fields of the cortex of neighboring brain gyri.

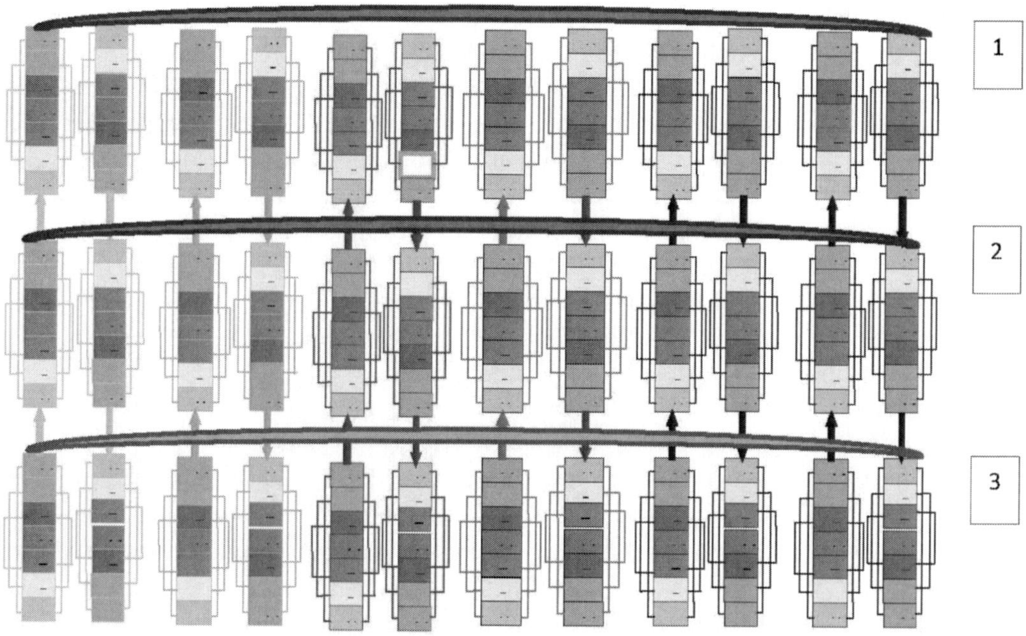

Figure 42. Information-commutation platforms (ICP) of the brain: 1 – central switchboard ICP; 2 – intermediate routing ICP; 3 – peripheral (registration and executive) ICP.

5. The cortex of the brain and cerebellum, which consists of a set of homogeneous NT ICM subscribers of the input information channels and the NT ICM receivers of the output information channels that are equally distributed throughout the brain gyri, represents the *central information-commutation platform* of the brain, which is the control center that coordinates the input and output information that comes from the subarachnoid and subdural spaces of the brain. Biologically active parts of NT in the area of the subcortical nodes of the brain, spinal cord and vegetative ganglias of autonomous nervous system form the *intermediate information-commutation platform* consisting of the combination of NT ICM receivers both of the input and output information channels and lines. It functions as the main switchboard for routing the information. The neuroreceptors of the brain (visual, auditory, sensory, etc.) are the *peripheral registration information-commutation platform* consisting of the NT ICM receptors of input information channels (lines) of the appropriate analyzers. The sympathetic and parasympathetic nervous system forms a *peripheral executive information-communicative platform* consisting of the NT ICM subscribers of the output information channels (lines) connected with the nerve-muscular segment of the locomotor system of a human and provides execution of the motor functions of the brain (speech, singing, walking, running, etc.). Central, intermediate

and peripheral ICPs function as the controllers of corresponding local areas of the brain, establishing the hierarchy of vertical control from the center to the periphery of the brain NT.

6. The general architecture of the brain's information structure is represented by intraneural (inside nerve tissue) ICPs, consisting of the information-communicative modules (ICMs) of NT formed from the information sectors (IS) of the cell systems which are part of these modules, as well as extraneural (outside of nerve tissue) holographic information (reflex and cognitive) registers (HIR), each of which have systemic vertical and complex horizontal commutation. In the systemic vertical commutation of the information at the level of the ICP, the brain works as a telephone switchboard and a router of the information along the NT ICM output and input information channels and lines. Vertical system commutation and information transfer inside the NT ICM always happens in the unvarying direction of inter-level interaction: from inductome to genome, transcriptome, proteome, metabolome, secretome, cell magnetome and the tissue magnetome and no other way. It provides the strict systemic directionality of vertical commutation of the information along the information channels and information lines only upwards or downwards. The horizontal complex commutation of the information at different levels of the NT ICM of the brain can be performed reciprocally at the level of the brain ICPs by the synapses between nerve cells forming special layers of neural networks and transferring information through intercellular gap junctions. The horizontal complex commutation of the information at the level of every NT ICM is performed largely at the biochemical level by the interaction of the cell secretomes of its structure. Spatial horizontal commutation at the level of extraneural HIRs is achieved due to the formation of holographic carriers of information in the form of holograms, and vertical commutation is provided due to the connection of reflected EMWs or EMWs that come through the holograms with the input information lines of different analyzers (motor, visual, auditory, sensory, etc.). The hologram formation is the fundamental biophysical mechanism of horizontal complex commutation of the extraneural registers and it provides the transfer of the information at large distances and connection of the regions of the brain due to holograms transferred with natural CSF flow without energetic expenses of the body.
7. The main neurodynamic processes of commutation and information routing in the extraneural HIRs of the brain happen at the holographic level in CSF over the surface of the brain in subarachnoid and subdural spaces. The unit of the information relations in extraneural registers is electromagnetic holograms of the IIMs formed by the interference, diffraction and composition of the scattered EMWs of cortical NT ICMs, input and reflected signals of the information lines of different analyzers.
8. The information in the intraneural ICP (inside NT ICM and between the levels of NT ICM) and extraneural registers of the brain cannot be transferred independently without the information carrier. Any information received by the brain from peripheral receptors does not disappear or interrupt. It circulates uninterruptable around the brain and is registered on the main cerebral (genome, proteome, transcriptome, etc.) and extracerebral (holograms, the pia and the arachnoid) material carriers of information automatically and in a distributed manner. In the uninjured pia and arachnoid mater in a healthy brain the information is recorded on these

information carriers automatically and is stored there almost forever (throughout the lifetime of a human or mammal) and can be reproduced when necessary to the appropriate extent.

9. The information in the brain is biochemically or biophysically transformed and modified at every information level and is packed in specific "transport containers" for its transfer by the information carrier specific for this level. At the level of inductome that includes resonance wave processes, the movement of elementary particles and atoms, the information carrier is the electromagnetic field of femta-frequencies (10^{-14}) range. At the level of genome the information carrier is DNA; at the transcriptome level the carrier is RNA. The information is carried by the proteins at the proteome and secretome levels, and by the proteins along with the fats and carbohydrates at the metabolome level. The electromagnetic waves of millimeter range become the carriers of the information at the level of the cell magnetome. While the information carriers at the level of neurons of the nerve tissue are EMWs of hertz range and the information is carried by the packages of impulse currents through the axon bodies.
10. The holograms' EMWs are the carriers of information at the level of extraneural registers. The ENWs leave the NT ICM subscribers and appear in the CSF intermeningeal space of the brain, where, due to composition, subtraction, diffraction and interference, they form new extraneural carriers of information in the form of EMW holograms, at which point they change their frequency-wave and amplitude characteristics. Due to the EMW interference, their reflection from the brain meninges and diffusion in the CSF in the subarachnoid and subarachnoid space, the transitory commutation information HIRs, represented as a set of universal holographic carriers of information, form around the brain. These sets of universal holographic carriers integrate specific regions of the brain NT ICMs located even at a large distance from each other, with the EMWs passing through them in different combinations, and thus, provide extraneural (outside the brain) three-dimensional spatial commutation of different parts of a whole brain.
11. Extraneural HIRs of the brain are formed between the meninges (pia, arachnoid and dura) in the areas where the information incoming to the brain is processed. Processing happens on the basis of the holographic principle and almost without energetic expenses of the brain spent on synthesis, analysis and calculations. The holographic principle in the information processing in subarachnoid and subdural spaces is realized due to extraneural anatomical formations of the brain: CSF, which fills intermeningeal spaces above the brain and fulfills the role of scattering lens for EMWs, splitting them into the object and reference beams; and the dura mater and the arachnoid mater, functioning as the reflectors of EMWs.
12. The arachnoid mater plays the role of a system administrator, a system disc and software for reflex activity in the extraneural HIR of reflex subscribers of the brain, as well as storage of all brain software that records the sequences of all algorithms, completed programs and system manipulations with IIMs. The mechanism of forming the system software algorithms is established by projecting the EMW holograms on the pia; they carry integrated electrostatic charges (ESCs), which leave traces on the arachnoid passing through it; the traces are the pia engrams transported

by holograms. The dura plays the role of the register of cognitive subscribers by reflecting the EMWs and comparing them with the data registered on the pia.

13. The role of the hard drive disc is played by the pia mater of the brain. On the one hand, the pia is a unique holographic membrane which covers the whole cortex of the brain, and on the other hand, it is penetrated by a large number of blood vessels (veins and arteries) that can immediately transfer the information from organs and tissues to the commutation mechanism of nerve tissue. Also, the fibers of the vegetative nervous system pass through the pia, permitting information control of all vegetative life of organs, tissues and vessels of the body.
14. The information-commutation processes in the extraneural registers of the brain develop in the CSF space around the brain mostly between the pia, arachnoid and dura. During extraneural processing of the information, several stages of the information-communicative processes can be distinguished: a) the stage of local automatized and algorithmyzed communication (reflex stage); b) the stage of distributed holographic communication (the stage of formation of the information images of the functional systems); c) the stage of memory formation (the recording and reproduction of holograms) on the pia surface; d) the stage of the formation of the systemic operation processes (intellect and cognition) by engrams on the arachnoid. So, all processes of automatized extraneural commutation of the reflex activity happen in the subarachnoid space of the brain and are limited by the volume of reflex information-commutation register, while the processes of the information commutation presented as EMW holograms in the subdural space are limited by the volume of cognitive information-communication register.
15. At the level of extraneural registers outside the parenchyma of the brain the function of an information carrier is fulfilled by the EMWs that carry ESCs. Interaction of the EMWs in the intermeningeal CSF space of the brain is achieved by interference, diffraction, imposition and composition and leads to the development of holograms that function as the main biophysical carriers. They integrate the information from tissue magnetomes of various information lines into one image, vesting the IIMs with three dimensions. The hologram, just as other biochemical carriers (DNA, RNA, proteins, etc.), is a fundamental integral biophysical material carrier of information at the extraneural level of consciousness. Reflected EMWs passing through a hologram carry the integrated ESCs to several receivers of the output information channels (lines) at once.
16. The main extraneural information channel in the body of humans or mammals is cerebrospinal fluid, which washes the brain and spinal cord in the intermeningeal space. The main extraneural information carrier is the pia of the brain and the arachnoid mater. The pia is a universal holographic membrane and functions as the main reservoir of memories. The arachnoid functions as the system administrator and manages the algorithms and system software recorded on it when the holograms pass over it and while they record on the pia.

The Main Principles of the Brain's Operation

Modular principle of the functioning of intraneural (inside the nerve tissue) architecture of the brain. A system-forming and communication-organizing information unit of intraneural ICPs of the human/mammalian brain is an ICM of NT, which is represented by a self-regulating multilevel information structure of NT, morphospecific to its location in the brain. The main functions of the NT ICM are the reception, transfer, accumulation, transformation and modulation (upregulation, downregulation or additional generation) of information. The NT ICM does not participate in the processing, analysis or synthesis of the information. Depending on topical localization in the 3D space of the human/animal body, the brain ICPs are subdivided into intermediate, peripheral registration and peripheral executive ones. The NT ICMs are subdivided into NT ICM receivers, NT ICM subscribers and NT ICM transmitters, depending on their functional meaning and their role in the information transfer. In different combinations all of them form input and output information channels, which collectively form the appropriate input and output information lines at the intra-organ level. Informationally, the cortex of the brain is a central controlling information-commutation platform that consists of the set of homogeneous NT ICM subscribers of the input information channels and the NT ICM receivers of the output information channels that are equally distributed in different gyri of the brain. Biologically active parts of the NT in the area of subcortical nodes, spinal cord and vegetative ganglias of autonomous nervous system form the intermediate *information-commutation platform,* which consists of combinations of NT ICM transmitters of both input and output information channels and lines. The main information mission of this platform lies in the switchboard functions of routing the incoming information. The neuroreceptive system of the brain (auditory, visual, kinesthetic, sensory, etc.) is the *peripheral registration information-commutation platform,* which consists of the NT ICM receivers of the input information channels (lines) of appropriate analyzers. Sympathetic and parasympathetic nervous systems form the peripheral information-communicative platform composed of the peripheral executive information-communicative platform of the NT ICM subscribers of the output information channels (lines) connected with the nerve-muscular segment of the human locomotor system and provides execution of the brain motor functions.

The intraneural ICPs of the brain NT are formed of the central, intermediate, peripheral executive information-commutation platforms and present open architecture of the bio-organic *switchboard*, which is equally distributed through the brain and spinal cord parenchyma and connected with brain periphery by the input and output information channels that are functionally united in the information lines. The open type of the brain architecture is conditioned by the exit of the information from the brain into the extraneural information-cellular space of the level of consciousness, located in the subdural and subarachnoid spaces of the brain, processing the information outside the NT of the brain and transferring the processed information to the NT ICM receiver of the cortical output information lines and channels of the brain.

Holographic principle of the operation of extraneural information registers of the brain. The extraneural information registers (ENIR) of the brain are located between the membranes (pia, arachnoid and dura maters) where the incoming information is processed. I would like to accentuate it again: *the information is processed, analyzed and synthesized not* *in the nerve tissue of the brain, but only in the ENIR of the brain; that is, outside its biological substrate*. Processing relies on the holographic principle and consumes almost no energy; the information is interrupted only in the subarachnoid and subdural spaces of the brain. The intermeningeal CSF space functions as the central processing unit of the brain supercomputer. The role of system administrator and system disk in the brain, as well as the keeper of all system software, is played by the arachnoid mater, which registers the sequence of all algorithms and executed programs. The algorithms of the system software are formed by the projection of EMW holograms of the subdural space on the pia by other EMWs, which carry the ESCs and leave traces on the pia when passing through it. These seem to be the engrams (traces) of the information images matrices transported by holograms. The role of the hard disk drive is played by the pia.

The principle of systematicity of vertical commutative connections and complexity of horizontal commutative connections in the brain. There exist two types of information commutative connections in the brain: systemic vertical and complex horizontal commutation. In systemic vertical commutation the nerve tissue of the brain works as a telephone switchboard and a router of the information throughout the modules of NT of the input and output information channels and lines within the framework of their intraneural ICPs. The vertical systemic commutation of the information inside the NT ICM always follows one direction of the inter-level interaction from inductome to genome, transcriptome, proteome, metabolome, cell magnetome and then tissue magnetome. This determines the strict systemic direction of the vertical commutation of the information along information channels and lines only upwards or downwards (afference or efference).

The horizontal complex commutation of the information at different levels of the NT ICM of the brain can be performed reciprocally at the level of the brain ICPs by the synapses between the nerve cells, forming special layers of neural networks. The horizontal complex commutation of the information at the level of each NT ICM is performed largely at the biochemical level in the interaction of cell secretomes of its structure. The horizontal complex commutation at the level of the ENIR is achieved due to the formation of connecting holograms between the input and output information lines of various analyzers (motor, visual, auditory, sensory, etc.). The hologram formation is the fundamental biophysical mechanism of horizontal complex commutation of the extraneural registers and it permits the transfer of information at large distances and the connection of the brain's regions due to hologram transfer with natural CSF flow without energetic expenses of the body.

Regulatory principle of the information organization of the brain. The information circulates in the brain continuously and cyclically, controlling the processes of homeostasis and sanogenesis in the brain. Regardless of the functional state of the brain (asleep or awake, excitation or inhibition, stress or rest, etc.), the brain never rests or relaxes; it provides for perpetual mobility of information. Even during sleep, the intensity, circulation and processing of the information in the brain does not decrease; only routing and commutation properties and connections change. Sleep functions as a switchboard and provides the commutation of the information inside every NT ICM and transmission from the dialog mode of the information relationship between central and peripheral NT ICM to the autonomous mode. During sleep the central, intermediate and peripheral NT ICM synchronize and regulate their autonomous work and information relationship both inside their tissue information structure and the information structure of every somatic cell. They test the correctness of functioning of inter-level information relations both inside the cell and inside the tissue, comparing them with their reference samples included in the program files of the genome of every cell and correcting the faults. It provides self-regulation and self-tuning inside every NT ICM and, if necessary, correction of defects in the inter-level and intra-level relationship of the NT ICM. Therefore, the time of sleep is individual for everyone. This time is necessary for the NT ICM system to test all its information levels and correct the errors. Due to the detection of faults in the level and inter-level relationship, the responsibility for the repair and construction of the cells and tissues in the genes of every cell system of the tested NT ICM are synchronically activated, which is accompanied by a targeted change of the magnetic field, transcriptome and proteome profile of the cells and correction of the faults. Two phases (sleep and wakefulness) of the brain's operation, on the one hand, provide for the relay-race principle, continuity and cyclicity of the reception, processing and storage of the information between the NT ICM, and, on the other hand, the opportunity of self-regulation, technical self-service, repair and self-restoration of every information level of the NT ICM.

Relay principle of information commutation in the brain. The information in the brain is a "relay baton" that is continuously transferred within the NT ICM from one level to the next and it is not lost at any of the levels. Information is transferred continuously through ascending information channels and information lines between NT ICMs by double-step electromagnetic package transfer from peripheral NT ICMs to intermediate NT ICMs (one step) and from intermediate to central ICMs (two steps), and, respectively, *vice versa* in descending information channels and information lines. The commutation and routing of central and peripheral NT ICMs are achieved via a two-step consecutive chain between the central, intermediate and peripheral NT ICMs, which are morphologically realized by a two-neuron reflex arch of the neurons of the chain of the main NT ICM located on the corresponding ICP. In the transfer of information at large distances it is modulated, coded and amplified if necessary by the static NT ICM transmitters located on its pathway. The morphological substrate of the NT ICM transmitters is tissue complexes of vegetative ganglia, tissue structures that provide the functioning of the brain interneurons, tissue structures of the NT in the projection of the nuclei of 12 pairs of cranial nerves, brainstem and pons cerebelli. The interactions of neuromagnetomes of different regions of the brain organize and commute the NT ICMs of the brain as a single central switchboard system, synchronizing the functioning of the central NT ICM, optimizing and regulating the parameters of the inter-level profiles of the brain cortex, and providing the timeliness of inter-level transfers of information by information channels and lines. The biophysical integration of the NT ICMs at the level of magnetomes in neural cells leads to synchronization and a coordinated reaction of various biochemical parameters of the downstream information levels (proteome, transcriptome, genome) and balance of information between different NT ICMs. Thus, the information is not interrupted and not violated; it only changes the information carriers and movement directions.

Modulation principle of the information setup of the brain. Modulation (lat. modulatio "rhythmical measure, melody") is the process of varying one or more parameters of the high-frequency carrier wave according to a low-frequency information signal (message). Regardless of the character, length or power of the information received by the NT ICM, information is modulated according to the phase, amplitude and frequency. The controlling (modulating) signal contains the transferred information and the role of the information carrier is played by a high-frequency wave, known as a carrier wave. So, modulation is the process of "mounting" information on a known carrier (DNA, RNA, proteins, EMW, etc.) of its information level. Due to modulation, the range of the low-frequency controlling signal is transferred to the range of extremely high frequencies. It permits the adjustment of the functioning of all NT ICM receiving-transferring devices to various frequencies to avoid interference. The modulation principle of NT ICM organization provides targeted traffic in information channels and information lines. The information moves through the NT ICM sequentially and in one direction from the inductome level to the level of tissue magnetome of the NT ICM. So, when the data are input to the information channel, they are received by the level of inductome of the peripheral NT ICM receiver, and at the exit is the level of tissue magnetome of the NT ICM subscriber. The modulation principle permits registration of the slightest input information which, passing through the NT ICM of the input information channel, can be amplified to be fixable and able to be processed by the NT ICM subscriber distant from the NT ICM receivers.

The channel of the information exiting the brain (lines of output information) has the same structural attributes as the channel (line) of the input information; and the information moves along it (including information line) in the same order (NT ICM receiver, NT ICM transmitter and NT ICM subscriber). Consequently, when the pia receives unimportant, or vague and unprocessed information (holograms) from the intermeningeal space, it is immediately sent to the magnetome-field level (level of inductome) of the NT ICM of output information channel (information lines), where it is enhanced both in the NT ICM receiver and the NT ICM transmitter. And, at the exit from the output channel (information line) its level of regulatory signal will have such level of tissue magnetome of NT ICM subscriber that it is able to send the signal to appropriate executive organs to perform the function. It permits the registration of even weak output information ("Just thought it's dangerous" due to audio- or video-registration), which can be amplified when coming through the information channel of the data input and then brought to the executive organs, which provide the execution of the requested function of danger evasion. This is the basic mechanism of intuition and presentiments. So, the modulation principle of the transfer of information conditions the movement of information from the periphery to the brain cortex by the input information channels and from the brain cortex to the executive structures by the output channels.

The mechanism for the modulation of information provides the transformation of the signals to increase the efficiency and interference immunity of the process of information transfer in the NT. Generally, the methods of modulation are based on the control of the signal parameters according to the information message. When the signals are modulated, their shape and spectral features change. The characteristics of the signal spectra are significant for communication systems of the brain because they permit the registration of weak, insignificant and currently meaningless information that was received (maybe occasionally) by the NT ICM receiver of the input information line. Passing through all information levels of the brain and output information channel, the information can be amplified to such a level that it can be realized by the executive organs at both reflex and intellectual levels. This mechanism serves to transfer the automatized mode of reflex activity into a conscious (intellectual) mode of control of this activity. The sensitivity of the NT ICM receivers and the strength of the ICM subscribers of the input and output information channels permits an immediate reflex response to any slight signal (the stage of automatic commutation). The information between the NT ICM channels of the input information data and input information channels moves with the help of the packages of information and is transferred at the morphological level by electromagnetic impulses through the nodes of

Ranvier from the neuron body by a transferring axon to a receiving neuron located inside the NT ICM. The synapses play the technical role of connectors to transfer package-impulse information.

Principle of internal and external electromagnetic "illumination" of the pia. The term "illumination" of the brain cortex was introduced by the 1962 Nobel Prize winner Francis Harry Compton Crick. The term describes the phenomenon quite accurately; it is manifested in the activation of a specific cortical area by the incoming information. However, it is the pia mater of the brain that is illuminated and not the cortex, as Crick thought. The activation and reproduction of memories in the brain are achieved due to the principle of external and internal illumination of mnestic engrams on the pia or the effect of the system engrams of the arachnoid. Holograms of the object are projected onto the pia as IIMs and are recorded on it as on a standard holographic medium in the form of mnestic holograms, and the IIMs are reproduced by illumination (activation) of the engrams from below by EMW-stimuli of the magnetomes of central NT ICM or by the electromagnetic effect of reflected electromagnetic waves from above. Accordingly, the position of efferent and afferent parts of the cortical terminals of the analyzers that receive excitations from the internal medium of the body (proprioreceptive, kinesthetic, motor, static and coordinatory), and the analogous parts of the analyzers receiving excitation from the environment, permits the momentary transfer and processing of all incoming information at holographic level and enables an immediate response to it.

Principle of the personalized volume of memory and intellect in the brain. One of the main principles of brain functioning is the accumulation and personalization of the memory volumes. Every object of the environment, actions and thought associated with the object has IIMs at the level of consciousness (ENIR) recorded on the surface of the pia during the development, education and training of a person/mammal and their number increases during a lifetime and the accumulation of experience. This information is registered by the brain on the pia and can be reproduced from it anytime, if the "hard drive" of the pia is intact. The information recorded on the pia forms a personalized and extremely individual volume of the intellect and memory operating at the information level of consciousness, according to the individual algorithms of the arachnoid, thus resembling the inquiries of the computer to the hard drive. Personal information received from internal and external sources is registered on the pia automatically and is evenly distributed on the surface of the information carrier. This method of storing information is extremely reliable, and in the case of mechanical or other injuries the individual data can be restored even by a small fragment of the preserved information carrier.

Register principle of simultaneous extraneural automatic processing of a large amount of data is another important principle of brain operation. The formation of holographic IIMs at the level of the field of consciousness helps to operate and process huge volumes of the data received both from internal organs of the body and from the environment "outside the morphological structure" of the NT of the brain. It opens up unlimited opportunities for the single-step processing of large data volumes, the simultaneous execution of a great number of motor actions and the automatic evaluation of incoming audial, visual, tactile (sensory), olfactory and other information without the involvement of additional memory resources and brain regions. The information level of the field of consciousness is formed as a result of various automatized and standardized manipulations with different IIMs performed by the central cortical NT ICMs. They can be described by several mathematical theories (control theory, automata theory, communication theory, image discrimination theory, etc.). But the information processing can be realized only in the extraneural registers of the information-communication organization (ICO) of the brain. Extraneural registers of the information processing are subdivided into the reflex information register (RIR), located in the subarachnoid space of the brain between the pia and the arachnoid, and the cognitive information register (CIR), located in the subdural space of the brain between the arachnoid and the dura.

The principle of the energy efficiency of brain functioning. The use of the mechanism of the extracerebral (outside the brain) holographic processing of information enables an unlimited number of simultaneous brain operations with no specific energy expenses of the human/mammal body for thinking, and provides the energy-efficient low-consuming formation of IIMs, saving additional energy resources and not involving them in the establishment of new information volumes of the memory for the recording, storage and reproduction of information. The memory resources on the pia do not demand energy and information capacity of the pia that has the size of up to 2200 cm^2 permits the recording of information equivalent to the contents of 22000 bibles. The pia is used by the brain as the hard disk to record, store and reproduce information without additional power consumption.

Such biological switchboard as the brain has all the attributes of Alan Turing's machine for data operation. It has the input and output channels. The role of the information input channel is played by the peripheral NT ICM receivers, located in the tissue structure of the receptor apparatus of the organism (receptors of eyesight, hearing, all receptors of different types of pain, temperature and proprioceptive sensitivity, etc.), that are connected with the NT ICM transmitter of the vegetative nervous system, spinal cord and subcortical cerebral structures and the NT ICM subscribers. The information in the brain is cyclic, just as in Turing's machine, but the information structure of the brain has an open architecture and can adapt at all information levels to the changing conditions of the inner medium of the body and changing factors of the environment.

We will conclude the chapter with a summary of the information discussed above:

1. The brain cortex is a switchboard and router of the signals in the brain and the intermeningeal space functions as the processor of the biocomputer. The main functions of the central NT ICM in the brain cortex are the management, commutation and routing of the information that circulates between the central NT ICM of the brain and peripheral NT ICM located in the solid organs, i.e., the organs of locomotion, vessels, sensory organs and in the autonomous nervous system. The NT parenchyma (gray and white matter) of the brain does not process input and output information. Analysis and synthesis occur outside the biological substrate of the NT of the brain. The NT of the brain functions as a switchboard to route and direct information for its processing and forwarding it for long-term storage. The central NT ICM subscribers of the input information lines and NT ICM receivers of the output information lines form the brain cortex. They are located close to each other and are integrated into cytoarchitectonic fields of the brain to provide optimal functional interaction of the signals. Hence, in certain cases the input-output lines can be commuted by synaptic contact between their cell components. However, the horizontal commutation of information predominantly happens extracerebrally and that is why it can be easily controlled by the "intellectual" holographic processing of

the information. The biological substrate of the brain that provides mechanical and information integration of central NT ICM involves the parts of the brain cortex united by the function. Morphologically, it is achieved by the location of cytoarchitectonic fields of the brain cortex. They excellently function as the switchboard (router) of input and output signals of the brain inside one analyzer (visual, motor, audial, etc.) and form the direction; that is, the route of the signal between interacting ICMs of NT. As a result of these interactions, the extraneural HIR of reflex activity of the brain forms and there the input signals from peripheral NT ICMs commute and the output signals to peripheral ICMs of NT are formed.

2. The morphological substrate of the brain HIR is the CSF space found between the membranes of the brain (the pia mater, the arachnoid mater and the dura mater) or, in other words, the subarachnoid and subdural spaces of the human/mammalian brain. The level of the consciousness field forms at the holographic information level of the brain, where the EMWs remain the main information carrier and the EMWs' interference results in the formation of holograms, the projection and registration of the image in the mind, and recording and reproduction at the holographic film-like surface of the pia. We would like to repeat that at the extraneural level the main transitory information carrier is a hologram, and the main permanent carriers of the information at this level are the pia and the dura. The holograms are carried by the natural flow of the CSF circulating around the brain and spinal cord in the subarachnoid and subdural space at large distances, so they can be projected to the pia during the CSF circulation over the convexital, lower and inner surfaces of the brain. The CSF circulation provides the transferal of the holograms around the brain's surfaces, as well as the projection and recording of the holograms on the surface of the pia, which covers the brain cortex and provides, if necessary, repeated recordings of the holograms on the pia during CSF recirculation. At every information level the information is adapted to the level, and may be specified, enhanced, decreased or modulated, but its quality and content remain unchanged.
3. Extraneural HIR (the processor) of the brain is located between the pia and the dura and is mechanically divided by the arachnoid mater into two interconnected reservoirs: HIR of reflexes and HIR of functional systems. The arachnoid in the area of the spinal cord fulfills mainly reflex functions for the ICMs of NT located in the spinal cord, and subdural space is filled with adipose tissue. This is conditioned by the fact that we do not need delicate holographic processing of the information there, as in the neocortical projection, and all options of reflex activity can be realized when the EMWs of the NT ICM transmitters are reflected from the arachnoid of the spinal cord. The information processes that happen in the HIR of reflexes can be described by the laws of the information theory as the algorithms of the theory of automata, and in the HIR of the functional systems the operation of the brain can be described by a range of information theories: the theory of communication, the theory of control, catastrophe theory, etc.

   The main information assignment of the arachnoid is the *reflection of the electromagnetic waves* from the NT ICM subscribers of the input lines and their guidance to the NT ICM receivers of output lines. The arachnoid mater provides for the controlled automatized work of the switchboard, represented as the brain cortex. The commutation of the EMWs in the HIR of reflexes happens automatically to provide the conditioned reflex activity. The automatism of the HIR of reflexes is also provided by the even frequency-amplitude parameters of EMWs of the tissue magnetomes of interacting NT ICM. The accuracy of the data transfer in the HIR of reflexes is conditioned by the vicinity of receiving-transmitting NT ICMs and morphological arrangements, such as fibrous walls between the pia and arachnoid that slow down the flow of CSF in the subarachnoid space, the stability of its surface structure and closely neighboring synapses between closely located NT ICMs. Part of the EMWs pass through the skull bones and can be registered in encephalography. It cannot be excluded that the interference of these extracerebral EMWs creates their own holograms outside the skull, but the projection of their IIMs through the skull bones is doubtful. However, these facts need additional research and examination.

4. The reflection of such electromagnetic waves from the dura mater provides a high throughput capacity of the arachnoid for CSF, as well as strong and extra-strong signals. However, passing through the CSF as if through the lens, the EMW scatters and divides into an object beam that carries the information image and reference beam. Interference of the scattered EMWs form holograms in the HIR of functional systems (subdural space), which project onto the pia and leave traces on the arachnoid passing through it. In other words, the arachnoid functions as the system disk where the traces (system engrams) of the holograms that pass through it form. The order and sequence of the established holograms are recorded on the arachnoid and stay there as an algorithm for the lifetime of a human/mammal.
5. The holograms of the brain form in the HIR of functional systems and leave their traces (mnestic engrams) on the pia passing through the arachnoid. Consequently, the pia is the memory reservoir that stores all images and events registered by the brain. The holographic surface of the pia is the main carrier and storage of the data at the level of the information field of consciousness, operating by this information carrier the brain forms memory, intellect and thinking, i.e., cognitive functions. Scattered object and reference EMWs of neuromagnetomes of central ICMs of NT interact in the three-dimensional liquid subarachnoid space of the brain filled with the CSF and limited by the pia from below and by the arachnoid from above. This causes the diffusion, interference and reflection of electromagnetic waves (when the CSF functions as the lens), reference and object EMWs of magnetomes that emerge due to their reflection from the arachnoid and the dura mater and development of the holographic effect from the object registered by peripheral ICMs of NT. The holographic principle of the brain's processing of the data is the reason why the brain parenchyma has such a well-known appearance with the gyri and fissures. The cause of such evolutionary morphological and adaptation changes was the necessity to maximally increase the contact surface of the exits of cortical analyzers (the surface of the pia is 220000 mm^{2}, and in the area of the neocortex 1600 cm^2) with the pia on the one hand, and, on the other hand, this advantage provided the maximal surface for the recording, storage and reproduction of the holograms on the pia and practically limitless memory volumes in humans and mammals. The principle of holography permits the use of the surface (convexital) parts of the brain covered by the pia and lower and lateral surfaces for processing and storage of the data. The gyri of the brain, washed by CSF (natural lens to scatter the EMWs), permit the use of the surface of the neighboring gyri as the reflector, or "mirror", to form both object and

reference EMWs necessary for holograms. Limited distances between the gyri and fissures of lateral and internal surface of the brain provide accuracy for projecting the holograms to the specific area of the natural holographic membrane (the pia) and easy restoration if necessary.

The proposed principles of the human/mammalian brain organization and operation help me as a neurologist to explain the range of clinical syndromes and as yet unexplained scientific evidence about the brain.

Chapter 7

THE METHODOLOGY AND TECHNOLOGIES FOR DEVELOPING 3D VIRTUAL MODELS OF THE BRAIN

ABSTRACT

This chapter is dedicated to the critical analysis of various models and simulations of the brain that have been recently developed by different consortiums, universities and private companies by the leaders in IT. These simulations range from mathematical models on the basis of the super powerful computing systems (Blue Gene/Q) to mathematical models as analogues of the artificial brain (SAPUN simulation). The simulations of the brain almost completely repeat the number of neurons and even synaptic terminals of the human brain, but they are not capable of the slightest intellectual effort. The structural organization of the brain is mimicked at different levels of available knowledge. Some researchers replicate the spatiotemporal architecture mimicking the spatial arrangement of the brain and the structure of its internal connections (the Blue Brain Project); others underpin the model with the results of diffuse-tensor MRI of the brain and DNA assays received in genome testing of the brain sections (the project of the Allen Institute for Brain Science), and still others want to get a morphological 3D substrate of a super-accurate model of the brain relying on the microscopic details of the brain's anatomy (the BigBrain Project). These models convincingly demonstrate that it is not the imaged structure of the brain that should be mimicked, but the information principle of its operation.

Keywords: information-commutation theory of brain, information channels, architecture of the brain, information-commutation modules of nerve tissue, memory, cognition, thinking, consciousness, block scheme of the organization of the human brain, information principles of the operation of the human brain

Is it theoretically and technically possible to develop a simplified 3D virtual computer model of a human/mammalian brain in health and in neurological disease? At first glance, the methodology for modeling and research of the brain simulators is already available and the solution is proposed according to the system approach, neural networks and synapses. This fact can be confirmed by the works performed by the IBM Corporation (USA). The IBM supercomputer BlueGene/Q Sequoia of Lawrence Livermore National Laboratory, LLNL, accomplished the calculations of the **mathematical model of the brain**, which consists of 10 billion neurons and 100 trillion connections between them, i.e., synapses. **To date this**

mathematical model is the largest simulation of the brain. However, it should be noted that the mathematical model developed by the IBM and LLNL expert teams is not exactly a brain model. It is the model of a calculating system based on 2048 billion neurosynaptic computer kernels, wherein IBM has implemented an absolutely new architecture of calculation systems that follow the principles of the brain's operation. IBM representatives have confirmed that their task was not to work out the complete simulation of the brain. According to them, they developed a mathematical model of an innovative module cognitive computing system, the architecture of which is far from that of von Neuman. This model approaches the complexity of the brain, which contains about 100 trillion synapses, and this value meets the requirements of the SyNAPSE (Systems of Neuromorphic Adaptive Plastic Scalable Electronics) program of the DARPA (the Defense Advanced Research Projects Agency) [148]. For the large-scale mathematical model the IBM experts relied on the architecture and structure of the neurosynaptic cognitive chip, which they presented a year earlier. These chips are based on the matrices of electronic analogues to the neurons and synapses, the connections between the neurons. In the model these neurosynaptic kernels were divided into 77 groups similarly to the regions of the brain. During modeling, all 530 billion neurons and 100 trillion synapses worked 1542 times slower then they work in reality. But the result is impressive if we talk about mathematical modeling on the calculating systems.

Just as many previous examples, this model had one goal, which was the development of a computer that operates like a human brain and is able to analyze diverse information from different sources. The development of such a computer is the final goal of the abovementioned SyNAPSE program. Besides, a future computer must be small-sized and low energy consuming, which is even harder to achieve than incorporating the necessary number of artificial neurons and synapses.

It is well known that computer functioning is provided by two components: hardware and software. On the whole, the hardware is a reasonably organized material, while biologically it is the structure of a body: organs of perception, executive organs and the brain. The structure of the body is the condition for software. The software in this context is comprised of conditioned and unconditioned reflexes, behavior patterns that help realize biological goals, i.e., survival. A program can be launched only if the appropriate hardware is available. For example, well-articulated speech is only possible if the proper vocal apparatus is present; flight is only possible if the wings are available and appropriately constructed, and rational thinking is possible only if the construction of the brain is appropriate. However, the human brain, i.e., the brain of Homo sapiens, has a huge potential for "advanced" software. As a lot of researchers note, it is quite possible to expand the use of the brain that we all have. Such a model demonstrates the connection between a material carrier (nervous system) and the ideal foundations (biocomputer software) for the mental activity of a human. The neurophysiologist John Lilly in 1968 published the book *Programming and Metaprogramming in the Human Biocomputer: Theory and Experiments,* in which he combined his neurophysiological research of the cortex with ideas of computer programming. According to Lilly, the program is the set of internally compatible instructions on signal processing, on the formation of the data and memorizing both of them and on the preparation of messages; it demands the usage of logical processes, processes of selection and storing addresses. Primarily, John Lilly thought that all adults were programmed biocomputers; this was inherent human nature, it could not be changed, and all humans are able to program themselves and others. Later he came to the conclusion that his brain was a giant biocomputer, and that he was a meta-programmer of this biocomputer, while the brain was located in the body and the mind was the means of programming [149]. According to the information-commutation theory of brain, the concepts of John Lilly are incorrect. Having no understanding of the structure of the brain, he attempted to give a metaphysical explanation to the material carriers of the data in the brain, but could not find them and escaped into abstract philosophy and fantasies. However, his search for a computing concept of the brain is still worth remembering.

The computing concept of the brain can serve as a good model for practical use, as was proven by the achievements of neuro-linguistic programming (NLP). NLP was initiated by John Grinder, a linguist, and Richard Bendler, a mathematician, psychotherapist and computer specialist, who studied the methods of efficient influence on human behavior. Currently the method is widely used in business, public management, sport, etc. In any case, when using computer analogies, we must keep in mind that the biocomputer and its operator are not identical.

Neurobiologists from the University of Waterloo (Canada) claimed that they had developed the most complex and the largest functional computer simulation of the brain known as Spaun (Semantic Pointer Architecture Unified Network). It is able to distinguish numbers, to learn them, to detect the sequences of numbers and to write them on paper using a robotized manipulating hand. The development of such simulation is a big step in brain modeling technology, as the simulation can mimic the real behavior of a human by modeling the physiological processes of the neurons and synapses. Chris Eliasmith, the author of the simulation, spent years studying the brain's structure and interactions between different functional parts of the brain. A book entitled *How to Build a Brain* was published to describe the structure of gray matter, dendritic connections and other details of the brain's anatomy [150]. As a demonstration example, Chris Eliasmith developed the SPAUN, the most complex simulation of the functioning brain.

With the help of an open source neurosimulator known as Nengo, Chris Eliasmith's team emulated the operation of 2.5 million neurons, distinguished according to the functions of the human brain regions (ganglias, thalamus, prefrontal cortex, etc.) [151, 152]. The brain simulation has virtual organs of sight and a robotized arm which is able to perform certain tasks of which previously no other brain model was capable. Unlike the IBM Watson and other systems, the SPAUN (Semantic Pointer Architecture Unified Network) was developed for the ultimately realistic modeling of human brain operation, and not to solve practical tasks. For example, the IBM team aimed at the development of an accurate space model in the Blue Brain project, but did not take into account the functional differences of the brain regions. The data were input through a digital 'eye' with a resolution of 28x28 pixels. No other ways to input the data were designed. The set of figures and signs that were transferred to the memory could be shown. The system perceived some signs as commands that should be fulfilled. The SPAUN puts down the results of the calculations with a mechanical 'hand'. Interestingly, the information is processed by a computer in a way similar to that of a human brain, as far as neurobiologists understand it. The system has a prefrontal area, basal ganglia, subcortical nuclei, thalamus, etc. The neurobiologists programmed the data processing to be as close to natural as possible. The visual signals are forwarded to the visual area of the cortex, and then to the thalamus. The thalamus is responsible for the distribution of the information to different areas of the brain cortex. The basal ganglia control the information flow through the prefrontal area and renew it according to the current needs. For example, if at the moment a meal must be cooked, then the necessary sequence of actions is loaded to the prefrontal area. In urgent cases, this information is erased and, for example, information about driving is loaded. The human is able to quickly switch from one task to another; he demonstrates extremely high cognitive flexibility, due to the basal ganglia and long-term memory. The simulation is divided into two main parts; one part is the simulation of the brain cortex, and the other simulates the main ganglia. The neurons of the simulation are connected in a physiologically realistic way, and the parts of the mathematical simulation interact in the same way as the parts of a real brain are supposed to interact according to the opinion of contemporary science. The scientists also entailed the SPAUN with limitations that were supposed to be characteristic of the human brain. For example, the system was not able to keep a very long sequence of signs in the short-term memory. Currently, neurobiologists are working on the mechanism of self-education and rerecording of the neurons in the 'brain' so that the SPAUN is able to reprogram itself and learn new tasks. So, to date, the SPAUN is the most complex and functional simulation of the human brain (Figure 43).

The SPAUN differs from other artificial "brains", such as IBM's Watson, primarily because it was originally designed to mimic human behavior and not to find solutions in ways similar to humans'. In designing Watson, the IBM team had the goal of providing an efficient solution to a specific set of tasks, search, analysis and decision making, but the methods for solving these tasks do not resemble the processes that happen in the brain at all.

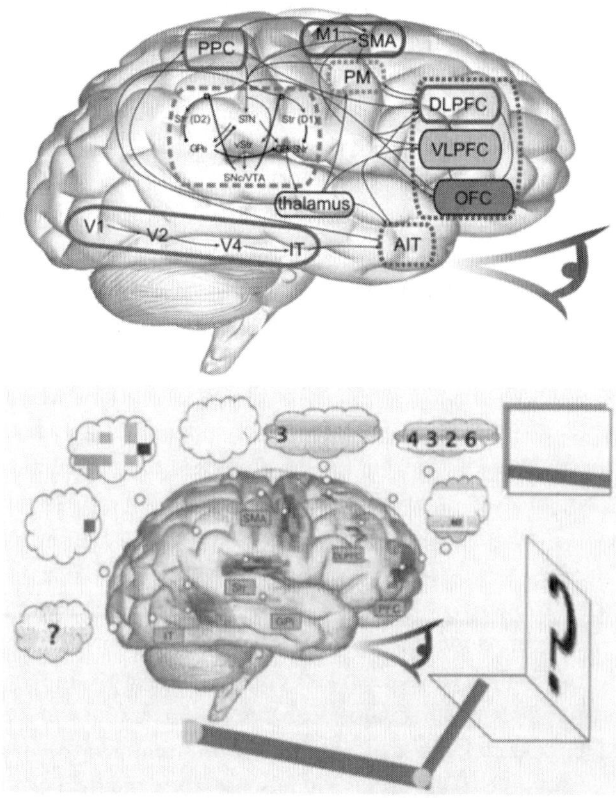

Figure 43. The principal scheme of the SPAUN (Semantic Pointer Architecture Unified Network), a functional computer brain model.

The SPAUN is able to really see such rows of numbers as 1-2-3; 5-6-7; and 3-4. Artificial neurons process the visual data and extract the images of the figures. This visual information is received by the cortex through known routes and the cortex is able to perform various manipulations with the data, such as a comparison of the data with images from the memory, copying and processing them. On the basis of the received and processed information the model can draw some logical conclusions and can independently find answers to some questions from the IQ test. "Depending on what's going on in the cortex, it takes information from one part of the cortex and routes it to a different part of the cortex. Every time it does that, it updates the state of the cortex, and tries to figure out what's the next best thing to do," Eliasmith said. "You can think of the basal ganglia as controlling the flow of information through the cortex, in order to solve different tasks. . . . This model is trying to address that issue of cognitive flexibility. How do we switch between tasks, how do we use the same components in our head to do all those different tasks?" he said.

"Still, Spaun has its limits – it is relatively simple, compared to real neural networks, and it is hard-wired, lacking the plasticity and adaptive capability human brains are known to possess." Eliasmith is working on updates that would allow it to learn new tasks and perceive instructions on a more complex level. He is even working on a program in which Spaun isn't given explicit instructions, but rather positive or negative feedback. "We would just tell it if it is doing a good job or a bad job," he said. "Eventually it would discover its own strategy for accomplishing its own task."

In its ability to mimic the physiology and related behavior of the brain, Spaun serves higher purposes for both neuroscience and computer science, Eliasmith said.

"It lets us understand how the brain, the biological substrate, and behavior relate. That's important for all sorts of health applications," he said. He can kill off neurons systematically and watch how their deaths affect performance, simulating the process that happens as people age, for instance. Or, Spaun can help other machines emulate brain function more accurately and more efficiently, Eliasmith says. "We can try to discover the algorithms being used by biology, and maybe understand the principles behind them, to build better artificial agents." [153]

The development of a virtual 3D simulation of the human brain based on the system approach was excellently demonstrated by the EPFL's Blue Brain Project in Switzerland. Neurocomputing simulations of the Blue Brain Project showed that the so-called brain waves were the side product of the functioning of ion channels on the neuronal processes. "We need a computer model because it is impossible to relate the electrical activity of potentially billions of individual neurons and the resulting brain waves at the same time," says EPFL scientist Sean Hill. "Through this view, we're able to provide an interpretation, at the single-neuron level, of brain waves that are measured when tissue is actually probed in the lab," says Sean Hill. Sean Hill and his team aimed to define the nature and possible functions of the so-called brain waves that emerge in the mammalian brain when the nervous cells work. The scientists have distinguished several types of such waves and each is expressed by a specific brain area and associated with a certain activity of the brain. So, we learned to evaluate the state of a human's health by these waves. The researchers of the Blue Brain Project designed a simulation of the brain that consisted of 12000 neurons and accurately reproduced the structure of one rat brain region. Observing its operation, the scientists noted that virtual nerve tissue issued impulses that were similar to the waves of live rodents. The researchers examined the operation of some of the simulation components and found that the brain waves emerged in the ion channels on the surface of dendrites. These channels are necessary for the exchange of electric signals between the neurons and one of the side-effects of their work is brain waves. According to the biologists, their model does not have 100% accuracy, but even so it can be used to study relations between different wave types and the functioning of the parts of a body. The Blue Brain simulation is designed to mimic the spatial structure of the brain and the structure of its internal connections, but it cannot mimic the behavior of a real brain, as Chris Eliasmith says. "These artificial brains don't actually do anything. They don't see, they don't remember, they don't recognize objects," he said. "They sit there and generate complex voltage patterns, but those complex voltage patterns aren't tied to behavior" [153]. The works of American and European neuroscientists along with the approaches and principles of the systemic organization of the brain underlie another computer simulation of the human brain, which was developed in the Allen Institute for Brain Science in Seattle (USA). The design of the computer map of the brain required over four years of fundamental research of the brain processes. The atlas of the human brain (Figure 44) is an interactive instrument of research which helps scientists to understand the functioning of the brain and the treatment of its disorders. The evidence used to develop the model was obtained through magnetic resonant imaging and diffusion tensor imaging. Allan Jones, the director of the Allen Institute for Brain Science, said that the brain was sliced and the tissue was used to read RNA. A quantitative read-out from the RNA was obtained on a DNA micro-array which took assays of the ~25,000 genes in the human genome. The data were systemized to develop a detailed map of the human brain. So, for example, the researcher is able to get a 3D image of any areas in the brain where the biochemical reactions are the most highly expressed [154].

The researchers detected an amazing agreement: 94% of all biochemical reactions in both hemispheres of the brain proceed identically, and at least 82% of human genes are responsible for brain processes. Allan Jones says it is not surprising. When we think about the complexity of brain functions and the various cell types found in the brain it does not look that amazing as the part of the genome is employed to support the brain.

Other researchers are also attempting to develop a map of the neuronal connections of a mouse brain which the MRI is not able to do. They turn brain samples into digital images of electronic microscope. The computer reads the digital images, compares the outlines of nervous cells and yields 3D photographic images. The mapping of the brain has limitless potential for human genetics and the manufacturing of new pharmaceuticals, which will be a significant step forward in the fight against brain diseases.

On June 21, 2013 the *Daily Mail* announced that for the first time in the history of science researchers had worked out a high definition 3D model of a human brain that was named the BigBrain. The BigBrain shows the anatomy of the brain in microscopic detail for the first time ever – at a spatial resolution of 20 microns. This is smaller than the size of one fine strand of hair and 250,000 times more detailed than current MRI brain scans [155].

Researchers from Germany and Canada took 7,400 individual slices from the brain of a deceased 65-year-old woman and plotted 80 billion neurons during the 10-year project.

Now the brain model is available online for free to help other scientists to develop the field of neuroscience.

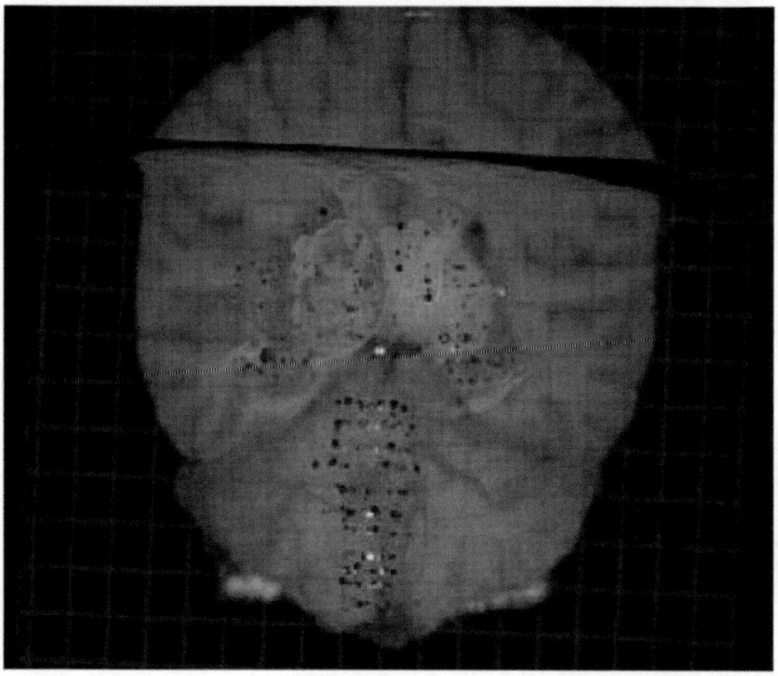

Figure 44. Computer atlas of human brain. The data used for the model were obtained in diffuse tensor MRI of the brain.

BigBrain provides a resolution much finer than the typical 1mm resolution from MRI studies.

Senior author Dr. Alan Evans, a professor at the Montreal Neurological Institute at McGill University in Montreal, Canada, said the project 'has been a tour-de-force to assemble images of over 7,400 individual histological sections, each with its own distortions, rips and tears, into a coherent 3-D volume.'

The sophisticated contemporary methods of image processing reveal an unprecedented look at the very fine details of the human brain's microstructure, or cellular level.

The detailed 10 trillion-byte cerebral atlas will be developed and accessed freely. It represents the structure of a human brain with a definition that exceeds 50 times all previously existing atlases.

Summarizing all of the abovementioned facts about brain simulations, we have to admit that the scientists have succeeded in the development of a model of an autistic brain: the model can do complicated calculations but is not capable of primitive intellectual activity, which is observed in cases of severe intellectual deficiencies. To my mind, the only way to develop an intellectual mathematical simulation of a human brain is to employ the technologies of extraneural processing of information on the basis of the proposed theory of the information-commutation organization of a human brain. This method will permit the development of energy-efficient technologies of calculations, neurocomputing equipment and neurorobotics.

Chapter 8

METHODOLOGICAL ERRORS AND SYSTEMIC ERRORS OF THEORETICAL NEUROLOGY IN THE DEVELOPMENT OF 3D VIRTUAL MODELS OF THE BRAIN

ABSTRACT

Contemporary data, tools and technologies that are used for the development of virtual simulations of the brain are discussed in this chapter, and the reasons for the failures in contemporary modeling of the brain, as well as the opportunities and promises of mathematical modeling as the main instrument for the development of multilevel information structures and 3D virtual models of the brain in health and in diseases of the central nervous system in theory. The systemic and methodological errors of neurobiologists in their specialty lead to systemic crisis in neuromathematics, biophysics and neuromodeling. The methodological approaches to the brain research are compared and analyzed: the methodology of the system multilevel approach of the HBP and the methodology of the information approach that we propose. The readers may decide whether we have succeeded in it. But the process of comparative analysis of these two ideologies, which basically differ in their matter and, at the same time, are similar in their manner, was very exciting. With the meticulousness and delight of a school teacher I picked out the inaccuracies and errors in the description of the structure of the multilevel system of the HBP methodology, and criticized colleagues for the impossibility and inexpedience of the systemic integration of biochemical, morphological, neurophysiological and cognitive data about the brain. A new information methodological approach is proposed, which permits representation of the multilevel research of the brain in the biochemical or biophysical normalized information values of the brain in their inter-level relationship and connections.

Keywords: reasons for the failures in the development of artificial intelligence and brain simulations, mathematical brain models, 3D virtual brain model, brain simulation, principles of 3D modeling of the brain

In the previous chapters we described the most important and significant models of the human and mammalian brains which, in some cases, can simulate the functions of the brain

(The Blue Brain Project), serve as a universal manual in anatomy, histology and immunohistochemistry, provide the model for trying new pharmaceuticals (the BigBrain project), model sophisticated calculations on the universal basis of supercomputer technologies (SPAUN model) and demonstrate commutative synaptic connections in the human brain (the Human Connectome Project and its map of neural network activity of the brain). However, none of the models can perform a hundredth part of the things that the brain of the most common human is able to do. What is the basic reason for the inefficiency and even primitiveness of the computer models of the brain? Most likely, the key reason for the failures in the development of an optimal model of the human/mammalian brain lies in the absence of the *functional theory of the structure and operation of the brain and the appropriate methodology to develop a computing model.* In other words, the reasons for the failures in brain modeling lie in the incorrect basic concepts of theoretical neurology on the brain structure and misunderstanding of the fundamental mechanisms of brain operation. Therefore, the design of the computer models presented in the current practice of theoretical neurology does not rely on the fundamental scientific theory or hypothesis that would explain the organization of the brain, but on the available practice and achievements of the mathematical calculations and innovative hardware and software as well as on the technical opportunities of contemporary neuromorphic equipment that mimics the functioning of separate elements of the brain organized as supercomputers consisting of microchips that imitate neurons, memristors technically analogous to synapses, methods to expand the processor cores and others. To date, these neuromorphic devices that imitate separate elements of the brain top all technological solutions in theoretical neurology.

The other, no less important reason for the failures in brain modeling is the absence of clear, accurate practical skills that would match the complexity of the brain in the therapeutic management of brain functions and targeted regulation of inner organs. In other sciences (biochemistry, biophysics, molecular biology, etc.) practice has permitted an understanding of the features of the studied object, but in theoretical neurology it adds up to general confusion and prevents us from deciphering the fundamental codes of the organization and structure of the brain. Unfortunately, in the past 100 years the specialists have not learned to empirically correct the activity of the brain, regulate asocial behavior or eradicate sociopathic motivations in people with behavior deviations. The societies of highly developed countries found a rather strange way out of the dead-end of social controversies and impotence in the face of immoral and asocial phenomena. It chose tolerance to the deviant states of mentally deficient people who suffer from sociopathic personality disorders. The societies of Europe and Northern America sacrificed their moral and ethical values to restore social balance between different social groups and groups of social minorities. The boundaries of the norm between mental health and disease are leveled off, although these deviations are the manifestations of organic diseases of the human brain and they demand therapy and not adaptation to their asocial and immoral behavior. The pathway of tolerance to the violations of the age-old ethical and moral traditions of a highly developed society is the way to degeneration and the disappearance of our civilization, and not to its progress and heyday.

Having no understanding of the organizational principles of the brain, we are not able to work out the ways to manage those members of society who violate ethical and moral rules. Unfortunately, the current levels of neurology and psychiatry demonstrate that we are able to generally suppress the functional activity of the human/mammalian brain, by the newest sedatives and antipsychotics, to bring the person to prostration and inability to manage their thinking or to activate emotions by antidepressants and psychostimulants, but are unable to generate specific disposition, orderly thinking and behavior in humans, to socialize them and make them adequate to their circumstances and surroundings. Society cannot cope with the criminality because we do not understand how the brain operates. The jails are full of sociopaths and their release can bring even more damage to the foundations of society. And the solution here is the search for the theory of the organization of the brain and its operation.

Apparently, the absence of theoretical knowledge about brain functioning in neuroscience does not enable physicians to learn how to treat basic neurological and mental diseases or, moreover, to set the tasks to the engineers and software programmers to model the disorders of the brain. The neurologists and psychiatrists treat nervous and mental diseases in humans with various pharmaceuticals, physiotherapy and surgery courageously and fearlessly, and sincerely believe that they understand what they are doing. Actually, knowing the anatomy of the brain does not help physicians in the therapy of nervous and mental diseases, and on the contrary, creates an illusion that they are right, and the administered pharmaceuticals are well-reasoned, though they violate brain regulation and the sanogenetic abilities of the brain. Without understanding the fundamental principles of the biological structure of the brain, and being unaware of the potential harm that we bring with our incompetent treatment, the conventional therapy of nervous and mental diseases disturbs the delicate balance of already disordered information-commutation relations in the brain. We will illustrate this with an example of conventional cerebroprotective treatment with Cerebrolysin (the pharmaceutical received from the nerve tissue of cattle) or Cortexin (the pharmaceutical received from the cortex of calves) for ischemic vascular or traumatic injuries of the brain and analyze this standard therapy from the standpoint of the information-commutation theory. It is possible that in administering standard therapeutic Cerebrolysin or Cortexin schemes for brain injury we are not able to realize the disastrous effects of the irreversible changes in the genome, transcriptome and proteome of different cells of the nerve tissue that are caused by the proteins of the mammals of different species. Unfortunately, all doubtful advantages of these drugs are canceled out by the harm that the therapy brings. On the one hand, it is associated with the immunological problems initiated by the introduction of foreign proteins to the patient, and on the other, it leads to mutations in the genome of the patient. In acute injury of the brain and destruction of nerve tissue a large amount of neurospecific antigens is expressed in the blood and they are neutralized by neurospecific antibodies. Therefore, the introduction of a large amount of xenogeneic antigens from Cerebrolysin or Cortexin in an acute phase of ischemic injury of the brain enhances autoimmune aggression in the nerve tissue of the injured brain and eliminates even more of the information-commutation modules of the nerve tissue than were eliminated by the injury alone. On the other side, when Cerebrolysin is administered in the subacute and chronic stages of brain injury, the neurologists and psychiatrists are motivated by its cerebroprotective, nootropic and neurotrophic effect on neurons. But they obviously do not understand that they can irreversibly harm the information-commutation modules of already injured tissue through the systematic administration of foreign proteins of mammals belonging to different species from the patients with disordered proteome of various cell systems of nerve tissue, thus destabilizing the genome of the majority of the nerve cells and promoting carcinogenesis, an accumulation of mutations of hereditary diseases and degenerative processes in these cell systems. According to the information-commutation theory of the brain, it becomes clear that in changing the protein profile of the cells of the nerve tissue we automatically affect the genome of these cells, as the relations of genome, proteome, transcriptome and metabolome are rigidly regulated by the reference genetic programs of neural cell systems. By changing the proteome profile of the cells of human nerve tissue by foreign proteins for the best of neurotrophic and nootropic reasons, we establish stressful conditions of tension for the regulation and sanogenesis of all information levels of the cell systems of the nerve tissue of the brain. This biological stress results in the adaptation of the cells of the nerve tissue to foreign proteins, which is, however, only possible due to the adaptive micro-mutations of the genome, which modify intracellular signaling and lead to new adaptive phenotypes of these cells. The administration of seemingly safe drugs and the consequent change of the proteins in the proteome of various cells of the nerve tissue (and not only neurons) leads to the modification of the main information-commutation properties in different modules of nerve tissue of the brain and thus, to hindered commutation by the information input and output channels (lines) manifested in disordered thinking and cognition. Vertical systemic disorders in receiving, transferring and processing the data in the NT ICM at different information-communication platforms lead to long-term failures and blocked sanogenetic mechanisms and, consequently, to atrophic processes in the morphological structure of the NT ICM, disintegration of horizontal communication of the cell systems of NT ICM and further progression of psychoorganic syndrome. Thus, inaccurate proteome-based therapy with conventional cerebroprotectors and nootropics targeted at the modification of the peptide profile of a nerve cell provides a more harmful effect than even the stressful action of the environment and the injury itself. I do not call for a rejection of all experience of the therapy of nervous diseases that has been acquired by contemporary clinical neurology. I insist on working out rigid algorithms of drugs administration on the basis of the information-commutation theory and their use as a guide with consideration of the basic mechanisms of the brain sanogenesis. To our big surprise, the brain possesses enormous durability so that it is able to cope with extreme loads on its information structures, despite our purposeful iatrogenic therapeutic actions and severe ischemic injury. However, one should note that, in disregard of good intentions and all efforts of the doctors to disorder information-commutation relations in the brain with the pharmaceuticals, the brain still comes off with honor from dangerous situations. Still, they leave their marks in the injured central, intermediate and peripheral information-commutation modules of the nerve tissue of the brain, as generally all such therapeutic interventions leave their traces in the human body. Hence, the results of our treatment fully match the level of our incompetence in the therapy of nervous diseases and in the knowledge of brain functioning. So we come to the eternal questions of the Russian intelligentsia: What shall we do?

Let us speculate about it, relying on the information-commutation theory of the human brain. The notions about the functioning of the brain in clinical neurology rely mostly on anatomical, histological, cytological, immunohistochemical and neuromorphological (magnetic resonant imaging and computer tomography) data and the data of the neurophysiological, psychophysiological and neuropsychological tests; that is, on morphofunctional systemic manifestations of the brain's structure and functioning. These systemic views of neurologists and neuroscientists are that very systemic error which is extrapolated to the level of clinical medicine and computation technologies. Translating the ideology of a model of a neuron as a biological system to the technique (neurocomputers, software based on neuromathematics and mathematical multilayer neural networks, memristors, etc.), we attempt to reproduce neural networks, protein networks, genome networks, networks of signal transduction pathways in the cells of the brain. But, unfortunately, it does not work. Errors in the theory and methodology turn out errors in the technologies and therapies.

As we have already said, the essence of the systemic methodological error of theoretical neurology and all methodologies of the system approach to the brain lies in the *fundamental dogma of clinical neurology* which incorrectly formulates the basic theoretical scientific concept that a neuron is the main information-commutation unit in the brain. Undoubtedly, the neuron is an important biological cell system, a frequently occurring morphostructural element of a human/mammalian nervous system, but it is only a part of the information-commutation module of the nerve tissue enabled as the key unit in the data transfer in the brain. We have discussed this issue in Chapter 5 of this book and would like to repeatedly stress that a neuron is only a tissue-specific somatic cell connected to other neurons by axons and dendrites. Connected neurons and their multiple synaptic contacts (synapses) form neural networks. There is an opinion that these very features of the neurons permit multilayer information network structures that are capable of integrating their activity and the establishment of functional systems that fulfill the main functions in the brain. Hence, when the networks were modeled as technical analogues of neurons and synapses to provide the foundation for all functional systems of the brain, they should have demonstrated how the main functions of the brain are realized. Unfortunately, nothing that was expected happened. The modeling of multilayer neural networks did not lead to the expected efficiency in the provision of the requisite functions. Having analyzed the results of multilayer neural networks, most of the researchers of neurocomputation [156] came to the conclusion that the statement that multilayer networks are able to realize the function is erroneous. It seems that the neurophysiologists and neurologists made mistakes too, when they said that the functional systems aimed at this result (accomplishment of the function) were the instrument for commutation in the brain [26, 157]. Previously, it was considered that for this the functional systems form highly specific engrams (compositions) from the neurons of different neural networks presented as specific neural clusters, and these engrams of neurons temporarily unite different brain regions and different layers of neural networks to fulfill specific cognitive and psychic functions. How true are these views about the formation of inter-neuronal engrams in the brain according to the information-commutation theory of the brain? How is it technically possible for the brain to immediately form the engrams between distant parts of the cortex? To my mind, it is impossible. The neurons are not able to form engrams either technically or technologically. For this, there should be strong transverse axonal connections between neurons in the brain's cortex, whereas they are almost absent in the anatomy of the cortex. There are systemic commutative vertical connections between the neurons of the brain's cortex and neurons of different levels of the NT ICM (central, intermediate and peripheral) which are regulated by their activity and are realized mostly at the biophysical level as the package-impulse transferal of data. Horizontal communication between the neurons functions predominantly at the level of synapses and is realized at the biochemical level involving mediators, neurotransmitters and growth factors. Hence, the idea of forming the engram of the functional system as the composition cluster of functionally united cortical neurons located in different parts of the brain does not stand up to scrutiny either practically or according to the theory of the information-commutation relations. However, the holograms that result from the interference and superposition of electromagnetic waves of the magnetomes of different parts of the brain that can be located at a distance permit the formation of the matrix of any informational image in the subarachnoid and subdural spaces and register it at the pia, which seems quite real and technologically feasible. Unfortunately, the available systemic concepts about the functioning of the neurons, neural networks and neural engrams are supported by various neurophysiologists, neuropsychologists and neurologists. These concepts do not contribute to our understanding of the brain. On the contrary, they confuse us in the 3D networks of neurons, genomes, proteins, RNAs, etc.

As we have noted before, the scientific views on the biological model of a neuron - that is, the neuron as a living cell with membrane, nucleus, organelles, nucleolus, signal transduction pathways and synaptic contact - lead to misunderstandings and an incorrect evaluation of the role and place of a neuron in the data transfer in the central nervous system. That is why the conceptual framework of the theory of information is mixed with the conceptual framework of neuroanatomy and neurophysiology. The neuroanatomists and neurophysiologists are convinced that anatomical structures (lobes, gyri, hemispheres) provide the transfer of data from one structure to another and that they are similar to the informational nature of the work that the brain performs. They are not discouraged by the fact that the main anatomical formations of the brain are separated by septa, CSF spaces, tentoria and others, so that the opportunity for direct interaction between them at the level of the brain's cortex is technically ruled out. Returning to the example of the telephone station, we would like to observe that regional formations in the brain are only separate blocks of commuting hardware and every person with common sense understands that the commuting hardware can be located at the station in any order, in case the principles of commutation and communication are observed and all station workers understand that commutation blocks are not the information; the information is in the conversations of the subscribers. A cell phone tower is important for the quality of the cell operator services, but it does not belong to the structure and content of the information. So when the information that is exchanged by the subscribers, the brand and the shape of cell phones, as well as the features of the cell phone tower and the switchboard stand are ranged equally for systemic analysis, we can hardly explain the principles of mobile phone communication. We must not combine the uncombinable.

A similar thing happened in contemporary neurology whereby biological and informational notions were mixed and the term "information" implies the connectome of the brain (axonal and dendritic connections in the brain, the map of the network of the brain), and neural cell, synapses, microcircuits of neural cell nuclei, brain regions, psychophysiological data, neurophysiological data and experimental psychological data. All these discrepant, multilevel, multi-scale and heterogeneous pieces of "information" about the brain, which the scientists are attempting to bring together into one system, seem to be able to explain the principles of brain operation to us. It is very similar to the mobile phone story, isn't it? This is the reason why it is almost impossible to understand the principles and mechanisms of the brain's operation and organization. Otherwise, within the past 50 years since this knowledge became available, one or other of the neuroscientists and neurologists around the world would definitely have been able to structure and systemize the data within the necessary system.

The example with mobile communication demonstrates the sequence of necessary and obligatory steps for the innovative development of any field of science. First, we have to develop a new paradigm of scientific thinking, which is able to initiate a new theoretical concept; then, we propose an appropriate method to realize this theory involving specific technologies, and only after this do the hardware and software find their practical implementation. However, to start working on these stages we badly need a contemporary neurological theory to understand the brain and to mathematically model the operation of the brain.

As the neuroscientists do not have any clear and definite concepts on how the brain operates, we do not have innovative concepts that would permit a new comprehensive theory of the brain's operation. Incorrect theoretical standpoints of the expert neurologists lead to the erratic neuromorphic development of technical analogues of this equipment. This is brightly illustrated by the inclination of the specialists in computing hardware to work on memristors; that is, equipment analogous to synapses. Undoubtedly, they permit the technical connection of different layers of artificial neural networks, but this does not provide for the expected breakthrough. The result has been the development of certain models of the brain that integrate thousands of neurons and multilayer neural networks; the artificial synapses number in the thousands too, but the results are feeble. This means that we chose the wrong direction. The scientists who support the hypothesis of neural networks as the top-priority brain theory have obviously made a mistake.

As a rule, results like this are conditioned by errors in the methodology. Let us look critically at the available methodology of the multilevel and multi-scale systemic analysis of the operation of the brain, which was proposed by the leading European theoreticians of neurology in the Human Brain Project. The methodology of the project is the collective result of the leading specialists and scientists of Europe. It was written by three hundred experts in neurosciences: neurologists, neuromorphologists, neurophysiologists, computer professionals, theoretical mathematicians, engineers and the top programmers. The methodology passed through the scientific and technical examinations of top neuroscientists and only after their approval did it receive the administrative and financial support of the European Commission. Moreover, the support of this methodology by American specialists can be clearly seen in their BRAIN Initiative, launched in 2013 by the US President. Hence, I presume that the methodology of understanding the human brain which is described in the Human Brain Project flagship report is the quintessence of the current state of the methodology and the academic level of global neuro-research and the highest bar of the achievements of contemporary sciences about the brain.

In Figure 6 we have already demonstrated the basic methodology of the system approach to our understanding of the brain, as shown by the Human Brain Project experts. One should especially note the way in which the information received in the brain research will be systemized. The system approach is the main methodology and pride of European scientists; they even have a separate section in the report named *Methodology*. It is necessary to take into account that the project developers consider this approach to be the mainstay for the development of the mathematical model of the brain. Figure 45 demonstrably compares the methodology of the system approach to brain research and our methodology of the informational approach to neuroscience research.

The lowest level of information in the Human Brain Project which is considered to be accessible for brain research is the genome of a neuron; that is, hereditary and programmed information. The specialists of the HBP did not mention that there exists a level of atomic information, a level of elementary particles and a magnetic field level of magnetic resonances, oscillations and torsion fields. The biophysical data did not seem to be related to precise research of the European genome and post-genome biochemical school. Then the experts distinguished the levels of post-genome information (RNA, transcriptome, proteome proteins, carbohydrates, fats and the rest of the metabolome proteins). These are extremely important informational levels of a nervous cell and their research is pivotal. We completely agree with the division of the information at these informational levels: genome, transcriptome, proteome and metabolome. However, then according to the project designers, the information is represented by the "synapse"; that is, the morphological formation that provides a connection between the neurons. What is the significance of the anatomical structure that provides the connection between the cells and the information that passes through it? To my mind, the relationship is the same as that between the brand of a cell phone and the principles of mobile communication. Where is the information in the synapse? The information in the synapse is transmitted by mediators and neurotransmitters that carry it from one cell to another. That is, the information carrier is the expressed secretome of a cell and not a biological arrangement that provides the connection with other cells. If we use the example of an electrical circuit again, information is the current that goes along the circuit, and not the cable or cable-connecting terminals. At this point, the differences between our approaches become obvious, as we think that only the secretome is the source of information at this level, and not the structure where it is produced. Further, at the next level of gathering the information from the brain we observe the same tendency to confuse the anatomical and informational notions. According to the European experts, the key structure of the nervous system is the cell; that is, the neuron. Meanwhile, it is apparent that the cell is only one element in the circuit and not its information. The element of the circuit transforms the information and transfers it further. For example, current intensity decreases or increases in every element of an electrical circuit, and so on. These very changes of the information parameters are significant, rather than the geometry (shape, size, angles) and density of the elements of the circuit. Therefore, the description of the visual parameters of the cell has no meaning for the informational significance, capacity and specific transformations of the data when they pass through the cell. Moreover, the consideration that the hereditary and programmed information, which is inherent to the cell genome, and gene expression correlate with the cell geometry and morphological plasticity does not stand up to scrutiny. Without any doubt, the shape of a cell is conditioned by its proteome and, accordingly, by its genome, but external appearance does not have any special significance to the informational content and internal relations and interrelations in a cell, or, if they do, it is extremely indirect. We think that the morphological structure of a cell is a complex manifestation of all of its information levels, but it does not give anything, if evaluated according to the informationology. Within the framework of our information approach we consider a nervous cell to include all of the abovementioned levels of a neuron (genome, transcriptome, proteome and metabolome) and to integrate the electromagnetic field which is formed by all of the biochemical machinery of the preceding levels of information; that is, its magnetome. Hence, the acquisition of information about the magnetome of these cells is more significant for modeling than studies of the shape, size and geometry of angles and sprouts of the nerve cell. At this level, we have considerable divergence from the methodology of the system approach of the HBP specialists.

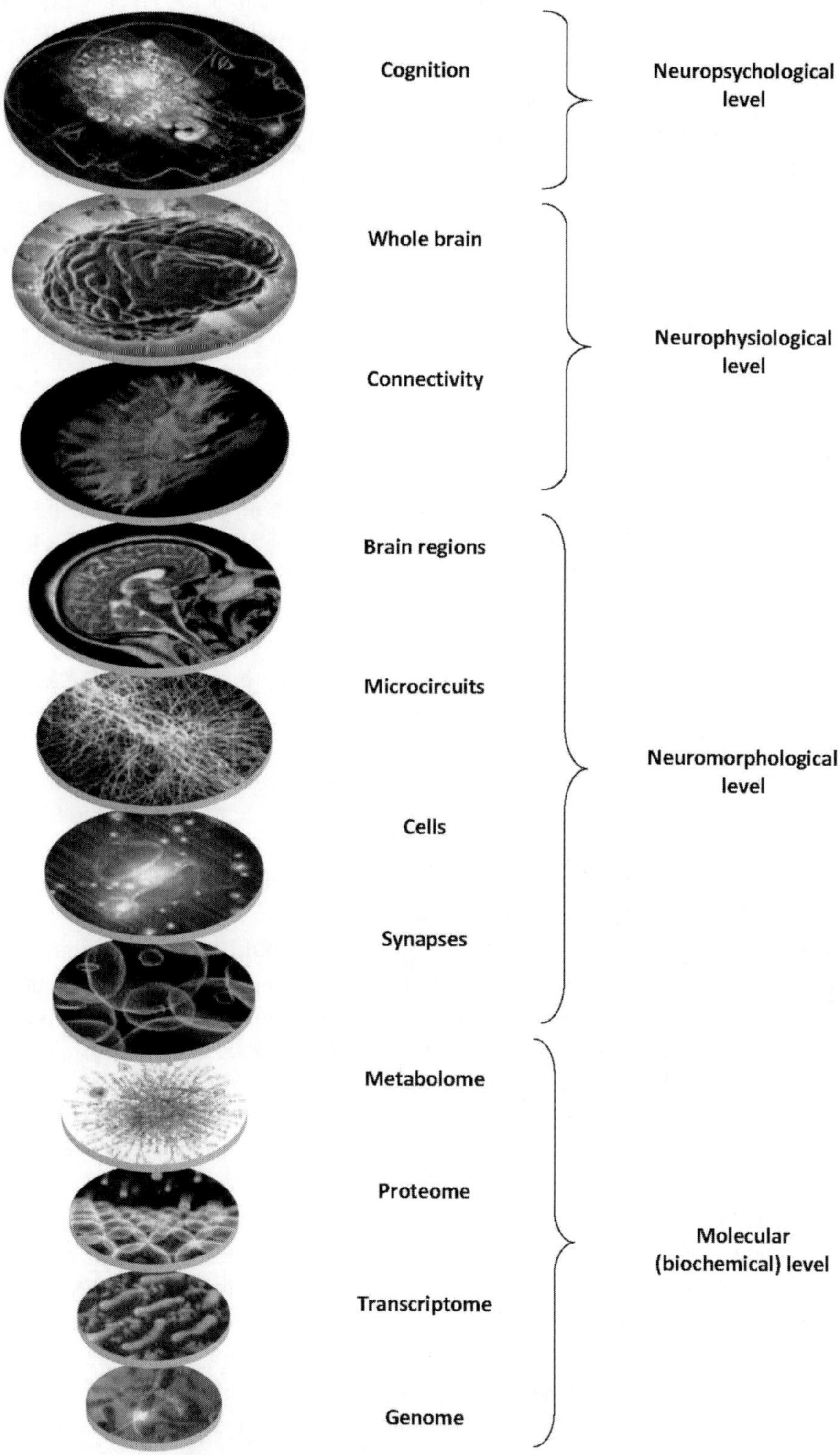
Cognition
Neuropsychological level
Whole brain
Neurophysiological level
Connectivity
Brain regions
Microcircuits
Neuromorphological level
Cells
Synapses
Metabolome
Proteome
Molecular (biochemical) level
Transcriptome
Genome

Figure 45.

Further, the morphological tendency in the system approach of the Human Brain Project to the study and analysis of the evidence about the brain does not change either. The next level of the system approach is cellular microschemes, which is the sets of the systems of cells that are anatomically united in the integral morphological formations in the brain (subcortical nodes, nuclei of cortical nodes, etc.) formed by means of cellular and molecular composition; these allegedly support the role of the cells in the cognitive sphere, and cell geometry and patterns of the selection of the synapses condition local synaptic connections (connectivity) in the models of microschemes (the HBP). The HBP researchers are convinced that electrophysiology, multi-electrode records and optogenetic tests will provide the information for the validation of the models of micro-schemes. However, the evidence received in these tests will not show how the information travels through the microschemes, or how it is related with upstream and downstream levels of the information. Here, the anatomy of the brain is opposed to the informational principles of its organization. In this case, the brand of the cell phone equals or is opposed to the character of the transferred data.

Undoubtedly, the studies of the switchboard, which consists of a set of micro-schemes, cannot present the informational content of this level. The authors of the Human Brain Project are convinced that morphological research with structural and functional MRI will permit such measures of the brain regions that can be used to develop the brain simulations. They think that information about cell architecture and brain tissue density, which is typical for specific brain regions, conditions the cell composition of the regions of the simulations. However, as previously stated, this information level unites anatomical and information terms and the associations of their scientific content are not clear for the analysis of the informationology of the research. It is not clear, either, how the distribution of the receptors, ion channels and other proteins will condition the neurochemical organization inside and between the brain regions, and, moreover, how information about the correlation of protein profiles, cognitive networks and genome variability will display neural mechanisms of the cognitive sphere. The relationship between the genome and neural mechanisms of the cognitive sphere cannot be traced here even theoretically.

In the opinion of the HBP specialists, "This work would map the architectures of different layers and areas of the brain, providing constraints for simulation and modeling by introducing area-specific information on the level of large cognitive systems and behavior". Besides, it remains unclear what important evidence can be produced by the diffusion tensor imaging (DTI) and fiber tracking which, of course, can provide evidence about the pathways and density of the fibers for the studies of connectivity inside and between the regions of brain. However, it is already well studied and described by the neuroanatomists of the previous century and hardly requires further elaboration. Yet, it remains an important issue for the analysts and developers of mathematical modeling. Still, even in the electrical circuit it is important to understand the principles of the elements' connections (series or parallel) and not the color of wires and the way they interlace, not to mention the brain. It is obvious that anatomical evidence about a whole brain received via multimodal sensor physiology and anatomy is hardly able to depict how different regions of the brain cooperate to form certain functions of the brain (perception, locomotion, awareness), or to help validate the simulations of the human brain. But what can these manifestations of higher nervous activity be "attached" to –anatomy again, the genome or proteome of the neuron? What is the relationship between synchronic scans of the brain's vasculature and the support of the cognitive sphere and the brain's metabolism? It all seems to be confused and united according to discrepant characteristics. It seems to me that at this information level we should study the relationships and interactions of the information structures of the nerve tissue that result from the interaction of magnetomes of different cell systems, which are the main elements of the tissue. Today, these are not merely words; it became possible with the development of computer magnetic encephalography.

Further correlations made by the HBP experts are also diverse, as they repeatedly propose visual research and the consequent integration of evidence at the level of the whole brain. We presume it to be methodologically incorrect. The integration of anatomical evidence at the level of the brain region will not result in anything significant because this information has been available for a long time already and some quantitative variations will hardly make a big change. But if we look at the information maps of the magnetomes of different brain regions and match them with the informational structures of the tissues located in the regions and then, with the help of neuro-mathematical methods and multilayered neural networks, integrate these data into databases that reflect the multi-layers and multilevels of the information, this could be both interesting and promising.

Regarding the brain as a whole, we have already described our views on the issue in Chapter 4. The brain of a human or a mammal, which consists of the information structures of its regions, emerges integral when these information systems are united by the pia mater, which belongs to the biological ICMs of NT of the cortex of these regions. The integration of the regions at the level of a whole brain does not happen after the integration of anatomical data as a whole, but it happens as a result of the holographic interaction of the magnetomes of these informational structures. Due to this, the holograms of the information image matrices are formed and they serve the informational link between all involved informational structures and the main regulator and synchronizer of the parameters of these structures to fulfill the function. Therefore, holographic IIMs have their own features, amplitude and frequencies and they can be measured; they have specific characteristics associated with the cognitive activity of humans. Only in this case would it be possible to trace the relationship between cognitive function and the genome and post-genome characteristics of the informational structures involved in its formation.

In Figure 46 we can see the difference between receiving the evidence in our approach and that in the HBP. We consider only natural formalized biophysical and biochemical processes to be informational. In the HBP the formalized natural biochemical and artificial morphological, neurophysiological and neuropsychological information, which was the result of the analysis of subjective relations of the researchers to the brain, ranked equally.

In the flagship report the authors of the HBP did not answer an important question: what is the key system-forming element of the system that they developed and why did they integrate heterogeneous information? What is the purpose of integrating the evidence from different levels and of differing quality? What is its benefit for the mathematicians who are trying to analyze a whole brain?

I am full of respect for the European and American neurologists in general, and for the separate researchers engaged in the project in particular. And it would be incorrect to criticize the proposed ideology and methodology as well as the authoritative opinions of the team of leading experts in clinical neurology and fundamental neuroscience about the issue of the understanding and modeling of the brain, if you are unable to propose your own idea. I have my own ideas on the improvement of the available methodology of computer modeling of brain and, accordingly, on the development of new technologies for knowledge acquisition and I have described them in Chapter 7. Still, I would like to comment on the methodological scientific platform of the HBP and provide several arguments that characterize its theoretical and conceptual weakness and certain inconsistency.

In my opinion, the team work dedicated to the development of the principles of brain understanding and research has a dramatic methodological and technological blunder associated with the stake made on the system approach that would prevent them from finding the solution in due time or would cause significant delay. Obviously, in three or five years the team will face a wall of insurmountable technological obstacles associated with the incorrect understanding of the mechanism of the brain's organization and operation, and this is absolutely logical and predictable.

So, what is the key methodological error of the theory of understanding the brain described in the HBP and the principles of its operation that are planned to be employed for the development of mathematical models? Let us abstract from the comparison of our methodological approaches and consider the biased attitude of provincial Russian scientists to the top European researchers. Let us admit that I am wrong with all my opinionated and orthodox thinking and the truth belongs to the European methodology of research. Let us take "the end" as a starting point; that is, the expected results of the realization of a large-scale scientific research, and what these fundamental and amazingly expensive projects of the brain research are supposed to bring.

The results that such a project is expected to obtain are the development of novel neuromorphic computer systems that operate in the image and likeness of the human brain: 1) the information and communication technologies and platforms, as well as a virtual computer simulation of brain: the goals of the HBP; 2) the development of the information neuro-technologies and biotechnologies of the brain-computer interface: the goals of the Brain Initiative; 3) a computer map of the activity of the neural network of the brain and the database of all connections in the brain: the goal of the Human Connectome Project.

Without any doubt, the authors of these projects suppose further use of the acquired informational neuro-technologies to form new markets of biotechnologies, development and introduction of the advanced highly technological simulations of the brain to medicine with the hope that they will help in the study of nervous diseases, develop new pharmaceuticals and solve the challenges of the brain-computer interface, as well as engaging the developed innovations to the military neuro-technologies for the defense in their countries. Highlighting the resulting information and communication technologies, the authors of the projects rely on the methodology of the system approach and not on the ideology and methodology of the mathematical theory of information. It is rather strange that the mathematicians and programmers followed physicians and brain researchers who do not know the basics of mathematical logic and the theory of communication developed by the father of the information theory, Claude Shannon; they did not study the theory of distributed processing of information by Eduard Yevreinov [158] and do not know the works of Norbert Wiener about cybernetics and informationology, or the automata theory and the theory of informationology. Otherwise, it would definitely set them thinking about how they could develop the information and communication platforms of the brain research and new approaches to the analysis and processing of multilevel and multi-scale information, if they ignore the framework of informationology.

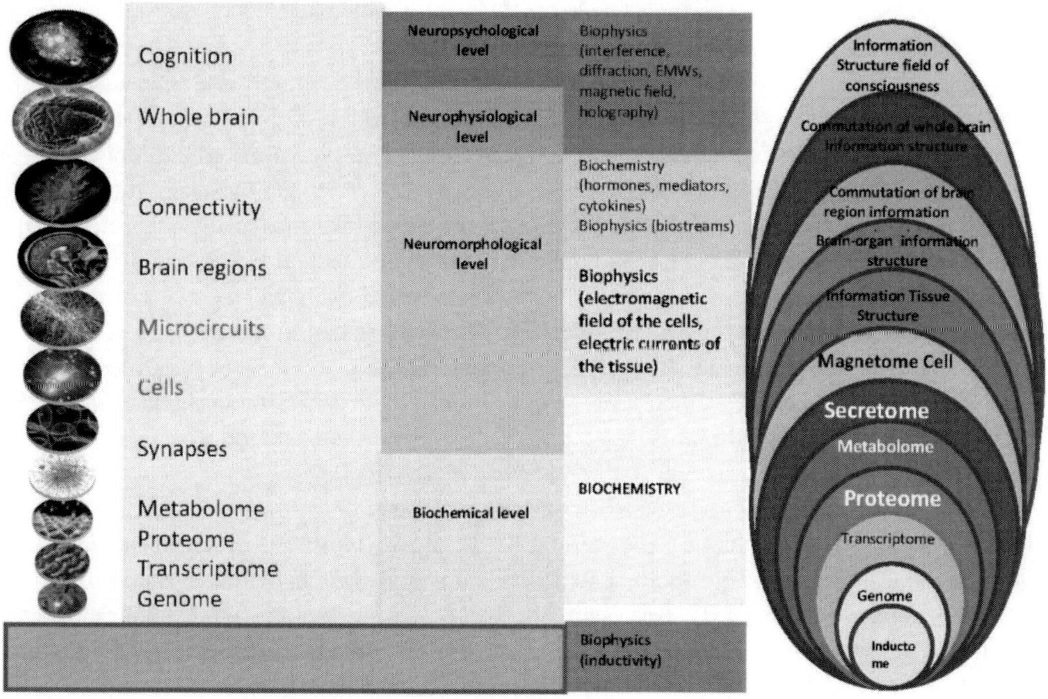

Figure 46.

Another reason for the failures and erratic scientific constructions in neurology lies in the discrepancy between the visual image of an object and the information structure and complexity of the studied object. To date, the principle of visualization to obtain and to process the information was the main engine for progress in neurology and other neurosciences. Everything that the researchers have seen with their eyes and registered as an image via medical computerized recording devices is considered information. Much better, if the picture, which is supposed to reflect the acquired information, could be multicolored by means of mathematical transformations of the shades of gray, or using fluorescent dyes. The information is acknowledged by the scientific community to be the most informative and advanced if it is colored with antibodies that are able to specifically stain any protein substrate in the mammalian/human brain, or if it is a computer image of the latest tomographic equipment. Other information, which cannot be evaluated visually, is perceived extremely skeptically and is considered non-demonstrative. On the one side, it was very convenient and obvious for the development of the methods of visualization in medicine, but, on the other side, we lose huge bulks of information that could be used for understanding the mechanisms of the operation of the brain and the development of new therapies of brain diseases. For example, a nice picture of the brain MRI has completely replaced the essence of the method, and, namely, the level of magnetization of certain brain structures. In general, contemporary journals treat everything that concerns biophysical information extremely skeptically and such research findings are only published as something "physical" which is barely informative for neurologists and neuroscientists. Misunderstanding of the biophysical processes of the brain by the biochemists (immunologists, geneticists, neurobiologists, molecular biologists, specialists working in cultural labs, proteomic labs, transcriptomic labs, etc.) who head all top-rated journals has led to a situation where all biophysical information is perceived as foreign to biology and medicine.

The third reason for the failures and methodological errors is the impossibility of juxtaposing information of differing quality and of different levels in one frame of reference. The methodology of the system approach is meant for the analysis of information of one level and for processing information which is quite homogeneous in its quality. Then, it permits the detection of important systemic patterns in one frame of reference using the rules of the theory of system control. As, for example, we can draw a chart of the interrelations of proteins in a cell of the system of genetic networks or describe the main proteins of the signal transduction pathways and learn to manage them. But when it concerns incomparable information belonging to different levels, this approach cannot unite it in a goal tree or a chart of logical structure, because there is no logic in the theory of systems, but there is the continuous flow of information, its transformation and the order of its transformation with the transfer from one level to another.

If we accept that everything that I described in Chapter 7 is a mistake, the principles of informationology still remain. The question is: What is the difference between the informational structure of the brain and spinal cord and the analogous morphofunctional system which is represented by the system approach? Can the main difference be reduced to additional mechanisms of information acquisition and elimination? Where is biological activity, the holographic nature of the mind, cognitive functions and others in this information structure? Let us try to understand it.

According to the system approach, the brain as a system consists of several functional systems (following Konstantin Anokhin and Konstantin Sudakov [26, 157]) and their structural elements are cell formations of different parts of nerve tissue, which consists of separate cells (neurons, astrocytes, oligodendrocytes and microglia), synapses between nervous cells, fibers of nervous cells, arterial and venous vessels. Different parts of nerve tissue form different regional structures with specific functions (brain lobes, brainstem, pituitary gland, hypothalamus, cerebellum, corpus callosum, etc.). Together they form a whole organ called the brain. That is the morphological (anatomical, histological, cytological) principle of studies that is taken as the basis for brain research, as well as psychophysiological and neuropsychological principles. Despite the legitimacy and appropriateness of the approach, it does not permit an evaluation of the internal relations and interactions of the elements of the brain system. Moreover, brand new molecular data of genome and post-genome technologies (transcriptomics, proteomics, metabolomics, etc.) can hardly stay within the framework of these systemic-morphofunctional views. Psychophysiology, psychology and neuropsychology are incomparable with the genome and post-genome evidence and need the interface between them to be developed.

Summarizing the abovementioned information, for both approaches information received by the researcher is the key system-forming factor at all levels of brain research. The transferal, storage and transformation of the information from level to level are the thing that is common to all available methodologies of brain research. Information as a universal generative basis of nature and society is the uncontested resource of scientific progress. In some fields (computer science, cybernetics) information is the measure used to eliminate uncertainty (entropy); in the information theory it is the number of received, processed and transferred messages (bits). In the newly appeared scientific field called synergetics (from the Greek *sineros* – working together) information means the measure of the organization (coherence, connection and orderliness) of the system is the condition (reason) for coherence of its composing elements which leads to a reduction of self-relations and self-organization of these elements and the reduction of the entropy of the system which, in turn, leads to the enhanced coordination and coherence of the system in general.

Natural information of the surrounding world is the primary reason for the emergence of living beings, the condition for their development and improvement. Information is the foundation of the relationships between people and nature; it is the substance of the relationships and emergence of an integral global information-cellular community. Information is a universal (omnipresent) field of relationships and reflections inside us, between us and outside us. Information is the universal generative foundation of the Universe. However, we must keep in mind that information can be natural or artificial. The term "artificial information" is represented as written material, acoustic information, radio- and tele- transmissions, computer and typographic books and everything man-made is the consequence of natural information manifested in the real world, our sensations and observations.

Hence, all of the above assumes that only natural and formalized information that is received from different levels of the nerve tissue and located in the key regions of the brain should be taken as the basis for a promising informational mathematical simulation of the brain. The key regions of the brain include all of the cortex of the brain and the cerebellum (the square of the cortex is 1600cm^2 and the thickness of the cortex 0.5 mm (0.05 cm) = 80 cm), 20 cm^3 of nerve tissue of subcortical ganglias, 10 cm^3 of the nerve tissue of the brain stem and pons cerebelli. That is, about 100 cm^3 must be included in the research. The information received from different informational levels of the studied object must be objective, valid and verifiable; only in this case can it be structured and systemized within the researched level according to its scale. The incomparable data and incommensurable terms cannot be integrated within one level. At every specific level the principle of systematicity of the integration of equisignificant and equivalent information must function. The principle of integration of the information received from a specific level must be obvious even to non-specialists.

The first for the analysis is the level of tissue-specific multilevel information structure that embraces several levels: wave-resonant, elementary particles and atomic. Previously, we have shown that the integral value of all these levels is the magnetization of the studied part of the nerve tissue that can be measured in the course of transformations of the data of magnetic resonant imaging of the brain. The information of this level is clear and not questioned; we called it the inductome of the nerve tissue. Management of the inductome opens up fantastic opportunities to manage the genome of the brain nerve tissue affecting the signal transduction pathways and to manage proteome. In other words, at the level of regulation of the inductome, one can manage proliferative processes and the differentiation of the cells and brain tissue; one can combat atrophic processes and suppress proliferative processes in the brain without the use of pharmaceuticals or physiotherapy. It can become a new novel filed in the therapy of nervous diseases, on condition of the right approach and rational effect on the information-commutation modules of the nerve tissue.

To construct the model, the information received from the level of genome must contain the profiles of genome DNA, the data of gene structure and other natural biochemical information obtained in gene sequencing. However, this information should not include theoretical concepts and schemes of geneticists about mutations or any logical speculations of the researchers, such as fanciful schemes of the search for genetic polymorphisms, etc. Artificial information on the characteristics of the level in the manner of the subjective analysis and sensations of the researcher must not be the object of structuring and integration of the data with objective formalized and standardized data of uniform biochemical tests. The methodology and formalization of the manner of obtaining natural biochemical evidence at the next post-genome levels (transcriptome, proteome, metabolome, secretome) must fully meet the demands that were described for genome level research. Additional morphological information should not be used to expand the informational continuum of the data of a certain level, or replace the biochemical data. One should follow the principle of homogeneity and stereotype of the information; we cannot use neurophysiological evidence from the cell and from inside the cell, or microscopic phenotypical characteristics of the cellular and sub-cellular elements in one row with biochemical data; that is, unite them and find correlations between them and the multilevel biochemical structure of these cell systems. Apparently, the microscopy and neurophysiology of the cells are an absolutely different and higher level of the information continuum and hierarchy and can be matched with the multilevel biochemical structure.

Therefore, I refused to obtain information from the artificially defined morphological level of synapses. Previously, I have already explained that it is inappropriate and inadequate to receive objective information from such a micro-anatomical structure as the synapse. So, in the methodology of the development of mathematical brain simulation involving the informational approach we propose the use of information released by the cell, i.e., by the secretome of a cell that permits the transfer of data from one cell to another, instead of the synapse. The content of natural information output by the cell (its secretome) or input through the synapse is more important from the informational point than the anatomical structure of the connector that links these cells.

Besides, I reject gathering the information about the cell as a biological object, its phenotype, geometry and staining opportunities by various dyes. These characteristics bring no valuable information, though the cells are the main structural element of life according to contemporary systemic views. At first glance, everything about the cell seems right. The cell is the basis of life on Earth. According to the systems theory, the cell is the thin line that separates animate objects from inanimate ones. Everything above the level of the cell in this system belongs to animate objects, and everything below is inanimate. But according to the theory of information, the cell is one of the elements of the scheme that processes the data, the goal of which is to acquire, to store, to transform or to transmit the information. Was an ordinary transistor of the 1960s the key element of an electric circuit that transmits the information (current) in the scheme of a wireless? Of course not. Over the course of time, its functions could be fulfilled by other radio components that work according to the same principles. For example, it can be replaced by a microchip based on microcircuits or nanotechnologies. This would be very small and more efficient. The main thing in the information scheme is the fact that the information element fulfills a necessary function. We would like to stress again that the principle of the informational influence of a cell on the flow of the information which is transferred through it is important for us. A somatic cell is only one of the options of the conversion element and information switchboard in the body. According to informationology, it is more important to understand what makes the cell a living body, what provides the work and interaction of different informational levels inside the cell and helps transmit the data from one level to another, both inside and outside the cell.

The electromagnetic field emitted by the intracellular structures, i.e., the magnetome of the cell, is that informational mechanism. That is, according to the theory of information, all informational levels, from genome to magnetome, present an informational structure that we define as a cell, from the anatomical viewpoint. But the magnetome is a system-forming factor in the hierarchy of the informational levels which provides for the target-oriented and coordinated movement of data between the levels and their management.

The next level of the mathematical modeling must be the acquisition of data from different parts of the nerve tissue to describe the tissue-specific multilevel informational structure. We do not think it practical for mathematical modeling to examine cellular "micro-circuits" or, in other words, the complexes of cells with various geometry that form the nerve tissue in different regions of the brain. All information about these structures of the studied system the authors of the HBP expect to obtain from electrophysiological tests, multi-electrode records, and cell mapping with the help of staining and optogenetic tests. The microelectrode records of bioelectrical activity of specific areas of the brain tissue are very interesting and spectacular, though it is not quite clear why we need this artificial information and how it can integrate all down- and upstream informational levels of the studied system: from genome to connectome and, moreover, to cognitive sphere. I think that to evaluate the informational level of tissue the electromagnetic features of the studied part of the nerve tissue must be examined; that is, the magnetome of a specific part of the nerve tissue. Now I will be able to map the magnetome of the human brain tissue using low-invasive technologies of computer magnetic encephalography.

Therefore, we have almost everything necessary to develop a primary information unit of the information-commutation module of the nerve tissue for our information simulation of the brain's operation; the information from various levels can be recieved, profiled and integrated in a multilevel information-commutation structure using cloud computing and neuromathematics. This very structure of a topically specific sample of nerve tissue is the main structural element of the brain's organization and operation.

According to the methodology of the informational approach, the next level of the informational knowledge that is necessary for understanding the brain's operation and for the development of mathematical models of the brain seems to be an integrated magnetome of the tissue that emerges due to the interactions and interference of the magnetomes of the cells (neurons, neuroglia, endotheliocytes and fibroblasts of the vessels, synapses, etc.) entering the anatomical entity of this part of the tissue, and not an anatomical formation of the elements of the nerve tissue that consists of the set of the nervous cells with various geometry. Integration of the informational layers of the cell elements of the tissue forms a specific integral composition that consists of the DNA profile of these cells (genome) with the normalized signal intensity (NSI) profile, gene expression of these cells (transcriptome), the profile of NSI of the proteins of these cells (proteome), the profile of the products of metabolism of the cells (metabolome) and the magnetomes of each of these cells (magnetome). Therefore, informationally, the key features and values of the magnetome of the studied sample of the nerve tissue will correlate with the characteristics of the genome, post-genome and magnetome levels of the cell components of the tissue.

Further research of the HBP experts is oriented toward the morphological and functional characteristics of the information about different regions of the brain with the help of structural and functional MRI. The researchers are convinced that MRI and fMRI permit the measurement of the brain regions, which can be used for brain simulation development. This is logical. But the question arises: What difference do the sizes of the brain lobes make to the informational principles of the brain's operation? Is one lobe smaller or bigger in different people and what is the difference between the geometry and tissue density of one person's brain lobe and those of another? For what element of the model is this necessary? The cell architecture and tissue density, which are characteristic of the specific region, condition the cell composition of the model's regions, as the HBP experts say, but these aspects have already been studied at the previous level. And it is still unclear how and why the distributions of the receptors, ion channels, signaling and other proteins, which are considered to condition neurochemical organization inside and among the brain regions, are being studied.

It seems to be reasonable to examine and describe the multilevel informational structure which is formed in a specific region of the brain at a specific moment. Or, in other words, we scale up the knowledge of the informational structure of different samples of tissue within one brain region and form the matrix of the information image (MII) of this brain region. This is done so that at the next stage these MIIs will be united into the integral informational structure of a whole brain that consists of the MIIs of its regions at a certain moment. It is not very important for us to know how these regions are connected technically because it is absolutely clear that there is an anatomical communication. But it is of key importance for us to know how these communication relations in the whole brain are activated at a specific moment and how this activated information structure can be presented in three dimensions. So, the research of the connectome (existing anatomical connections between the regions of a whole brain), which is proposed in the HBP, has significant fundamental meaning for the personalization of anatomical data in the connectome structure, but it is of minimal informational importance for the mathematical modeling of the brain. The principle of the informational relations in the whole brain must be replicated and not the color, appearance or thickness of the nervous fibers that connect its regions. Meanwhile, the functional methods of brain research (functional MRI and PET) can show the activity of the brain structures, at least, in the area of the brain's cortex, so that we can try to relate this activity with the multilevel informational-commutation structure. In other words, a functional MRI of the brain will help us to find out how the lights on a switchboard turn on and we can make implicit judgments about the processes inside the switchboard. This is probably not what we want to get.

According to the HBP specialists, the pinnacle of brain research is the study of the cognitive functions of the brain. But this information is artificial and subjective. We consider the research of the biophysical informational level of the field of consciousness to be the top informational level of the brain. This logically follows from the main principles of the brain's operation and its organization. Consequently, the cognitive functions of the brain can be related only to dynamic holographic matrices of the information images, but not to the results of encephalography or magnetoencephalography.

Chapter 9

THE METHODOLOGY FOR DEVELOPING A 3D SIMULATION OF THE BRAIN USING THE INFORMATIONAL APPROACH

ABSTRACT

The methodology and the principles for the 3D modeling of the human brain on the basis of the information-communication theory and information approach are represented in this chapter. The author analyzes the advantages of the information approach as related to the development of the virtual 3D models of the brain of a new type. The main sources of the information that is necessary for the multilevel mathematical modeling of the brain are determined. In the chapter the author describes how to translate the theory of brain modeling to practice. It is very important to correctly estimate the role and meaning of the mathematical model for understanding the clinical picture of the nervous and mental diseases, for the development of new computing equipment and the solution of the issues of biological computer science. Using simple examples, the author explains methodological errors in the brain modeling and proposes optimal technological solutions for the development of mathematical simulations of the brain, ways to answer the challenges and to overcome unsolved issues. The chapter shows that the neurons and neural networks are overrated in brain modeling, while the role of the microenvironment of the neuron that forms the module of the nerve tissue is underestimated. For contemporary simulations of the brain, only one leading parameter of the brain is taken into account, and the relationship of life-time data about the brain tissue that can be received by various imaging techniques (CT, MRI, PET, MEG, EEG) with the genome and post-genome values of the specific site of the brain tissue is omitted. If stated once, the model of the interrelationship of molecular disorders and imaging tests of the nerve tissue of the brain permits the prediction of disease by any information level of the tissue. The new molecular-wave approach to the brain modeling in various disorders is proposed. Moreover, the author makes several theoretical propositions and conclusions about the methods and technologies for the biomanagement of the functions of a healthy and a diseased brain and possible novel approaches to the therapy of the diseases of the central nervous system.

Keywords: information mechanisms of the development of the symptoms of brain injury, brain concussion, Parkinson's disease, cortical atrophy, neurocomputing technologies, superneurocomputer, neural interface, brain-computer interface, brain-like computer systems

In this chapter we will consider an opportunity for the practical application of the information approach and the information-commutation theory in the development of an alternative 3D virtual simulation of the human/mammalian brain in health and in disease. What benefits can the methodology of the information approach and our unified theory of the brain give to the development of a new type of virtual simulation of the brain? First, the methodology has already proposed a novel model of the information structure that consists of the information-communication modules of nerve tissue and can be used to simulate different configurations of the information structure of all nerve tissue of the brain. It provides a real alternative to a biological model of a neuron. Second, the use of the information simulation of the ICM of NT of the brain permits the registration, mapping and profiling of experimental data of every information level of the studied cell systems of the nerve tissue. Third, with the help of the advanced technologies of neurocomputing mathematical programming it is possible to receive the summarized mathematical simulation of the ICM of NT of the studied sample of the nerve tissue using the received objective information about each information level. A completely digitalized structure of the ICM of NT of any part of the brain enables the use of the ICM of NT in the development of a neuromorphic artificial architecture of the brain that will be close to biological and will consist of different ICMs of NT.

The received digitalized information structure of ICMs of NT can be installed on the multilayered neural networks that mimic neural systems of the nerve tissue of the brain. As a result, the picture is similar to that in a living brain: multilayered, multi-qualitative and multi-component biological information about the structure of a specific brain area is introduced into the multilayered neural network of that area of the brain. This structure has severe restrictions in the interaction of the levels, which are conditioned by hereditary features, i.e., by genome level. The information in this neural network is transformed and integrated into a new information body; namely, an information matrix of neural tissue (IM of NT) of the specific part of the brain nerve tissue. It can be modeled anytime and we can see how different information levels of the specific zones of the nerve tissue of the brain change their biochemical, biophysical and functional activities; for example, under the influence of a pharmaceutical. The IM of NT reacts to the external and internal information in the synchronized interrelated response of every level, and this response is of key importance to all other levels. The IM of NT does not depend on the morphological connections between neurons, neuroglia and vascular cells in the nerve tissue, or on the number of sinuses between them, but it demonstrates the unity and opposition of the changes in the information flow through the biochemical substance with its biophysical and functionally active manifestations. The cells as biological objects, synapses as the means of their connection, the combination of cell nuclei as specific morphological substrate are not related to the information that flows through them, so their geometry and phenotype can be ignored informationally for the sake of increasing the objective information significance of the results of profiling different levels of the multilevel system of the examined sample of nerve tissue.

It should be noted that the number of neurons and neural layers, synapses and connections between them plays almost the most important role in all mathematical simulations of the brain. How important and how objective is this information? Let us draw an analogy between the brain modeling and the electrical design project of a house. Are we interested in the number of wires and terminals that are necessary for the assembling? Then, why are we so concerned about the number of synapses for brain modeling? What difference does the brand of the sockets, switches, terminal blocks and circuit substrate make for the quality of current conductance? These details are necessary only at the stage of project assembling and only to the narrow group of people involved. What is the importance of the number of the terminals (synapses) between the wires used in the project? Does it matter what color and what length the wires (connectome) are that are used to join the main elements of the electric circuit? What difference does it make how many resistors (cells of neural matrix) are used to make the circuit function? It is the internal properties of the wires - internal characteristics of the terminals that would not lead to the short-circuit failure and resist the power surge - that are really important. And, of course, the main and strictly guided order of connections (communicative connections) between the elements of the scheme matter.

Returning to the information model of the brain, the commutation of the information structures of specific areas of the nerve tissue is most significant for the development of the virtual model of the brain. We can choose the way proposed by the HBP to study the communication connections of the information structure within the brain regions (brain lobes, basal ganglia, cerebellum, etc.) and of the brain on the whole, but we should not restrict ourselves by the communication connections and information structure of one nervous cell, a neuron. Contemporary technologies are rough and imperfect so far and do not permit examination of all information levels using one cell. I repeat myself, but it is extremely important. This is associated with the technological characteristics of contemporary genome and post-genome research of the cell systems. For example, for genome analysis we need to study the DNA of at least two million cells. For the microarray of gene expression (transcriptome) we need no fewer than 2.5 or 3 million cells in order to receive the requisite number of RNAs for complete transcriptome analysis, while 2 to 4 million cells are necessary for proteome analysis. This number of cells is used to prepare the lysate, which is tested for all known proteins. To study metabolome and secretome we also need a rather large number of pure cell cultures that counts as much as 10^6 of the cells. Hence, to study the information structure of a neuron the researchers need no fewer than 10 million homogeneous "pure" cultures of neural cells. Where can we get them? And do we really need the data received from pure cultures of neurons? It has nothing to do with the real situation. We need the data from a real information-commutation module of the nerve tissue sample.

From the standpoint of theoretical neurology, the development of the information structure of a separate neuron will have an important fundamental and academic meaning in the future, but it has no practical meaning for neuro-research aimed at the development of the virtual model of the brain. We would like to repeat that the information structure of the nerve tissue in specific functionally important ICMs of NT (brain cortex, cerebellum, basal ganglia, brainstem, etc.) and their communication are of fundamental significance for the development of the information models of the brain. The standard procedure for resuspending the tested sample of the nerve tissue with trypsin will separate the tissue in cells, and help us receive the complex of all cells and morphological elements of the studied sample of the nerve tissue of the brain: the bodies of neurons of different types (motor, sensory, proprioceptive, etc.) and of different types, various types of neuroglial cells (astrocytes, oligodendrocytes, microglia, etc.) different types of synapses that provide for the communication between cells, neural fibers, vascular cells (endotheliocytes), cells of the connective tissue and extracellular matrix (fibroblasts, fibrocytes, myocytes, etc.). However, it is not necessary to do this, because for the bioinformation analysis we need all proteins, RNAs, DNAs, carbohydrates and fats of this part of the tissue and they can be received by working directly with the sample of the nerve tissue.

The information structure of all examined nerve tissues received from a specific part of the brain form the information structure of neural tissue and its research will result in the complete transcriptome profile of gene expression, general proteome profile of all proteins available in this tissue sample, etc. Due to the genetic research of the sample of the nerve tissue, we can receive a general genetic map (genome) and DNA profile (genome profile), but we need not detect mutations in it. These data are irrelevant at this stage. The main parameters of the summarized metabolome profile of the tissue sample can be obtained from the available biological material of the studied brain tissue using MRI mass-spectrometry. The metabolome of the tissue sample can be evaluated and digitalized according to the accumulation and metabolism of glucose in the nerve cells of this sample of the nerve tissue with life-time methods of positron emission tomography (PET) of the brain. This method permits evaluation of the process of utilization of the glucose by the level of the radioactive glucose accumulation in this part of the brain. Profiling of the metabolome data of the studied sample of the nerve tissue can be very important for the development of the information matrix of this information-commutation part of the nerve tissue. The magnetome of the studied tissue sample can also be examined in live objects in magnetoencephalographic mapping of the brain. The inductome of the brain of the trial subject can be calculated according to the results of the MRI and then mapped and profiled in a digitalized way. Now PET scans permit the correlation of the functional activity of the brain with the localization of anatomical formations of the brain when the PET scans are linked to multilevel spiral computer tomography. Hence, localization of the studied sample of tissue will be verified by the data of multi-slice spiral CT. Modeling of the real information images of the ICM of NT on the real anatomy of the brain of the trial subject (human or mammal) permits the development of a personalized 3D simulation of the brain of the studied human or mammal.

All of the data received in the research of the ICM of the studied sample of the nerve tissue of the brain can be integrated into one virtual information image (VII) of this sample of the brain tissue using cloud neurocomputing technologies. Only neurocomputation technologies and neurocomputation mathematics can integrate such heterogeneous data on the basis of neural network-driven integration of the data. This is their distinction and uniqueness. For this, the technologies to develop narrow-focused databases can be used or standard neurocomputation technologies to integrate multi-scale, multi-qualitative and multilevel data can be applied. The superneurocomputer will help to form the digital matrix of the VII of the area of the ICM of NT, receive the mathematical model of this area and detect the patterns, relations and interactions of different information levels in the general structure of the tissue area both between the levels and under the influence of internal and external factors. These neurocomputation technologies are the method of choice in the processing of such data.

It seems possible to “attach” the information matrices of the VIIs of different ICMs of the nerve tissue of the brain to the personal features of anatomical structures of the subject’s brain, because the PET data can already be linked to the anatomy of the brain received in spiral CT or, which is better, MRI. This can now be achieved by means of the standard computer processing of the data using the methods of MRI and PET correlated with spiral CT. With the help of standard technologies of 3D modeling we can receive a 3D virtual model of a whole brain of the object that permits topically oriented distribution of the matrices of the VIIs of the tissue information structures in the brain. The 3D model of the VIIs of the information structure of the brain that reflects the activity of different regions of the brain can be received using the technologies of superneurocomputation for modeling the information structures of different areas of the nerve tissue of the brain. The general scheme of brain modeling should include an extraneural unit of data processing and an intraneural unit of receipt, transmission and modulation of the data. Intraneurally, the VIIs of different areas of the ICMs of NT should be placed in the computer model according to the chart of the brain structure, shown in Figure 41. This will be the complete biochemical and biophysical information that characterizes the VIIs of the object at the intraneural level in norm (intraneural VII). The primary task of this stage of research is to detect the patterns of interaction and interrelations of the information levels inside every tissular structure. At this stage all available relations between the levels of one information system must be detected, along with the interaction of identical levels of different remote information structures (the proteome of one structure with the proteome of other structures; the proteome of one structure with the magnetome of another and the secretome of a third structure). We can study the interaction of the areas with the highest functional activity that is characterized by the change of various information levels and their influence on the neighboring and remote proteome-magnetome changes in the part of the brain tissue.

Further, the mathematical modeling software must model the exit of electromagnetic waves (EMWs) from the ICM-subscribers into the subarachnoid and subdural spaces, the interference of the EMWs and formation of the holograms in the extraneural space of the brain; that is, the formation of the information images of the VII. We need to receive the information matrices of the holograms of extraneural VIIs in different functional states of the subject: sleep, walk, purposeful movements of hands and legs, visualization of images, tests for counting, logic, writing, etc. The result of this work will be the 3D maps of the information structures of the brain and the correlation of interdependence of the extraneural and intraneural VIIs in different physiological states of the brain. As the next stage of the research we can link the state of the information structure of extraneural VIIs to the manifestations of higher psychic and cognitive functions of the trial subject. Thus, we would be able to answer the eternal questions of the neurologists and neurobiologists about the influence of the genome on cognitive functions and *vice versa*.

How can the theory be translated into the development of a personalized 3D virtual simulation of the brain in trial subjects? Let us consider the plan and the main stages for the development of a model of the human/mammalian brain. Before the fundamental research of the brain in humans or animals is initiated, it is necessary to approve and authorize the plan and general program of the research, as well as the main trial protocols at the meetings of the Scientific Board and Ethic Committee of the research center that conducts the trial. Without their approval the neurological research will appear illegitimate and ethically inappropriate. The moral and ethical issues of neuro-research are as important as the genome and post-genome research.

When the ethical and legal issues of brain research are solved, we have to decide upon the personal subjects of the research and the methods of the subject's research. Undoubtedly, the subject of the research is one and the same: the brain. But in every case it differs in size and generic features: in one case it is the brain of a rat (mouse); in another it is the brain of a primate (monkey); in the third – the human brain. The choice of the trial subject depends on the primary goals of the researcher. The brain of a rat or a mouse is convenient for the studies of different biochemical information levels (inductome, genome, proteome, transcriptome and metabolome) in the information tissular structures of the brain. It is better to use the brain of the primate in cases where it is necessary to find correlations between biochemical and biophysical information levels (magnetome, proteome, transcriptome, genome and inductome) in the information structure of the brain tissue.

If we map all information structures of different parts of the nerve tissue of the brain and the development of a 3D virtual model of the information structure of the brain, then the brain of the primate will be the best choice as its size is close to the size of the human brain and it can display the main patterns of how different information levels of the brain interact. Having detected the basic patterns of the information structures of nerve tissue, we can extrapolate the results that were received in the primate's brain to the information structure of the human brain by analogy. The brain of a healthy person can be taken from the donor of the organs for the research. However, in this case we need the informed consent of the donor's relatives for the trial, approval of multiple ethical issues and compliance with many regulations (specialized transplant team, approval of the public institution for the research, etc.) specific to the transplantation procedures. The brain of a neurological patient for morphological, genome and post-genome research can be recovered right after the registration of the biological death of a patient in terminal stages of neurological diseases. The first thing that must be done for the development of the research program and protocols is to define the methods and biomedical technologies that are necessary to develop the information structures of the nerve tissue of the brain that will be further employed in the mathematical modeling of the brain. As far as we plan to receive the information structure of specific areas of the brain tissue, it would be practical to clinically examine the mammal (a mouse, a rat, a monkey, a donor) for visual signs of an organic defect of the nerve tissue (paralysis, paresis, strabismus, gait disorder, etc.) and defects in locomotion. For a primate or a human, a detailed neurological examination is necessary and the neurological status must be registered in the file of neurological examination and the digital visual control of the advanced neurological examination of a primate or a human must be done.

After neurological examination (of a rat, a monkey or a human), the general clinical tests of the subject's organs and systems are performed, including the biochemical testing of blood and neurophysiological testing (EEG, EEG cerebral mapping and electroneuromyography), as well as radiological testing (chest X-ray and brain CT) to verify complete health or nervous disease in the subject. The neurological diagnosis must be confirmed: in one case we must be sure that the subject's brain is intact and in the other to confirm the diagnosis by contemporary methods of clinical and paraclinical diagnostics.

The next stage of the examination must be the specialized computer diagnostic and functional examination that will be used for the development of localized information structures of the areas of the brain. The contrast enhanced MRI of the brain should be done to the subjects. The mice (rats) are scanned with 7 Tesla MRI. The trial monkeys and humans (neurological patients and volunteers) must be scanned with no less than 3 Tesla MRI.

The specialized examination for the development of the information structures of the brain will be continued by functional MRI of the brain with specific functional tests set in the approved protocol of the research (standard hand movements, tests for logic and counting, writing, etc.).

The third specialized method is the positron emission tomography (PET) of the brain associated with 64-slice computer tomography of the brain. This test will help evaluate the changes in radioactive glucose metabolism in the examined areas of the brain and help to correlate the PET results with the morphological substrate and anatomical formations of the subjects' brains. The obligatory stage of the specialized examination includes several functional tests during PET that are described in the approved protocol of the research (purposeful movements of hands and legs, visualization of images, tests for counting, logic, writing, etc.).

The fourth obligatory method of examination must be the magnetoencephalography (MEG) of the brain of healthy and diseased primates and humans. This test permits mapping the activity of the magnetic field of the nerve tissue of different structures of the brain with the accuracy of localization of the magnetic activity focus reaching 10 mm. The obligatory stage of the specialized examination includes several functional tests during MEG that are described in the approved protocol of the research (purposeful movements of hands and legs, visualization of images, tests for counting, logic, writing, etc.).

After the completion of diagnostic and functional tests of the brain the research proceeds to the morphological stage. After the decision on the necessity of morphological tests, the trial rats and primates are sacrificed according to the appropriate regulations established in the research center. All issues related to recovering the brain for the research from the donor are agreed with the head of the transplant team according to the guidelines.

At this stage the brain is removed from the skull of the trial mammals or humans and the standard transplantation solutions, such as *Custodiol* that are used in the transplant practice for perfusion and flushing of donor organs for their protection and preservation, are perfused under high pressure into the major vessels of the brain. When the perfusion of the brain is completed and the arterial and venous blood is washed away from the brain vessels, the brain substrate of the nerve tissue is cut into cubes of 1 cm^3. Every cubic centimeter of the nerve tissue extracted from the brain is placed into perfusion solution and labeled indicating its localization using coordinates of the 3D computer plan of the studied brain or on the appropriate 3D model of the brain map.

Every piece of the extracted and labeled tissue of the brain must be examined histologically and cytologically for their localization in the brain to be confirmed. Then the nerve tissue of the studied area of the brain is divided into 4 parts by lengthwise dissection of the studied sample of the tissue; each of them will be used to prepare the samples for genome and post-genome research. The first part of the cube of the nerve tissue is resuspended into the cells (no less than $2x10^6$) with trypsin and is used for RNA tests, and then the microarray complete transcriptome research of the 25000 genes expression is done. The second part of the tissue sample is used for cell lysate (no less than $3x10^6$) of the nerve tissue for microarray proteome research of 9000 proteins. The third part of the tissue sample is used for MRI spectroscopy of the cells of the tissue and evaluation of the cell metabolism. The third part of one tissue sample will be used to sequence nuclear DNA and genome research as the genome is one for a whole organism. In other probes this part of tissue sample will be used for extended biochemical analysis to profile the secretome of the cell: profile of the cytokines, neurotrophins, mediators in the tissue, etc.

Having completed the stage of collection of the material, the results of morpho-functional research (MRI, PET, CT and MEG) and the data of genome and post-genome information-structural tests of all samples of the nerve tissue are forwarded to the laboratory of the bioinformation analysis where they are first grouped according to the principle of their localization in the brain. Then the IT specialists systemize the available information and systemize the data received from different information levels of the brain tissue sample and then, with the help of mathematical modeling, integrate the data on every sample of the nerve tissue into information structures of the nerve tissue of the brain.

Then the data are mathematically modeled using neurocomputing, and thus, the information from these levels is integrated in one information matrix of the VII. Upon that, the specific mathematical limitations and coefficients are introduced so that all levels are tightly interrelated and interdependent. As a result, every information structure of the studied sample of the brain tissue reflects heterogeneous experimental data of eight information levels: inductome, genome, transcriptome, proteome, metabolome, secretome, cell magnetome and the level of magnetome of the brain tissue sample. Therefore, every examined sample of the brain tissue that was extracted from the labeled area of the brain will have its specific virtual information image and the coordinates in the three-dimensional space of the brain.

Today the technologies for the 3D modeling permit the placement of the information from the VII matrix of the specific tissue sample in the virtual space of a computer model of the brain as consistent with their reallocation in the biological brain; that is, to provide their true localization on the 3D virtual model of the brain. Placement of the information integrated into matrices of the examined areas of the nerve tissue in the three dimensions of the virtual brain and their integration into the global information structure of the brain gives a multidimensional and multilevel impression about the localization of the information in the brain and, accordingly, results in the development of the information image of a certain functional state of the brain. Therefore, the information approach to the development of the virtual model of the brain helps to integrate heterogeneous, multilevel and multi-scale information arrays as well as interconnecting the information from different brain regions in one global extra- and intraneural information structure of a whole brain. It seems that the studies of the information relations between the information structure of a whole brain and the information received in neurological examination or topical diagnostics of the disease, psychic, neurophysiological, neuropsychological and experimentally psychological examination of the subject can be correlated because these information arrays reflect the functioning of the brain as one integral system.

Chapter 10

THE FUTURE OF THEORETICAL NEUROLOGY IN CLINICAL MEDICINE, THE MATHEMATICAL MODELING OF THE BRAIN AND THE DEVELOPMENT OF A BRAIN-COMPUTER INTERFACE

ABSTRACT

In this chapter the author demonstrates the clinical proofs of the information-communication theory of the brain, using such nosological examples as brain concussion, degenerative-dystrophic diseases of the brain, Parkinson's disease, etc., and discusses the near future of theoretical neurology. The information-communication theory gives logical and clear answers to the complicated questions of neurology, and helps to understand such complicated, although absolutely common, processes as sleep, wakefulness, simultaneous control and performance of several functions by the brain, and to answer many other questions that bother every neurologist and psychiatrist with their complexity and ambiguity. The author sets forth his own point of view on the reasons and systemic mechanisms for the development of the range of neurological syndromes of nervous and mental diseases. The author explains some of the clinical phenomena manifested in the disorders of memory and cognition from the perspective of his new information-communication theory of the brain. The chapter briefly outlines the history of the development of neurocomputing technologies and presents a novel concept for the practical realization of scientific achievements in theoretical neurology and opportunities for translating the theory to mathematics, computer science and artificial intelligence developments. The chapter briefly discusses available solutions of the brain-computer interface and the advantages and limitations of the microchip implantation to the mammalian brain. For the first time, the author writes about the methodology and technology of the non-contact remote microwave radioengineering effect on the human brain.

Keywords: future of theoretical neurology, reasons and systemic mechanisms for the development of neurological diseases, neural interface, brain-computer interface, artificial intelligence

In this chapter we would like to understand what theoretical neurology, and specifically, the information principles that we postulated, can give to clinical medicine. We will study the opportunities and reality for the practical application of the unified mathematical model of the brain functioning in clinical medicine, consider the mistakes of the experts in the development of a brain-computer interface, and look at what we can offer to the engineers and programmers for the development of new architectures of computation devices.

So, how can our information-communication theory of the brain help a practicing neurologist in the explanation of the well-known facts of clinical neurology? To begin with, we will consider such a widely spread neurological pathology as traumatic brain injury (TBI) and look at its symptoms from the stance of the information theory. Disordered consciousness or the loss of consciousness in acute TBI is the hallmark of the disease. If consciousness is not lost, the clinical diagnosis is doubtful. Why does a brief or long-term loss of consciousness develop in brain concussion? Clinical neurology gives a simple answer to this question. It is considered a characteristic symptom in terms of nosology and it results from minor micro damages (micro contusions) and micro hemorrhages in the brain caused by minor shock affecting the skull or bones of the spinal column. The neurosurgeons also have their explanations for the mechanism of brain injury: the coup injury occurring under the site of impact or the countercoup injury of the brain on the opposite area associated with cerebral contusions. At first glance it seems correct. But why is it that we can lose consciousness and turn off reality for several seconds, and sometimes even for a minute, in the absence of any pronounced organic change confirmed on the MRI, and then again remember and understand everything? If the reason for this was interneural axonal injuries (damage to neural circuits, synapses and synaptic contacts), then consciousness would not be restored in a few moments. Recovery of these connections would take years of neurorehabilitation and not seconds. However, our scientific and pathophysiological understanding of TBI changes if we acknowledge that reflexes and cognition have an extraneural mechanism, i.e., at the level of the intermeningeal space of the brain, and follow the previously described mechanisms. A shift of the brain in the skull, even by several millimeters, disorders the localization of reflected EMWs from the ICM subscribers at the moment of the shock, so that they miss the ICM receivers of the output information lines to the brain cortex. So the displacement of the brain leads to the short-term disorder of cerebral electromagnetic commutation connections between different regions of the brain and disordered records of the data on the pia, which is accompanied by the loss of consciousness. *The consciousness of a human or animal exists at the definite moment when horizontal and vertical information-commutation connections of different areas of the brain at the intraneural and extraneural (reflex and cognitive) levels in subarachnoid, subduralspaces and brain parenchyma register on the pia mater.* Disordered algorithms in the recording of these connections at the moment of injury do not leave recorded video-, audio-, motor- or sensory IIMs on the pia. So the memories of the events associated with the injury drop out. The explanation is simple, clear and obvious and does not cause any philosophical disputes or questions such as ‘what are memories’, ‘what is consciousness’, etc. The duration of the loss of consciousness is the time taken for the brain to restore its initial position after the injury and to reestablish new extraneural and intraneural vertical and horizontal commutation connections between various information channels and lines found in different areas of the brain.

Memory disorder is the key symptom in the clinical picture of both acute and chronic TBI. The events of retrograde amnesia (loss of memory of the events preceding the injury) or anterograde amnesia (loss of the ability to create new memories for events after the injury) are characteristic of TBI, accompanied by micro hemorrhages or micro ischemias in the brain parenchyma as well as edema and swelling of the brain. However, the pathogenesis of memory disorders remains unclear [10]. Current clinical neurology and neurosurgery explain the symptoms of memory disorders by two-lateral damage of limbic system, particularly, medial regions of the temporal lobe (especially hippocampus), thalamus, hypothalamus, reactivity of nerve tissue, an inflammatory response to micro injuries, swelling of the injured brain and frequent subarachnoid or micro-parenchymatous hemorrhages. To a certain extent this is true, but it does not explain the reason why patients develop retrograde and anterograde amnesias, or why in some cases the memory disorder is short-term, and in some long-term. According to the proposed information-commutation theory of the brain, on the one hand, edema and swelling of NT in the brain block information transfer through the NT ICMs of the brain cortex and the exiting of information to ENIR of magnetomes of various analyzers. On the other hand, even a small subarachnoid hemorrhage in the acute TBI affects the transparency of the CSF, and consequently disrupts its information properties due to the sedimentation and adhesion of blood elements on the pia, arachnoid and dura. The processes in the formation of the IIMs in the ENIR depend on the number of cell elements of blood in the intermeningeal space. Both processes lead to disordered consciousness, such as obnubilation, a soporific state, or even coma. It is conditioned by the disorder of the process of EMW hologram formation in the subarachnoid and subdural space. Certainly, if the events of the period that preceded the injury were not recorded, they cannot be reproduced and that is how the retrograde amnesia is formed. As soon as the blood cells in the CSF lyse (although the CSF remains xanthochromatic), consciousness is restored almost at once, despite high protein levels in the CSF. Blood in the CSF caused by injury leads to swelling and edema of the brain; that is, to the failures of signal commutation in the information lines and channels of the brain ENIR. The failures in commutation are accompanied by disorders in the formation of the cortical NT ICM magnetome and impeded registration of IIMs on the pia. Regression of cortical swelling and restored conductance through the ICMs of the cortex results in the restoration of tissue magnetomes and, consequently, to the restoration of extraneural processing of the information in the brain and awareness. The period after the injury and before the restoration of the record on the pia will be anterograde amnesia. If some part of the pia was injured (micro hemorrhages under the pia, ischemic foci, vessel damage, damage to the pia), the events previously recorded on the pia become impossible to reproduce, which is frequently manifested in retrograde amnesia. The mechanism of transitory global amnesia (TGA) seems to be explained by an isolated spasm of the vessels in the pia occurring in stress, a shocking decrease of body temperature akin to diving in an ice-hole, which leads to loss of orientation in the space and inability to register events on the pia. That is why orientation in personality remains intact and neurological deficit is absent in TGA. After the spasm is released, the orientation and mnestic function of the patient restore rapidly. Therefore, conventional neurology and neurosurgery explains the disorders of consciousness and memory in the TBI as disordered conductance in the brain cortex, but exactly how this happens is as yet not clear, whereas the information-commutation theory offers an explanation as to the development of memory and consciousness disorders of different severities. Severe disorders of consciousness are directly associated with the inability or difficulty in the formation of holographic images in the intermeningeal space of the brain filled with the blood cells, which can also lead to the disrupted permeability of the pia and the arachnoid for the CSF and disorder the scattering property of EMWs issued by magnetomes of the NT ICM of input and output information channels (lines) of the brain. The collision of EMW magnetomes with the elements of blood disorders conditioned and unconditioned reflexes. That is why at the initial stages of coma the reflexes fade, and in atonic coma they disappear completely. The absence of extraneural closure of reflexes characterizes depression of consciousness. Blocked information at the level of cortical NT ICM leads to the absence of reflex closure in subarachnoid and subdural spaces. This is the answer to the question that was left unanswered by clinical neurology and relied on the suppositions about inhibition and loss of reflexes due to edema and disorder of the synaptic connections.

Diffuse adhesion of blood elements on the pia causes failures in memorizing current information and disorders in the restoration of past information in the acute stage. Swelling of the brain parenchyma and cortex leads to disorders of current memorizing associated with edema of the pia. If the elements of blood in the subarachnoid and subdural spaces of the brain are not lysed - for example, blood clots are formed - scars and adhesions develop between the arachnoid and the pia. Clinically, these would manifest as intellectual-mnestic disorders in chronic TBI cases. They can deteriorate due to the deformation of the pia and disorders of its holographic properties, i.e., structural distortions of available holographic imprints of memory engrams on the pia. Obviously, an outdated diagnostic method for TBI, called pneumoencephalography, which was used to diagnose arachnoiditis and adhesions of cerebral meninges by air or gas injections into subarachnoid space, or, occasionally, to separate adhesions between the pia and arachnoid, was extremely traumatic for the pia and for the long-term memory. So, it becomes clear why these manipulations resulted in memory loss that finally led to rejection of the procedure.

Information-commutation theory explains the paradox of neurology and psychiatry: Why does a hysterical attack not lead to a loss of consciousness and amnesia, while an epileptic attack is always accompanied by lost consciousness and memories about the events during the attack? The fact is that in hysteria the extraneural and intraneural links between different regions of the brain are not disconnected, as happens in the epileptic seizure, and, on the contrary, new commutation connections are formed in the brain, in the form of the matrix of information images of a behavior act of a staged attack. An epileptic attack is accompanied by a short-term disintegration of the majority of commutation connections of the brain due to the series of electric impulses from the brain cortex and the reflex spasm of the pia vessels. This explains the loss of memory in epileptic seizure and preserved memories in the hysterical paroxysm.

Subarachnoid and subdural hematomas in TBI lead to a whole range of psychopathological syndromes, varying from slight disorders of thinking and understanding to deep coma. Micro hemorrhage into the brain or white matter resulting from even slight injury (concussion) of the brain entails edema and swelling of the tissue components of the information channels (information channel mistake) around the hemorrhage focus, and disordered information signal conductance by output and input channels manifested in thinking difficulties and severe cerebral asthenia. Hence, the reason for cerebral asthenia is the hindered transfer of information through the information levels of the NT ICM of the brain.

The proposed information-commutation organization of the brain explains the nature of these symptoms as global disorders in the formation of holographic information images in the subarachnoid space, which can lead to severe disorders of the commuting capacities of cortical NT. Thus, it can be argued that any subarachnoid or subdural hematoma must be removed immediately and, regardless of the size or type of compression, a hematoma under the pia may not be left. The consequences of its preservation in the brain are a thousand times more serious than the potential complications from the surgical intervention. This thesis radically changes the existing strategies for surgical interventions in TBI. Even the slightest subdural hematomas must be removed, and in the event of a subarachnoid hemorrhage, it is extremely important to organize the evacuation of blood elements from the subarachnoid space, by cytophereis of the CSF, for example. This approach will permit the avoidance of severe complications of TBI, and significant mnestic disorders in future, as it is ubiquitously known that the brain injury is not dangerous by its presence but in terms of its consequences.

Clinical comprehension of the pia as the main information carrier of memory in such a biological super-computer as the brain and its main resource that provides for manipulations with memories gives a novel understanding of memory disorders and complete amnesia in transitory ischemic attacks and stroke. According to the new theory, a disorder of the blood supply in the vascular pool leads to an ischemic focus in the brain NT and angiospasm in the area of the pia. An angiospastic or angioparalytic state of the arterioles of the pia in a cerebrovascular crisis leads to deformation and the impossibility of reproducing information from the pia, and the situation deteriorates further as a result of disordered information conductance along the input and output channels. The mechanism of such memory disorder seems obvious and allows for the development of a novel therapeutic strategy to treat mnestic disorders.

The mechanism of global amnesias developed since minor doses of clonidine, an antihypertensive agent, have always seemed unclear. Clonidine (2-(2.6-dichlorophenylamino) imidazoline) used to be widely used in the criminal sphere in Russia in the '90s and hundreds of people with full amnesia still stay in psychiatric hospitals for a very long time. Clinically, their organs and systems are functioning normally and their encephalograms are almost within normal range, but their mnestic functions in the brain are lost, while intellectually intact. It would be interesting to study chronic memory disorders such as global amnesia and coma in clonidine overdose. Clonidine is an antihypertensive drug which specifically affects the neurogenic regulation of vascular tone. Clonidine stimulates the peripheral α1-adrenoreceptors and provides short-term pressor action. But, coming through the blood-brain barrier, it stimulates α2-adrenoreceptors of vascular motor centers, reduces the flow of sympathetic impulses from the CNS and releases noradrenaline from the nerve terminals, thus providing sympatholytic action. To date no research has offered a valid explanation regarding the psychopathological disorders and long-term and sometimes irreversible memory loss caused by the drug. However, the information theory of the brain can explain the memory loss and comatose state associated with clonidine. Clonidine overdose mostly affects the pia mater, which has considerable vasculature and vegetative innervations, rather than the brain NT or its major vessels. Angioparalysis of the pia causes it to sag (shrink), leading to coma and amnesia due to an inability to register information and disordered geometry of the surface hologram membrane of the pia.

Interestingly, changes in the geometry and elastic properties of the pia explain the toxic action of alcohol abuse on the memory. Initially, alcohol causes vasodilation of vessels in the pia, straining it and leading to an extremely precise recording of the events; then, alcohol causes the spasm of the pia vessels, leading to the loss of memory of the events associated with the alcohol abuse.

A similar explanation of memory loss can be given for the symptoms of atrophic degeneration associated with atherosclerosis in the brain cortex. Atherosclerosis of small branches of the pia makes its vessels rigid, interfering with its plasticity (we forget names, words, telephone numbers, but can remember them with an effort), and the progression of atrophic processes leads to the degeneration of cortical neural layers closely connected with the pia, causing distortion and misshape of this delicate "hard drive" of our memory. Such initial manifestations of cerebral sclerosis as a staggering and unstable gait result from the dislocated EMWs during the formation of the reflex arc of the motor analyzer.

Senile degenerative processes in the brain's cortex are accompanied by the psycho-organic syndrome of Walther-Buel's triad, comprising poor memory and decreased understanding, and affecting instability. Clinical neurology and psychiatry explain the psycho-organic syndrome in this pathology by atrophic processes in the brain NT, although they give no explanations for how it forms. Information commutation organization of the brain explains the development of such symptoms by considerable expansion of the CSF space between the arachnoid and the pia in the projection of the frontal lobes in the systemic atrophic process. Under such circumstances, the diffusion patterns of magnetome EMWs of cortical ICMs and the formation of holograms are disordered, as well as their localization on the arachnoid and registration on standard ICM receivers and the pia, leading to weakened memory and understanding and an unstable gait. We can force ourselves to restore forgotten information, but it is not remembered by itself. We can consciously control our gait, but our usual gait, which is based on reflexes, is difficult. That is, we can intellectually control the conditioned reflex activity of the brain and are able to activate mechanisms of walking, memory and attention. The interconnection of the frontal cortex with the limbic system of the brain is well known and disorders at the level of channel information exchange can be accompanied by emotional disorders, thus explaining the development of affective disorders and emotional lability.

Currently, hereditary or acquired genetic defects have been detected in every neurological and psychiatric disease. However, according to the proposed information-commutation theory of the brain, genomic mutations have their manifestations in the transcriptome of nerve cells, i.e., in all signal transduction pathways of an NT cell and in the cell proteome, so that they change the phenotype of the affected nerve cells and change the wave and field processes in NT. This opens up a whole range of novel post-genome methodological approaches to the diagnosis and treatment of nervous and mental diseases. The therapies can involve correction of the proteome profile of NT by peptide engineering, or a targeted change of the NT magnetic field (inductome), i.e., a change in the magnetization of pathological NT or cell magnetomes. New therapeutic opportunities for mental diseases can be found in MRI-directed changes in brain tissue magnetization, according to the information-commutation organization theory of the brain perceived as organic (genome-post-genome) diseases of information-communicative properties of NT ICMs in the brain, and not as mental or personality disorders.

The mechanisms and principles of brain operation put forward here explain the development of global amnesias in transitory disorders of blood supply of the brain and strokes. The slightest disorders in the blood supply of the cortical regions in different pools of the brain affect the blood supply in the pia, primarily, and not the state of the gray matter of the brain NT. Steal syndrome leads to the "desertion" of minor branches of the vessels in the pia, disintegration of the information between organ periphery, and transitory paresis of the pia.

The mechanisms and principles of brain operation that we have described can provide an explanation for the development of Alzheimer's disease. Disorders at the level of the genome of cortical neurons lead to disorders in the transcriptome and proteome of the NT ICM receiver of output information line and/or NT ICM subscriber of input line. An accumulation of amyloid in the cortical neurons is a standard manifestation of an imbalance in neuron proteome profiling. A standard channel mistake is formed, and the conductance along cortical NT ICMs and, consequently, the regulatory principle of brain operation becomes disordered. Genetic damage makes the neurons of NT ICM unable to compensate and restore independently, leading to the severe disagreement of information transfer along the output and input information lines, hologram record defects and global mnestic disorders on the pia. In an attempt to restore the proteome balance in NT ICMs, the neurons release excessive protein. The easiest way to restore the intracellular proteome and genome balance in the injured neuron is the simple division of the cell in order to eliminate its pathological components. Therefore, Alzheimer's disease is not a true disease of the brain, but a primitive method of compensating for neurons with a disordered proteome profile. Consequently, the neurons prepare to divide, get rid of unnecessary synaptic contacts and, as a result, become the reason for the disintegration of the cortical NT ICMs, and then of the whole nervous system at the level of cortical NT ICMs due to crude information disorders of information reception/transfer. This concept could radically change the methodology of treatment for this disease.

The information-commutation theory of the brain sheds light on the mechanisms of hallucination and the range of mental diseases involving metabolic disorders of the brain, reactive psychoses and schizophrenia. Hallucinations (auditory, visual, tactile, etc.) are formed IIMs that have not found complete materialization on definite cortical NT ICMs in corresponding analyzers, owing to communication errors of various brain regions, i.e., IIMs materialized on other incidental analyzers. Disorders of algorithmization and programming of IIMs on the arachnoid are an explanation for delusional disorders. And, most important, this demonstrates why the outcome of most mental diseases is psychoorganic syndrome and dementia, which result from disordered data conductance along NT ICMs. I am convinced that the accurate analysis of genome-post-genome disorders of the information levels of the NT ICMs of the brain can help to specify the mechanisms of hallucination and psychopathological syndromes in the cases of mental diseases. Modeling these diseases relying on the open principles of brain organization and functioning reveals a great number of new approaches to the therapy of neurological and psychiatric diseases.

In this chapter we explain only the most frequent symptoms of nerve diseases viewed from the standpoint of the information-commutation theory of the brain and theoretical neurology, but this methodological approach can be widely used to analyze any nerve and mental disease, as well as in forensic psychiatry. All information received by a human through the receptor analyzers is registered on the brain membranes automatically, so the development of the technology to read holograms recorded on the pia of the affected party can make a significant contribution in crime detection and investigation.

New methodology of the brain information-commutation theory permits the development of a technical task for the information-commutation model of the brain's organization and operation, which will be based on the realization of the information principles of the brain's operation, and will not be built only on the brain's anatomy or visualization of morphological data. It will not copy the system mechanisms of the brain connectome. In this work we rely on the objective evidence and facts received in our research and neurological experience. Also, we revise available practices to realize this model on the basis of the available medical equipment and Russian supercomputers.

As we have already mentioned, most experts - usually, the specialists in sciences (physicists, mathematicians, chemists) - who start to work with the principles of the brain's functioning and to solve the tasks of brain modeling, have to face certain challenges when they go deep into the issues of contemporary neurosciences, listening to the leading neurologists and neuroscientists who believe in the morphofunctional approach as the main methodology of brain research and who recommend neuroanatomical schemes. Up to now the "neuromorphic" approach - that is, copying the morphological structure of the brain in program software and neurocomputing - and directly mimicking the topical principle of the functions localized in the brain for mathematical modeling have not led to anything valuable. The task seemed to have been set incorrectly and the views of the neurologists on the work of the main structural elements and a whole brain appeared erratic, leading to unsuccessful mimicking of the morphological structure of the brain (shape of hemispheres, distribution of cytoarchitectonic areas through the cortex, etc.) or modeling only of the internal connections of the brain. Unfortunately, this does not lead to success, but only contributes to the fact that these simulations are unable to fulfill the hundredth part of the human brain's performance.

Let us accept it *a priori* that the principles of the information setup and operation of the brain are methodologically correct and universal. What do we have to do to establish such a model of the brain's operation that would illustrate that the principles we stated really function both in real life and science? First, we have to clearly determine the object and understand what brain functions we want to model to demonstrate them at work and what we want to create to amaze the scientists, the neighbors and everybody around us with the miracle of the operating brain, as well as to prove our hypothesis? Second, the model must find rather simple technical realization on the basis of already available technologies and reflect the principles of functioning and not the anatomy of the brain. Therefore, we will avoid repeating the morphofunctional and topical structure of the brain and will try to develop an averaged model of multilevel information structure of the brain. Actually, we do not need to fundamentally mimic all areas of the brain's cortex. The information modules are identical, and it is no coincidence that many researchers in the theoretical neurology have noted the monotonous structure of the cortex. Knowing the information relations in one part of the brain, they can be replicated to other areas of the brain. Let us look attentively at the cytoarchitectonic map of the brain's cortex. We can distinguish the regions of visual cortex in the occipital brain and combine this part of the cortex with them. We can model the areas of the frontal cortex on them as the frontal cortex is responsible for thinking. Or we can model the part of the motor cortex located in the projection of the post-central and pre-central gyri in the left in right-handed people with standard NT ICM subscribers and NT ICM receivers. Therefore, we do not need samples of all of the regions of the NT cortex; we can use only one, though it must be studied at all information levels (inductome, genome, proteome, metabolome, secretome, magnetome). Each of these levels must be digitalized in averaged digital values: the magnetism of NT should be profiled with MRI; the DNA of the tissue should be profiled at the genome level; the RNA should be profiled at transcriptome level; the proteins should be profiled at the proteome level, the expressed hormones, mediators and neurotransmitters in this region of the NT must be profiled too, and the activity of radioactive glucose in these regions must be registered with PET.

The NT ICM subscribers of the output and NT ICM receivers of the input information lines located in the basal ganglias of the brain and spinal cord (according to the scheme of the pyramidal pathway) must be studied similarly. To analyze the peripheral NT ICM receivers of the input information line and the NT ICM subscribers for visual functional system, the commutation area of the retina NT with optical nerve must be studied. Such multilevel biophysical and biochemical (genome and post-genome) evaluation of this NT ICM can be used to receive the modules that also can be used to model the reception of the motor functional system in the brain. To model the NT ICM receiver of the motor functional system it would be sensible to take the NT of one vegetative ganglion and study it in detail as we have described previously. For the information analysis of intellectual activity it seems practical to take one sample of the tissue of basal ganglia or brainstem, appropriately, and model it as the example of the NT ICM transmitter.

The multiprofile virtual information images (VII) of each of the examined NT ICMs must be obtained, when all data profiles of the information levels of various NT ICMs are received, using program technologies of neuromathematics, based on multilayered neural networks; and the interaction patterns between the levels must be detected in these information modules.

So, what, even theoretically, will a unified block scheme of a neuromorphic simulation of the functioning brain look like? It seems that the key structural element of it must be a multilevel NT ICM that conducts data in one direction (from magnetic field to magnetome levels) and that is capable of compensating and restoring information relations of the levels inside the module. As the NT ICM is the main information structure that provides information reception, its transfer, modulation, inter-level transfer and, if necessary, inter-module transfer of information from receptors to the brain periphery (brainstem, spinal cord and autonomous nervous system), and then to the brain cortex and cerebellum, two (input and output) information lines consisting of 100 information channels each, must be composed from the NT of every brain region. And they should become the central elements of this block scheme. The analogues of receiving equipment (video, audio, dynamometer, etc.) that register the information from outside must be arranged at the terminals of certain groups of the information channels (per 20 pieces) of the input information line. The executive structures (robotic arm, robotic hand, robotic extremities) must be located at the terminal of every group of the information channels of the output information line. The NT ICM subscriber, NT ICM transmitter and NT ICM receiver must be found in every information channel of output and input lines, and each of the NT ICM subscribers, NT ICM transmitters and NT ICM receivers should receive an electromagnetic signal of the object image from peripheral NT ICM receivers at the input terminal, and at the output terminal there is the output electromagnetic signal linked to the signal magnifier. The information between the NT ICM subscriber, NT ICM transmitter and NT ICM receiver of both output and input information lines must be transferred in the impulse packages imitating the transmission of the impulses along the nervous fibers that consist of the neural axons. The central NT ICM subscribers of input lines and NT ICM receivers of output lines must be united in one technological platform (but not connected or commuted between each other) according to the principle of integration of the input and output channels of specific functional systems (video, audio, motor, etc.) and their interaction (commutation) at the level of the magnetomes of the NT ICM subscribers must be emulated with program methods relying on the holographic principle along with the receiving interference holograms that carry integrated data masses. The program software must also emulate the input of the holographic information on the NT ICM receivers of various channels of the output information line, which will be completed with executive organs, such as, for example, a robotic arm.

The other important part of the simulation must be the emulation of the record and reproduction of holographic masses of the data on holographic membranes. The information received as masses of holographic data must be recorded by laser techniques on a framed holographic membrane or on a screen that models a holographic membrane. To enhance the resources of the recording device the membrane can be stretched on a wavy surface that models the gyri of the human brain. This will allow for a significant increase in the amount of the recorded information. Besides, the technology of equal distribution of all incoming information on a screen surface must be considered. It can be emulated by the uniform movement of the membrane under the laser beam. The reproduction of holograms can be imitated by the holographic membrane lighted by the second laser on the basis of the information masses received from the biotechnological platform, from the areas imitating the frontal cortex.

Hence, we have claimed the basic parameters of the technical task for the working model of the brain. But this brings up the question, what for? However, the question of how to employ this model rationally and demonstrably should be forwarded to the neuromathematicians, neuropsychologists and neurophysiologists. Today one can say that this model helps to explain the mechanism of the development of new samples of neuromorphic energy-saving computation devices, as well as to work out a novel human/animal brain-computer neurointerface. Here we would like to dwell on this in a little more detail.

Miguel A. L. Nicolelis and his team in their work "Extracting kinematic parameters for monkey bipedal walking from cortical neuronal ensemble activity" showed that the recent achievements in the development of the "brain-machine" interface (BMI) demonstrate the feasibility of upper-limb neuroprosthesing, but the BMIs were not evaluated as the means to restore walking ability [159].

The researchers demonstrated that continuous records from the ensembles of cortical neurons can be used to predict the kinematics of bipedal walking in rhesus macaques – both offline and in real time. Linear decoders extracted 3D coordinates of the leg joints and leg muscle electromyograms from the activity of hundreds of cortical neurons. As more complex patterns of walking were produced by varying the gait speed and direction, larger neuronal populations were needed to accurately extract walking patterns. Extraction was further improved using a switching decoder which designated a submodel for each walking paradigm. The researchers are convinced that one day the BMIs might allow severely paralyzed patients to walk again.

Nicolelis gave a lecture at TEDMED (2012), in which he used the example of the interface between a monkey named Aurora staying in the US and an automatized orthograde robot from Kyoto, Japan [160]. The interface permitted the robot to walk, relying on the registered algorithms of movement in the monkey's mind. The registration improved when the switching decoder was used that denoted the submodel for each paradigm of walking. Nicolelis hopes that the interface will help restore walking in paralyzed patients.

However, the question remains: Can the human brain control robots directly without the body? Without any doubt, the interface is possible and Nicolelis proved that with his outstanding experiment, when the smart monkey from the USA first learns to control its virtual projection and then, a robot in Japan, and the control is achieved through the power of thinking. It was spectacular but not very convincing. Most of the work in this sphere remains closed, and it is hard to check what is true and what is not at a half-globe distance. In his lecture Nicolelis gave no details, and his vague and unclear information did not explain the principle of the interface. "The kind of neuroscience that I do and my colleagues do is almost like the weatherman. We are always chasing storms. We want to see and measure storms – brainstorms, that is. And we all talk about brainstorms in our daily lives, but we rarely see or listen to one. So I always like to start these talks by actually introducing you to one of them.

Actually, the first time we recorded more than one neuron – a hundred brain cells simultaneously – ***we could measure the electrical sparks of a hundred cells in the same animal***, this is the first image we got, the first 10 seconds of this recording. So we got a little snippet of a thought, and we could see it in front of us.

I always tell the students that we could also call neuroscientists some sort of astronomer, because we are dealing with a system that is only comparable in terms of number of cells to the number of galaxies that we have in the universe. And here we are, out of billions of neurons, just recording, 10 years ago, a hundred. We are doing a thousand now. And we hope to understand something fundamental about our human nature. Because, if you don't know yet, everything that we use to define what human nature is comes from these storms, comes from these storms that roll over the hills and valleys of our brains and define our memories, our beliefs, our feelings, our plans for the future. Everything that we ever do, everything that every human has ever done, does or will do, requires the toil of populations of neurons producing these kinds of storms" [160].

If Nicolelis and his team used highly sensitive hydroacoustic sensors, then it would possibly permit the registration of a magnetic field of the brain, as acoustic waves belong to one of the ranges of electromagnetic oscillations. If they used magnetic encephalography, it would be no less interesting and exciting. But, as I understand from their other works, they use microchip implants for electroencephalography of the brain resulting in cerebral mapping, so there is nothing new in it.

About a decade ago, a large number of national and international researchers after several fundamental neuro-research studies rejected EEG and evoked biopotentials recorded from the scalp for the management of the human brain and then stopped using the EEG bioelectric potentials for brain bioregulation. To my mind this is right, as EEG seems to be the "echo of a stadium" or, to be exact, the "echo of the sky over the stadium" which is used to judge the score of a football match, and evoking potentials from this echo is like shooting in the dark. All we can get from the EEG or EEG cerebral mapping is the detection of the focuses of seizure activity in the brain. Today the most advanced research teams that are working on the neurointerface are concentrating on brain-implantable microchips and brain feedback systems. Only this technology permits obtaining real information from the nerve cells of the brain cortex and sending it back. But the technique has a major disadvantage that cancels all its advantages. The work of the team of Andrew Schwartz, a neuroscientist and one of the leading experts in the neurointerface from the University of Pittsburgh, showed that scarring processes around microchips lead to fading signals and stop functioning in about a year. They demand removal and the consequences of leaving them in the brain are harmful for nerve tissue. Obviously this novel approach requires updating and to my mind it is methodologically incorrect. In a discussion with Andrew Schwartz in 2013 in Romania, he mentioned that they had spent over a quarter of a billion dollars in 6 years and had even translated their invention to humans, but they still failed. In their work they relied on the 70-year-old methodology of Vvedensky and Ukhtomsky and are proud of it. But this is the methodology of the beginning of the last century. Schwartz mentioned that they felt they were in a dead-end and, so far, were unable to find the way out. He felt that the way out lay in using biocompatible materials for micro-chips electrodes. Anyway, they showed us a good example. They have developed amazing software that permits the activation of a robotic arm's operation by thinking. To be exact, it is not thinking, but a commutation algorithm of the image maintenance that they are attempting to replicate with software [161].

Both Andrew Schwartz and Miguel A. L. Nicolelis came to the conclusion that expanded image presentation is not necessary to control a robotized device. It is enough to establish a virtual body, a projection, a monkey or a human avatar. Monkeys and people can be trained to interact with avatars or to perceive an avatar as the performer from the first person and control its hand and leg movements with the brain.

In both groups the animals and humans were trained to control such projections and to examine the objects of the virtual bank. These objects look identical but when the avatar touches the surface of one of them, the brain receives an electric signal, and informs the brain of what was touched. Four weeks later the brain gets used to processing a new signal and develops a new sensor channel; it can even be called a new sense. Hence, the brain is freed and now it can send motor commands to control an avatar. The feedback signals are processed immediately by the brain without the skin being involved.

Undoubtedly, this research into the neurointerface of the brain and computer must be continued because it is opening new avenues for the formation of nonexistent virtual senses and perceptions that do not exist in reality, permitting a controlling influence on the brain of animals or humans. The main thing is to observe the issues of ethics and morals, as so far the ethics of such experiments in humans seems doubtful.

The information-commutation theory that we proposed throws a new light on the issue of the human brain-computer interface. Obviously, in the light of the information-commutation theory the encephalogram presents the registration of chaotic EMWs that come outside the skull and, registered in the scalp, they hardly reflect the real situation in the human/animal brain. Therefore, the information value and accuracy of algorithms based on the EMW "echo phenomenon" seem inexact and arbitrary. Besides, according to the unified information-commutative theory the brain can be controlled using the technologies of resonant wave influence on the basis of the changes in the tissue magnetization in the requisite area of the cytoarchitectonic field of the brain in the projection of the necessary analyzer. In this way, the holograms of certain movements can be developed on the basis of the magnetization of certain tissue in the area of precentral gyri of the brain using common MRI. If, later on, this pixel information is presented in voxels and then formed as the holographic result of the field characteristics of the motor area of the brain, then the specific holograms of exact movements can be modeled using neuromathematical program software. And, correlating these holograms, or, to be exact, map charts of magnetization with the automatized systems of robot control, they can be easily translated to controlling signals. And, on the other side, knowing map charts (holograms) of brain magnetization in precentral gyrus in specific motor actions (automatic walking, running, writing, etc.), we can cause movements in a person, independent from their will, just by changing the magnetization of the brain in this area. Analogous algorithms can be realized using magnetoencephalography data and using hydroacoustic units.

CONCLUSION

In the concluding part the previously stated evidence is summed up and the proposed information-communication theory of the brain and the methodology of the information approach is discussed as related to neuro-research as an alternative to the conventional system approach; its advantages over the systems approach along with the results and theoretical hypotheses received with this methodology are analyzed. The proposed theory explains to the neurologist the range of facts and their physical and information content that were left unexplained by contemporary clinical neurology and psychiatry. This concluding chapter outlines the future applications, the concepts and developments resulting from the application of the information approach to practical clinical neurology and other neuroscience. The author suggests speaking of craniomorphic computer systems of the data processing that model the internal structure and operation of the mammalian head, as distinct from the brain-like computer systems that mimic the brain. New horizons and future paths for neuro-research are set forth.

Keywords: information-commutation theory of the brain, theoretical neurology, alternatives in neuroscience, craniomorphic (head-like) computer systems, new horizons for neuroscience

Dear reader! If you are reading this concluding part, then, obviously, you are not a clinical neurologist from an academic neurological or neurosurgical institution, but just a person who is not indifferent, but interested in brain research. Otherwise, you would have put the book aside at the very beginning and thought it to be anti-scientific nonsense. But you did not do that and felt interest in what I can reach in my theoretical reasoning, and I hope I lived up to your expectations. I have gone so far that I have scared myself with my novel views on the functions of old and well-known anatomic formations in the brain. It is possible that I am mistaken in some things. Maybe I was too radical in my revision of conventional theories of the brain and neurobiology. But I am sure that I am right in my conviction that the brain is a fantastic tool with the function of an organic switchboard. And when you stand in front of such a switchboard at the telephone station and look at all those lights from automatically switching relays and cells, you must have the same feeling when you look at the work of the brain during functional MRI or PET. In this case, you also observe the relay and cells of the organic switchboard being turned on and off, though you do not realize it.

It seems extremely important to me to state the fact that the brain is able to process information outside of nerve tissue with the help of holography. Thus, the brain does not spend much energy on the sophisticated system of calculations and it permits the simultaneous implementation of various functions. We showed that the thought is material and has its information coordinates (genetic, transcriptome, proteome, biophysical), its "sources" in the human organism. It explains the scientific basis of the influence of words on the human consciousness and subconsciousness and opportunities for psychotherapy and hypnosis to affect the somatic state of organs and systems. So, we presume, that "in the beginning was the Word" as the information carrier and this is stated by the information-commutation theory of the brain that we proposed. We wanted to demonstrate how one can understand the nature of subconsciousness, and when one starts to understand the principles of its organization, it becomes clear how it can be influenced.

Without any doubt, the book reflects my personal and rather unconventional views on theoretical neurology, information-commutation theory, and the main principles of the information organization and functioning of the brain, as seen by a neurologist. It so happens that the main theoreticians in the sphere are not doctors of neuro-specialization (psychiatry, neurology, neurosurgery) or neurobiologists, but experts in exact sciences and engineers: software engineers, biophysicists and mathematicians who are developing their complicated and multi-component mathematical theories. Their understanding is very hard even for a well-trained neurologist, if possible at all, without specific training. This paradox of our time is characteristic. As neurobiologists, neuroanatoms and neurophysiologists are unable to propose any sensible theory that would explain the brain's organization, this work can be done instead by mathematicians, physics and chemists, who can apply their knowledge to explain the laws and patterns of brain work. Certainly, we need to know the rules and patterns of brain functioning, we need formulas of its unique multi-structural and multidimensional functioning, but we should not reject age-old anatomical and physiological evidence; in my book I wanted to show that the new views of a neurologist on the brain from new methodological standpoints can open up new functions in previously known anatomical formations.

For the first time we said in this book that the pia mater is the storage of memory in the brain, and the arachnoid mater is a system drive in which the software is recorded. It sounds riotous: the idea that the pia is necessary to excrete brain wastes and the CSF is the brain's "urine", and here we offer a new perception of anatomy. We consider the arachnoid mater is viewed as the main system drive of the brain, and not a broad ligament that fixes the brain and prevents it from falling. We arrived at this idea in the analysis of the information structure of the work of tissue modules of the brain and not due to genial speculations. As soon as it becomes clear that the information is electrons, resonances, frequencies and oscillations, it becomes obvious that such an ephemerous thing as information must have its carrier. It is not able to move wherever it wants; there should be something to carry it. Information is like an egoistic child who changes parents and nurses; he commands them but nobody can refuse him - everybody accepts the situation, regardless of whether they are happy or not. The information circulates between the human and the medium, as well as inside a human, sometimes going outside into the environment. That is why everything in our body is so well adjusted to gathering information, processing it, selecting the necessary piece and then sharing it. The genius of our Creator is obvious; the information comes from the space and goes away to the space. But we need to understand the established and genetically confirmed (by evolution) means of information transfer for medicine and for our modest information needs of existence on Earth. This is why - when we understand that the information carrier at the inductive level of nerve tissue (resonant, magnetic field, level of elementary particles, atomic) is the magnetic field; at the level of genome is DNA; at the level of transcriptome the carrier is RNA; at the proteome level the information is carried by the proteins; and at secretome level by protein complexes (hormones, mediators, neurotransmitters) - we become convinced that at the level of nervous cell and nerve tissue magnetome the information must have its carrier, too. It becomes clear that the information changes its carrier after the level of biochemical transfer, and electromagnetic waves become its new transportation. Therefore, there exists a rigid order and direction of the information transfer from the biophysical field level through the levels of genome and post-genome transporters to biophysical ones, i.e., electromagnetic waves. This important principle of changing vehicles helps us to understand the reason for it. The information-communication module of nerve tissue is the main information unit that helps to "increase" the minimal data to the level permitting its perception and processing, to modulate its quality and power. The information channels can be easily composed to get information channels, and, if necessary, information lines, because the information follows through the module only in one specified direction. When we understand that the brain has a clear principle of formation of the input and output information lines, it becomes obvious that electromagnetic waves carry the information to the subarachnoid and subdural spaces surrounding the brain. The CSF is not the "brain urine" anymore but the information bus to transfer large data volumes on the one hand, and the lens to scatter and reflect the waves, on the other hand. That is, the brain has a real technical opportunity, and not just a virtual one, to form the basis of holography: object and reference EMWs. The waves have nowhere to go and stay in the intermeningeal space, contacting the arachnoid they reflect, continuing their pathway, reflecting from the dura mater and interfering with each other establish new transport systems of the data transfer in holograms.

In the book we expressed many hypothetical questions about the organization and functioning of the brain, and each one demands additional examination and research. I have proposed an alternative view on the existing concepts in the sphere. I proposed the rejection of the range of conservative notions and dogmas: "the neuron is the main information unit of the brain", "the brain is a hologram", "memory is distributed through the neural network", "neurons and synapses determine the formation of functional systems of the brain", "the cognitive function of the brain forms in the cortex", etc. I offered an alternative point of view which is clear to me as a neurologist, and, hopefully, will be clear to neuromorphologists, neurophysiologists and neuroanatoms. I proposed an alternative view that gave me the answers to numerous questions which conventional neurology and psychiatry were not able to answer. I am grateful for the time you spent reading my book and I would be happy to answer any questions about new science, theoretical neurology, the framework of which I have attempted to state.

REFERENCES

[1] The Human Brain Project. A Report to the European Commission. Lausanne, Switzerland: The HBP-PS Consortium; 2012. Available from: https://www.humanbrainproject.eu/documents/10180/17648/TheHBPReport_LR.pdf/18e5747e-10af-4bec-9806-d03aead57655. Accessed November 30, 2014. Report.

[2] Jibu, M; Yasue, K. Quantum Brain Dynamics and Consciousness. An Introduction. Amsterdam, the Netherlands: John Benjamins Publishing Company, 1995. Book.

[3] Pribram, KH. Quantum holography: Is it relevant to brain function? *Information Sciences*, 1999, 115(1–4). Journal article.

[4] Taylor, JG. On the neurodynamics of the creation of consciousness. *Cogn Neurodyn*. 2007 June, 1(2), 97-118. Journal article.

[5] Labouvie-Vief, G. Dynamic integration theory: Emotion, cognition, and equilibrium in later life. In: Bengston, VL, Gans D, Pulney NM, Silverstein M, editors. Handbook of theories of aging. 2nd ed. New York, NY, US: Springer Publishing Co, 2009.

[6] Obama's 2013 State of the Union Address. The New York Times [Internet], 2013 Feb 12 [cited 2013 Feb 12]; Available from http://www.nytimes.com/2013/02/13/us/politics/obamas-2013-state-of-the-union-address.html. Newspaper article.

[7] National Institutes of Health. Brain Research through Advancing Innovative Neurotechnologies (BRAIN). *Working group Interim Report*, 2013. Available from http://www.nih.gov/science/brain/. Report.

[8] Duus, P. Topicheskiy diagnoz v nevrologhii: anatomiya, priznaki, simptomy [Topical Diagnosis in Neurology: Anatomy, Physiology, Signs, Symptoms]. *Moscow: Vasar-Ferro*, 1995. Russian. Book.

[9] Turing, AM. Computing machinery and intelligence. *Mind.*, 1950, 59, 433-460. Journal article.

[10] Shtulman, DR; Levin, OS. Nevrologhiya: Spravochnik praktisheskogo vracha [Neurology: A Guide for Medical Practitioner]. *Moscow: MED Press-Inform*, 2008, Russian. Book.

[11] Alzheimer's Association. 2015 Alzheimer's disease facts and figures. *Alzheimer's and dementia.*, 2015 March, 11 (3), 332–384.

[12] Bryukhovetskiy, AS. Klinichesaya onkoproteomika: personifitsirovannaya provioopukholevaya kletochanya terapiya [Clinical oncoproteomics: personalized anticancer cell therapy]. *Moscow: Poligraf Plus*, 2013. Russian. Book.

[13] International Association of Neurorestoratology. Beijing Declaration of International Association of Neurorestoratology (IANR). *Cell Transplant.*, 2009, 18, 487.

[14] Hawkins, J. How brain science will change computing [Internet]. *TED*, 2003. Available from: http://www.ted.com/talks/jeff_hawkins_on_how_brain_science_will_change_computing.html. Accessed July 12, 2012. Web page.

[15] Crick, F. Thinking about the brain. *Scientific American.*, September 1979, pp. 219-232. Journal article.

[16] Pavlov, IP. Dvadtsatilerniy opyt obyektivnogo izucheniya vysshey deyatelnosti (povedeniya) zhivotnikh [Twenty years' experience of the objective observations over higher activity (behavior) of the animals]. *Moscow: Nauka*, 1973, Russian. Book.

[17] Ukhtomsky, AA. Dominanta kak rabochiy printsip nervnykh tsentrov [Dominance as the working principle of nervous centers]. *Leningrad: Nauka*, 1978, Russian. Book.

[18] Davidovskaya, NA. Neoriya kompleksov v neiropsikhologicheskom aspekte [Neuropsychological aspects of the theory of complexes]. *Smalta.*, 2014, 3, 36-42. Russian. Journal article.

[19] Pribram, K. Languages of the Brain: Experimental Paradoxes and Principles in Neuropsychology. N.Y. : Prentice Hall/Brandon House, 1971. Book.

[20] Holonomic brain theory [Internet]. 2015 [cited April 4, 2014]. Available from: https://en.wikipedia.org/wiki/Holonomic_brain_theory. Web page.

[21] Einstein's brain [Internet]. January 21, 2005 [cited January 2014]. Available from: http://phys.org/news/2005-01-einsteins-brain.html. Web page.

[22] Anokhin, PK. Biologhiya i neirophisiologhiya uslovnogo refleksa [Biology and neurophysiology of condioned reflex]. *Moscow: Meditsina*, 1968. Russian. Book.

[23] Feighenberg, IM. Veroyatnostnoye prognozirovaniye v deyatelnosti mozga [Probabilistic prediction in the brain activity]. 1963, 2. Russian. Journal article.

[24] Simonov, PV. Teoriya otrazheniya i psikhophisiologiya emotsiy [The theory of reflection and psychophysiology of emotions]. *Moscow: Nauka*, 1970. Russian. Book.

[25] Simonov, PV. Emotsionalniy mozg [Emotional brain]. *Moscow: Nauka*, 1981. Russian. Book.

[26] Sudakov, KV. Funktsionalniye sistemy [Functional systems]. *Moscow: Izdatelstvo RAMN*, 2011. Russian. Book.

[27] Sperry, R. Brain bisection and the neurology of consciousness. In Eccles J, editor. Brain and conscious experience. New York: Springer Verlag, 1966. Book section.

[28] Ornstein, RE. The right mind: Making sense of hemispheres. *New York: Houghton Mifflin Harcourt*, 1997. Book.

[29] Benson, F; Zaidel, E. The dual brain: hemispheric specialization in humans. New York; The Guilford Press, 1985. Book.

[30] Khomskaya, ED. Neiropsikhologhiya [Neuropsychology]. Moscow: Izdatelstvo Moskovskogo Universiteta, 1987. Russian. Book.

[31] Luria, AR. Vysshiye korkoviye funktsii i ikh narusheniye pri lokalnikh porazheniyakh mozga [High cortical functions and their disorders in local injuries of the brain]. Moscow: Prosvescheniye, 1989. Russian. Book.

[32] Luria, AR. Mozg i psikhicheskiye protsessi [The brain and psychic processes]. Moscow: Izdatelstvo MGU, 1990. Russian. Book.

[33] Strangman, G; Heindel, WC; Anderson, JA; Sutton, JP. Learning motor sequences with and without knowledge of governing rules. *Neurorehabil Neural Repair.*, 2005 June, 19(2), 93-114. Journal article.

[34] Başar, E; Başar-Eroglu, C; Karakaş, S; Schürmann, M. Oscillatory Brain Theory: A New Trend in Neuroscience. *Engineering in Medicine and Biology Magazine.*, 1999 May/June, 3, 56-66. Journal article.

[35] Başar, E; Başar-Eroglu, C; Karakaş, S; Schürmann, M. Gamma, alpha, delta, and theta oscillations govern cognitive processes. *Int J Psychophysiol.*, 2001 January, 39(2-3), 241-248. Journal article.

[36] Jibu, M; Yasue, K. Quantum Brain Dynamics and Consciousness. Amsterdam: John Benjamins Publishing Company, 1995. Book.

[37] Beck, F; Eccles, JC. Quantum aspects of brain activity and the role of consciousness. *Proc Natl Acad Sci U S A.*, 1992, December 1, 89(23), 11357-11361. Journal article.

[38] Czarnecki, R. The Quantum Brain: Theory or Myth [Internet]? [cited Jan 2014]. Available from: http://serendip.brynmawr.edu/bb/neuro/neuro98/202s98-paper3/Czarnecki3.html 1998. Journal article.

[39] Globus, GG; O'Carroll, CP. Nonlocal neurology: beyond localization to holonomy. *Med Hypotheses.*, 2010 November, 75(5), 425-432. Journal article.

[40] Keppler, J. A new perspective on the functioning of the brain and the mechanisms behind conscious processes [Internet]. *Front Psychol.*, 2013, April 30 [cited 2014, September]., 4, 242. Available from: http://www.ncbi.nlm.nih.gov/pmc/articles/PMC3639372/. DOI: 10.3389/fpsyg.2013.00242. Electronic article.

[41] Andrus, VF. Razmyshleniya o formirovanii "dush" (prizrakov) i "fantomov" (privideniy) fauny i flory s tochki zreniya neitronnykh nauk [Reflections on the formation of "souls" and "phantoms" from the viewpoint of neutron sciences] [Internet]. 2013, May 19 [cited 2014, Jan]. Available from: http://www.elit-cons.com/files/RU/reflections_ru.pdf. Russian. Web page.

[42] Reimann, MW; Anastassiou, CA; Perin, R; Hill, SL; Markram, H; Koch, C. A biophysically detailed model of neocortical local field potentials predicts the critical role of active membrane currents. *Neuron.*, 2013, July 24, 79(2), 375-90. Journal article.

[43] Natarajan, R; Huys, QJ; Dayan, P; Zemel, RS. Encoding and decoding spikes for dynamic stimuli. *Neural Comput.*, 2008, September, 20(9), 2325-2360. Journal article.

[44] Sarajedini, A; Hecht-Nielsen, R; Chau, PM. Conditional probability density function estimation with sigmoidal neural networks. *IEEE Trans Neural Netw.*, 1999 October, 10(2), 231-238. Journal article.

[45] Freeman, WJ. Definitions of state variables and state space for brain-computer interface: Part 1. Multiple hierarchical levels of brain function. *Cogn Neurodyn.*, 2007 March, 1(2), 3-14. Journal article.

[46] Freeman, WJ. Understanding perception through neural "codes". *IEEE Trans Biomed Eng.*, 2011 July, 58(7), 1884-1890. Journal article.

[47] Capolupo, A; Freeman, WJ; Vitiello, G. Dissipation of 'dark energy' by cortex in knowledge retrieval [internet]. *Phys Life Rev.*, 2013, March [cited 2014, Jan]. 10(1), 85-94. Available from: http://sulcus.berkeley.edu/wjf/FY%20Dissipation%20of% 20%E2%80%98dark%20energy%E2%80%99%20by%20cortex%20in%20knowledge%20retrieval.pdf. DOI: 10.1016/j.plrev.2013.01.001. Electronic article.

[48] Cauller, LJ. The Neurointeractibe Paradigm: Dynamical Mechanics and the Emergence of Higher Cortical Function. In: Hecht-Nielsen R, McKenna T, editors. Computational Models for Neuroscience. *Berlin: Springer*, 2003. Book section.

[49] Kosslyn, SM; Ganis, G; Thompson, WL. Neural foundations of imagery. *Nat Rev Neurosci.*, 2001 September, 2(9), 635-642. Journal article.

[50] Cauller, LJ; Kulics, AT. The neural basis of the behaviorally relevant N1 component of the somatosensory-evoked potential in SI cortex of awake monkeys: evidence that backward cortical projections signal conscious touch sensation. *Exp Brain Res.*, 1991, 84(3), 607-619. Journal article.

[51] Cauller, LJ; Connors, BW. Synaptic physiology of horizontal afferents to layer I in slices of rat SI neocortex. *J Neurosci.*, 1994, Feb, 14(2)751-762. Journal article.

[52] Taylor, JG. On the neurodynamics of the creation of consciousness. *Cogn Neurodyn.*, 2007, 1, 97-118. Journal article.

[53] Favorov, O. The Cortical Pyramidal Cell as a Set of Interacting Error Backpropagating Dendrites: Mechanism for Discovering Nature's Order. In: Hecht-Nielsen R, McKenna T, editors. Computational Models for Neuroscience. *Berlin: Springer*, 2003. Book section.

[54] Freeman, WJ. Performance of Intelligent Systems Governed by Internally Generated Goals. In: Hecht-Nielsen R, McKenna T, editors. Computational Models for Neuroscience. *Berlin: Springer*, 2003. Book section.

[55] Hecht-Nielsen, R. A Theory of Thalamocortex. In: Hecht-Nielsen R, McKenna T, editors. Computational Models for Neuroscience. *Berlin: Springer*, 2003. Book section.

[56] Markram, H. The Blue Brain Project. *Nat Rev Neurosci.*, 2006 February, 7(2), 153-160. Journal article.

[57] McKenna, T. The development of Cortical Models to Enable Neural-based Cognitive Architectures. In: Hecht-Nielsen R, McKenna T, editors. Computational Models for Neuroscience. Berlin: Springer, 2003. Book section.

[58] Sutton, JP; Strangman, G. The Behaving Neocortex as a Dynamic Network of Networks. In: Hecht-Nielsen R, McKenna T, editors. Computational Models for Neuroscience. Berlin: Springer, 2003. Book section.

[59] Taylor, JG. Towards Global Principles of Brain Processing. In: Hecht-Nielsen R, McKenna T, editors. Computational Models for Neuroscience. Berlin: Springer, 2003. Book section.

[60] Taylor, JG; Taylor, NR. The Neural Networks for Language in the Brain: Creating LAD. In: Hecht-Nielsen R, McKenna T, editors. Computational Models for Neuroscience. Berlin: Springer, 2003. Book section.

[61] Zemel, R. Cortical Belief Networks. In: Hecht-Nielsen R, McKenna T, editors. Computational Models for Neuroscience. Berlin: Springer, 2003. Book section.

[62] Zemel, RS; Mozer, MC. Localist attractor networks. *Neural Comput.*, May, 2001, 13(5), 1045-64. Journal article.

[63] Friston, K. A Free Energy Principle for Biological Systems. *Entropy.*, 2012, Nov, 14(11), 2100-2121. Journal article.

[64] Knill, DC; Pouget, A. The Bayesian brain: the role of uncertainty in neural coding and computation. *Trends in Neurosciences.*, 2004, December 1, 27(12), 712-719. Journal article.

[65] Huang, GT. Is this a unified theory of the brain[Internet]? New Scientist. May 28, 2008 [cited 2014, Feb]; Available from: http://www.fil.ion.ucl.ac.uk/~karl/Is%20this%20a%20unified%20theory%20of%20the%20brain.pdf. Electronic article.

[66] Taylor, JG; Taylor, NR. Analysis of recurrent cortico-basal ganglia-thalamic loops for working memory. *Biol Cybern.*, May, 2000, 82(5), 415-32. Journal article.

[67] Taylor, NR; Hartley, M; Taylor, JG. The micro-structure of attention. *Neural Netw.*, 2006, November, 19(9), 1347-1370. Journal article.

[68] Carnegie Melon University. Carnegie Melon neuroscientist proposes new theory of brain flexibility [Internet]. 2007, Nov 15 [cited 2014, Feb]. Available from: http://www.eurekalert.org/pub_releases/2007-11/cmu-cmn111507.php Web page.

[69] Just, MA; Varma, S. The organization of thinking: What functional brain imaging reveals about the neuroarchitecture of complex cognition. *Cognitive, Affective, & Behavioral Neuroscience.*, September 2007, 7(3), 153-191. Journal article.

[70] Wallis, C. Study Advances New Theory of How the Brain Is Wired [Internet]. 2013, June 27 [cited 2013, Dec]. Available from: http://news.columbia.edu/brainwiring. Web page.

[71] Constantinople, CM; Bruno, RM. Deep cortical layers are activated directly by thalamus. *Science.*, 2013, June 28, 1591-1594. Journal article.

[72] Baev, KV. A new conceptual understanding of brain function: basic mechanisms of brain-initiated normal and pathological behaviors. *Crit Rev Neurobiol.*, 2007, 19(2-3), 119-202. Journal article.

[73] Zyga, L. Professor finally publishes controversial brain theory [Internet]. 2008, November 19 [cited 2014, Jan]. Available from: http://phys.org/news/2008-11-professor-publishes-controversial-brain-theory.html. Web page.

[74] Roy, A. Connectionism, Controllers, and a Brain Theory. *IEEE Transactions on Systems, Man and Cybernetics, – Part A: Systems and Human.*, November 2008, 38(6), 1434-1441.

[75] Crown, E. New theory challenges current view of how brain stores long-term memory [Internet]. 2005, Jan 14 [cited 2013 Nov]. Available from: http://www.eurekalert.org/pub_releases/2005-01/nu-ntc011405.php. Web page.

[76] Routtenberg, A. Long-lasting memory from evanescent networks. *Eur J Pharmacol.*, 2008, May 6, 585(1), 60-3. Journal article.

[77] Ramirez, S; Liu, X; Lin, Pi-A; Suh, J; Pignatelli, M; Redondo, RL; Ryan, TJ; Tonegawa, S. Creating a False Memory in the Hippocampus. *Science.*, 2013, July 26, 341(6144), 387-391. Journal article.

[78] Fingelkurts, AA; Fingelkurts, AA; Neves, CF. Natural world physical, brain operational, and mind phenomenal space-time. *Phys Life Rev.*, 2010, June, 7(2), 195-249. Journal article.

[79] Fingelkurts, AA; Fingelkurts, AA. Alpha rhythm operational architectonics in the continuum of normal and pathological brain states: current state of research. *Int J Psychophysiol.*, 2010, May76(2), 93-106. doi: 10.1016/j.ijpsycho.2010.02.009. Electronic article.

[80] Neftci, E; Binas, J; Rutishauser, U; Chicca, E; Indiveri, G; Douglas, RJ. Synthesizing cognition in neuromorphic electronic systems. *Proc Natl Acad Sci U S A.*, 2013, Sep 10, 110, E3468-3476. doi: 10.1073/pnas.1212083110. Electronic article.

[81] Inside Paul Allen's Quest To Reverse Engineer The Brain [Internet]. *Forbes.*, 2012, Sep 18 [cited 2014, Jan]. Available from: http://www.forbes.com/sites/matthewherper/2012/09/18/inside-paul-allens-quest-to-reverse-engineer-the-brain. Web page.

[82] Herper, M. Microsoft Co-Founder Paul Allen's Health Philanthropy [Internet]. *Forbes.*, 2012, Nov 29 [cited 2014, Jan]. http://forbesindia.com/printcontent/34221. Web page.

[83] Leon, SP; Knock, SA; Woodman, MM; Domide, L; Mersmann, J; McIntosh, AR; Jirsa, V. The Virtual Brain: a simulator of primate brain network dynamics. *Front. Neuroinform.*, 2013, June 11, 7, 10. doi: 10.3389/fninf.2013.00010.

[84] Vityaev, EE. Komputernoye poznaniye [Scientific discovery and computational cognition] [Internet] [updated 2014, Jan 15, cited 2014, Feb]. Available from: http://www.math.nsc.ru/AP/ScientificDiscovery/pages/Chapter_9_80.htm. Russian. Web page.

[85] Vityaev, EE. Ptintsipy raboty mozga, soderzhaschiyesya v teorii funktsionalnykh sistem PK Anokhina I teorii emotsiy PV Simonova [The principles of operation of the brain contained in the theory of functional systems of Anokhin PK and theory of emotions of Simonov PV]. *Neiroinformatika*, 2008, 3(1), 25-78. Russian. Journal article.

[86] An Overview of the Human Genome Project [Internet] [updated 2012 Nov; cited 2014 Jan]. Available from: http://www.genome.gov/12011239. Web Page.

[87] Human Proteome Project [Internet]. 2015 [cited 2015 Apr]. Available from: http://www.thehpp.org/. Web Page.

[88] US scientists relieved as Obama lifts ban on stem cell research [Internet]. 2009 March 10 [cited 2014 March]. Available from: http://www.theguardian.com/world/2009/mar/10/obama-stem-cell-research. Web Page.

[89] New Armed Forces Institute of Regenerative Medicine to Lead Way in Caring for Wounded [Internet]. 2008 April 17 [cited 2014 Jan]. Available from: http://www.defense.gov/releases/release.aspx?releaseid=11842. Web Page.

[90] The Human Connectome Project [Internet]. 2009 [updated 2015 June; cited 2015 July]. Available from: http://www.humanconnectome.org. Web Page.

[91] Marcus, G. The three-billion dollar brain [Internet]. 2013, March 12 [cited 2014 April]. Available from: http://www.newyorker.com/news/news-desk/the-three-billion-dollar-brain. Web Page.

[92] Fact Sheet: Over $300 Million in Support of the President's BRAIN Initiative [Internet]. 2014, Sep 30 [cited 2014 Dec]. Available from: https://www.whitehouse.gov/sites/default/files/microsites/ostp/brain_fact_sheet_9_30_2014_final.pdf. Web Page.

[93] Terentyev, AA; Moldogaziyeva, NT; Shaitan, KV. Dinamicheskaya proteomika v modelirovanii zhivoy kletki. Belok-belkoviye vzaimodeistviya [Dynamic proteomics in the modeling of a living cell. Protein-protein interactions*]. Uspekhi biologhicheskoy khimii.*, 2009, 49, 429–480. Journal article. Russian.

[94] Ferrell, JE. Q&A: Cooperativity. *J Biol.*, 2009, Jun 17, Vol. 8(6), 53._doi: 10.1186/jbiol157. Electronic article.

[95] Shaitan, KV. Energheticheskaya poverkhnost' i dinamika konfrontatsii molekul [Energy Surface and Conformation Dynamics of Molecules]. *Russian Journal of Electrochemistry.*, 2003, 39(2), 198–204. Russian. Journal article.

[96] Milo, R. Dynamic proteomics in mammalian cells: capabilities and challenges. *Mol Biosyst.*, 2007 Aug, 3(8), 542-6. Journal article.

[97] Trinkle-Mulcahy, L; Lamond, AI. Toward a high-resolution view of nuclear dynamics. *Science.*, 2007 Nov 30, 318(5855), 1402-1407. Journal article.

[98] Mayer, BJ. Protein-protein interactions in signaling cascades. *Mol Biotechnol.*, 1999 Dec 15, 13(3), 201-213. Journal article.

[99] Houtman, JC[1]; Barda-Saad, M; Samelson, LE. Examining multiprotein signaling complexes from all angles. *FEBS J.*, 2005 Nov, 272(21), 5426-5435. Journal article.

[100] Terentyev, AA, Moldogaziyeva NT. Strukturno-funktionalnoye kartirovaniye α-fetoproteina [Structural-functional mapping of α-fetoprotein]. *Biokhimiya*, Feb 2006, 71, 157-172. Russian.

[101] Zaretsky, JZ; Wreschner, DH. Protein multifunctionality: principles and mechanisms. *Transl Oncogenomics.*, 2008 May 15, 3, 99-136. Journal article.

[102] Ghaemmaghami, S; Huh, WK; Bower, K; Howson, RW; Belle, A; Dephoure, N; O'Shea, EK; Weissman, JS.Global analysis of protein expression in yeast. *Nature.*, 2003 Oct 16, 425(6959), 737-41. Journal article.

[103] Parrish, JR; Gulyas, KD; Finley, RL. Jr. Yeast two-hybrid contributions to interactome mapping. *Curr Opin Biotechnol*, 2006 Aug, 17(4), 387-93. Journal article.

[104] Stumpf, MP; Thorne, T; de Silva, E; Stewart, R; An, HJ; Lappe, M; Wiuf, C. Estimating the size of the human interactome. *Proc Natl Acad Sci U S A.*, 2008, May 13, 105(19), 6959-6964. Journal article.

[105] Venkatesan, K; Rual, JF; Vazquez, A; Stelzl, U; Lemmens, I; Hirozane-Kishikawa, T; Hao, T; Zenkner, M; Xin, X; Goh, KI; Yildirim, MA; Simonis, N; Heinzmann, K; Gebreab, F; Sahalie, JM; Cevik, S; Simon, C; de Smet, AS; Dann, E; Smolyar, A; Vinayagam, A; Yu, H; Szeto, D; Borick, H. An empirical framework for binary interactome mapping. *Nat Methods.*, 2009 Jan, 6(1), 83-90. Journal article.

[106] Cusick, ME; Klitgord, N; Vidal, M; Hill, DE. Interactome: gateway into systems biology. *Hum Mol Genet.*, 2005 Oct 15, 14 Spec No. 2, R171-181. Journal article.

[107] Mika, S; Rost, B. Protein-protein interactions more conserved within species than across species. *PLoS Comput Biol.*, 2006 Jul 21, 2(7), e79. Electronic article.

[108] Causier, B. Studying the interactome with the yeast two-hybrid system and mass spectrometry. *Mass Spectrom Rev.*, 2004 Sep-Oct, 23(5), 350-367. Journal article.

[109] Puig, O; Caspary, F; Rigaut, G; Rutz, B; Bouveret, E; Bragado-Nilsson, E; Wilm, M; Séraphin, B.The tandem affinity purification (TAP) method: a general procedure of protein complex purification. *Methods.*, 2001 Jul, 24(3), 218-229. Journal article.

[110] Rigaut, G; Shevchenko, A; Rutz, B; Wilm, M; Mann, M; Séraphin, B. A generic protein purification method for protein complex characterization and proteome exploration. *Nat Biotechnol.*, 1999 Oct, 17(10), 1030-1032. Journal article.

[111] Ho, Y; Gruhler, A; Heilbut, A; Bader, GD; Moore, L; Adams, SL; Millar, A; Taylor, P; Bennett, K; Boutilier, K; Yang, L; Wolting, C; Donaldson, I; Schandorff, S; Shewnarane, J; Vo, M; Taggart, J; Goudreault, M; Muskat, B; Alfarano, C; Dewar, D; Lin, Z; Michalickova, K; Willems, A. Systematic identification of protein complexes in Saccharomyces cerevisiae by mass spectrometry. *Nature.*, 2002 Jan 10, 415(6868), 180-183. Journal article.

[112] Zhou, M; Veenstra, TD. Proteomic analysis of protein complexes. *Proteomics.*, 2007 Aug, 7(16), 2688-97. Journal article.

[113] Domon, B; Aebersold, R. Mass spectrometry and protein analysis. *Science.*, 2006 Apr 14, 312(5771), 212-7. Journal article.

[114] Eilbeck, K; Brass, A; Paton, N; Hodgman, C. INTERACT: an object oriented protein-protein interaction database. *Proc Int Conf Intell Syst Mol Biol.*, 1999, 87-94. Journal article.

[115] Xenarios, I; Salwínski, L; Duan, XJ; Higney, P; Kim, SM; Eisenberg, D. DIP, the Database of Interacting Proteins: a research tool for studying cellular networks of protein interactions. *Nucleic Acids Res.*, 2002 Jan 1, 30(1), 303-305. Journal article.

[116] Bader, GD; Betel, D; Hogue, CW. BIND: the Biomolecular Interaction Network Database. *Nucleic Acids Res.*, 2003 Jan 1, 31(1), 248-50. Journal article.

[117] Breitkreutz, BJ; Stark, C; Reguly, T; Boucher, L; Breitkreutz, A; Livstone, M; Oughtred, R; Lackner, DH; Bähler, J; Wood, V; Dolinski, K; Tyers, M. The BioGRID Interaction Database: 2008 update. *Nucleic Acids Res.*, 2008 Jan, 36(Database issue), D637-40. Journal article.

[118] Teyra, J; Doms, A; Schroeder, M; Pisabarro, MT. SCOWLP: a web-based database for detailed characterization and visualization of protein interfaces. *BMC Bioinformatics.*, 2006 Mar 2, 7, 104. Journal article.

[119] Teyra, J; Paszkowski-Rogacz, M; Anders, G; Pisabarro, MT. SCOWLP classification: structural comparison and analysis of protein binding regions. *BMC Bioinformatics.*, 2008 Jan 8, 9, 9. Journal article.

[120] Spirin, S; Titov, M; Karyagina, A; Alexeevski, A. NPIDB: a database of nucleic acids-protein interactions. *Bioinformatics.*, 2007 Dec 1, 23(23), 3247-3248. Journal article.

[121] Gong, S; Yoon, G; Jang, I; Bolser, D; Dafas, P; Schroeder, M; Choi, H; Cho, Y; Han, K; Lee, S; Choi, H; Lappe, M; Holm, L; Kim, S; Oh, D; Bhak, J. PSIbase: a database of Protein Structural Interactome map (PSIMAP). *Bioinformatics.*, 2005 May 15, 21(10), 2541-2543. Journal article.

[122] Shannon, CE. A Mathematical Theory of Communication. *The Bell System Technical Journal.*, July, 1948, October, 27, 379-423, 623-656. Journal article.

[123] Wiener, N. Cybernetics Or Control and Communication in the Animal and the Machine. Cambridge, Mass: MIT Press, 1948. Book.

[124] Korotenkov, YuG. Formalizovannaya informatsiologhiya [Formalized Informationology]. Moscow: Mezhdunarodnoye izdatelstvo Informatsiologhiya., 2005. Book. Russian.

[125] Simonov, PV. Teoriya otrazheniya i psikhophisiologiya emotsiy [The theory of reflection and psychophysiology of emotions]. Moscow: Nauka, 1970. Book. Russian.

[126] Simonov, PV. Emotsionalniy mozg [Emotional brain]. Moscow: Nauka, 1981. Book. Russian.

[127] Hinton, GE; Andreson, JA. Parallel Models of Associative Memory. Hillsdale, New Jersey : Lawrence Erlbaum Associates Publishers, 1981. Book.

[128] Atick, JJ; Redlich, AN. Toward a theory of early visual processing. *Neural Computation.*, 1990, 2, 308-320. Journal article.

[129] Atick, JJ; Redlich, AN. What does the Retina Know about Natural Scenes [Internet]? Neural Comput, 1992 [cited 2014, Feb]; 4, 196-210. Available from: http://www. cnbc. cmu.edu/cns/papers/Atick-Redlich-NC92.pdf. Journal article.

[130] Baddeley, R; Hancock, P; Foldiak, P. editors. Information theory and the brain. New York: Cambridge University Press. 2000. Book.

[131] Bryukhovetskiy, AS. Transplantatsiya nervnikh kletok i tkanevaya engineeriya mozga pri nervnikh bolezniakh [Transplantation of nerve cells and tissue engineering of brain in nerve diseases]. *Moscow: ZAO Neurovita*, 2003. Russian. Book.

[132] Devyatkov, ND; Golant, MB; Betskiy, OV. Milimetroviye volny i ikh rol' v protsessakh zhiznedeyatelnosti [Millimeter waves and their role in the life activity]. *Radio i svyaz'*., 1991. Russian. Book

[133] Kanchjen, C. BioSVCHsvyaz' [(BioSHFconnection]. Information package on the conference in non-traditional aspects of natural sciences. *Tomsk*, 1992. Conference paper.

[134] Venkataramanan, M. *Darpa's 5 Radical Plans for Military Medicine [Internet].*, 2011 [updated 2011 March 01; cited 2013 Jan]. Available from:

[135] Neymark, YuI. Mathematical models in Natural Science and Engineering. *Berlin-Heidelberg: Springer Verlag*, 2003. Book.

[136] Karlov, VA. Nevrologhiya. Rukovodstvo dlya vrachey [Neurology. Manual for doctors.]. *Moscow: Meditsinskoye Informatsionnoye Agentstvo*, 2002. Russian. Book.

[137] Sandrigailo, LI. Anatomo-klinicheskiy atlas po nevropatologhii [Anatomic clinical atlas in neuropathology]. *Minsk: Vysheishaya shkola*, 1978. Russian. Book.

[138] Duus, P. Topicheskiy diagnoz v nevrologhii: anatomiya, fiziologhiya, priznaki, simptomy [Topical Diagnosis in Neurology: Anatomy, Physiology, Signs, Symptoms]. *Moscow: Vasar-Ferro*, 1995. Book. Russian.

[139] Kandel, ER. The molecular biology of memory storage: a dialog between genes and synapses. *Biosci Rep.*, 2004 Aug-Oct. 24(4-5), 475-522. Journal article.

[140] Friston, K; Kilner, J; Harrison, L. A free energy principle for the brain. *J Physiol Paris.*, 2006 Jul-Sep. 100(1-3), 70-87. Journal article.

[141] Friston, KJ; Stephan, KE. Free-energy and the brain [Internet]. Synthese. 2007 Dec 1 [cited 2014 Jan]. 159(3), 417–458. Available from: http://www.ncbi.nlm.nih.gov/pmc/articles/PMC2660582. doi: 10.1007/s11229-007-9237-y. Electronic article.

[142] Friston, K; Mattout, J; Trujillo-Barreto, N; Ashburner, J; Penny, W. Variational free energy and the Laplace approximation. *Neuroimage.*, 2007 January 1. 34(1), 220-34. Journal article.

[143] Memory [Internet]. 2002 June 01 [cited 2013 Dec]. Available from: https://www.google.ru/url?sa=t&rct=j&q=&esrc=s&source=web&cd=3&cad=rja&uact=8&ved=0CC4QFjACahUKEwjz79uOqPvGAhXKBiwKHb6yDeA&url=http%3A%2F%2Fhighered.mheducation.com%2Fsites%2Fdl%2Ffree%2F0072562013%2F46857%2Fspb2_ch07.pdf&ei=MiS2VfOOLMqNsAG-5baADg&usg=AFQjCNHt8KmThxdkeYMa9PoyTG1DzS6cAw&sig2=xDP_C0cPeeomhj7OTIWIMg&bvm=bv.98717601,d.bGg. Web Page.

[144] Off-Axis "Leith & Upatnieks" Holography [Internet]. In Benton SA, Bove VM Jr. Holographic imaging. *New Jersey: John Wiley & Sons, Inc.*, 2008 [cited 205 Jan]. Available from: http://onlinelibrary.wiley.com/book/10.1002/9780470224137. Book section.

[145] In-Line "Denisyuk" Reflection Holography [Internet]. In Benton SA, Bove VM Jr. Holographic imaging. *New Jersey: John Wiley & Sons, Inc.*, 2008 [cited 205 Jan].

Available from: http://onlinelibrary.wiley.com/book/10.1002/9780470224137. Book section.

[146] Luria, AR. O yestestvenno-nauchnikh osnovah psikhologhii [On scientific fundamentals of psychology]. In Smirnova AA, Luria AR, Nebylitsin VD, editors. Yestestvennonauchniye osnovy psikhologhii [Scientific fundamentals of psychology]. *Moscow: Pedagoghika*, 1978. Russian. Book.

[147] Vygotskiy, LS. Myshleniye i rech. [Thinking and speech]. *Moscow: Nauka*, 1934. Russian. Book.

[148] DARPA SyNAPSE Program [Internet] [updated 2013 Jan 11; cited 2014 Dec]. Available from: http://www.artificialbrains.com/darpa-synapse-program. Web Page.

[149] Lilly, JC. Programming and Metaprogramming in the Human Biocomputer: Theory and Experiments. New York: Three Rivers Press/Julian Press, 1987. Book.

[150] Eliasmith, Chris. How to Build a Brain. A Neural Architecture for Biological Cognition. Oxford University Press, 2013. Book.

[151] Bekolay, T; Bergstra, J; Hunsberger, E; Dewolf, T; Stewart, TC; Rasmussen, D; Choo, X; Voelker, AR; Eliasmith, C. Nengo: a Python tool for building large-scale functional brain models [Internet]. *Front Neuroinform.*, 2014 Jan 6 [cited 2014 Feb]., 7, 48. doi: 10.3389/fninf.2013.00048. Electronic article.

[152] Eliasmith, C; Stewart, TC; Choo, X; Bekolay, T; DeWolf, T; Tang, C; Rasmussen, D. A large-scale model of the functioning brain [Internet]. *Science*, 2012 Nov 30. 338, 1202-5. doi: 10.1126/science.1225266. Electronic article.

[153] Boyle, R. Meet Spaun, The Most Complex Simulated Brain Ever [Internet], 2012 November 30 [cited 2014 Feb]. Available from, http://www.popsci.com/science/article/2012-11/meet-spaun-first-computer-model-complex-brain-behavior. Web Page.

[154] Lehrer, J. *The Human Brain Gets a New Map.*, 2011 April 12 [cited 2014 Dec]. Available from: http://www.wired.com/2011/04/the-human-brain-atlas/. Web Page.

[155] Woollaston, V. Scientists create the world's first high-definition 3D model of a human brain. Daily Mail [serial online]. 2013 June 21 [cited 2014 Dec]; Sect. Science. Available from: http://www.dailymail.co.uk/sciencetech/article-2345661/Scientists-create-worlds-high-definition-3D-model-HUMAN-BRAIN.html. Newspaper article.

[156] Galushkin, AI.Neironniye seti. Osnovi teorii [Neural networks. The fundamentals of the theory]. *Moscow: Goryachaya Liniya –Telecom*, 2012. Russian. Book.

[157] Anokhin, KP. Obshiye principy kompensatsii narushennykh funktsiy i ikh fisiologhisheskoye obosnovaniye [General principles of compensation for disordered functions and their physiological validation]. The proceedings of the conference in defectology. Moscow: APN RSFSR, 1956. Russian. Conference paper.

[158] Yevreinov, EV; Kosarev, YuG. Odnorodniye univesralniye vichislitelniye sistemy visokoy proizviditelnosti [Homogeneous universal calculation systems of high productivity]. *Novosibirsk: Nauka*, 1966. Russian. Book.

[159] Fitzsimmons, NA; Lebedev, MA; Peikon, ID; Nicolelis, MA. Extracting kinematic parameters for monkey bipedal walking from cortical neuronal ensemble activity [Internet]. Front Integr Neurosci. 2009 Mar 9 [cited 2014 Dec].; 3, 3. Available from: http://www.ncbi.nlm.nih.gov/pmc/articles/PMC2659168. doi: 10.3389/neuro.07.003.2009. Electronic article.

[160] Nicolelis, MA. A monkey that controls a robot with its thought. No, really [Talk on the Internet], 2012 Apr [cited 2014 Feb]. Available from: https://www.ted.com/talks/miguel_nicolelis_a_monkey_that_controls_a_robot_with_its_thoughts_no_really?language=en. Web Page.

[161] Wang, W; Collinger, JL; Degenhart, AD; Tyler-Kabara, EC; Schwartz, AB; Moran, DW; Weber, DJ; Wodlinger, B; Vinjamuri, RK; Ashmore, RC; Kelly, JW; Boninger, ML. An electrocorticographic brain interface in an individual with tetraplegia. *PLoS One [Internet]*., 2013 Feb 6 [cited 2014 Dec]; 8(2). Available from: http://www.ncbi.nlm.nih.gov/pmc/articles/PMC3566209/. doi: 10.1371/journal.pone.0055344.

AUTHOR'S CONTACT INFORMATION

Prof. Andrey Bryukhovetskiy, PhD, MD
Director
Neuro Vita Clinic of Restorative
Interventional Neurology and Therapy, Russia
Fax: +74993249339
Email: neurovitaclinic@gmail.com

INDEX

D

E

F

G

H

I

J

K

L

M

N

O

P

Q

R

S

T

U

V